Dedication

Many people have helped in this project; I would like to thank Caroline Jackson for all her support and proof-reading, Joe Jackson, Di, Nigel, Emma and Angela for help with the photographs.

This Book is inspired by and dedicated to my friends at the Ludlow Survival Group. Particular thanks to Dave and Maureen D, Tim & Gill Anderson, Jason F, David C, Hugh & Fi, Andy and Nix W and my colleagues at EMAS.

This book owes much to the contributions of Dr Craig Ellis, thanks also to Gareth Mallon for his excellent Chapter on ECG Interpretation.

Updates

If you were like to receive information on updates, corrections and new editions. Or if you have any suggestions for new content. Please email me at;

Chris.breen@aol.co.uk

Contents

INTRODUCTION 5
CHAPTER 1 EXAMINATION OF PATIENTS 6
CHAPTER 2 ASSESSING CHILDREN AND THE ELDERLY 32
CHAPTER 3 FRACTURES & SPINAL TRAUMA 49
CHAPTER 4 DISLOCATIONS 62
CHAPTER 5 WOUNDS AND BURNS 64
CHAPTER 6 HEAD, CHEST AND ABDOMINAL TRAUMA 78
CHAPTER 7 ROAD TRAFFIC COLLISIONS (RTCS) 83
CHAPTER 8 JOINTS, MUSCLES, TENDONS AND LIGAMENTS .. 86
MEDICINE SECTION 102
CHAPTER 9 ALLERGIC REACTION 103
CHAPTER 10 RESPIRATORY & CARDIAC 104
CHAPTER 11 ABDOMINAL ASSESSMENT & ILLNESSES 130
CHAPTER 12 NEUROLOGICAL PROBLEMS 152
CHAPTER 13 COMMON INFECTIOUS DISEASES 171
CHAPTER 14 DIABETES 177
CHAPTER 15 POISONING 180
CHAPTER 16 SHOCK 181
CHAPTER 17 EAR, NOSE AND THROAT (ENT) 187
CHAPTER 18 EYE PROBLEMS 198
CHAPTER 19 DERMATOLOGY 201
CHAPTER 20 MINOR MEDICAL PROBLEMS 207
CHAPTER 21 MEDICATION 208
CHAPTER 22 VACCINES (IMMUNISATION) 227
CHAPTER 23 ENVIRONMENTAL PROBLEMS 229
CHAPTER 24 BITES, STINGS AND PARASITES 232
CHAPTER 25 CLINICAL OBSERVATIONS &TESTS 238
CHAPTER 26 DENTAL PROBLEMS 245
CHAPTER 27 SEXUALLY TRANSMITTED DISEASES (STD) 248
CHAPTER 28 OBSTETRICS AND GYNAECOLOGY 250
CHAPTER 29 NUCLEAR BIOLOGICAL & NERVE AGENT WARFARE 258
CHAPTER 30 GUNSHOT WOUNDS, EXPLOSIONS & TACTICAL CONSIDERATIONS 270
CHAPTER 31 TRIAGE 274
CHAPTER 32 NUTRITION 276
CHAPTER 33 MENTAL HEALTH 285
CHAPTER 34 ECG INTERPRETATION 290
APPENDIX 1 GCS 315
APPENDIX 2 MEDICAL TERMINOLOGY 317
APPENDIX 3 FURTHER READING 318
INDEX 322

Clinical Assessment and Diagnostic Skills for Nurses, Paramedics and ECPs
2nd Edition

By Chris Breen, RGN, Paramedic
& Dr Craig Ellis (MD)

Copyright © 2011-12 by Chris Breen, Dr Craig Ellis

Cover art and design © Chris Breen

Book design by Chris Breen

All rights reserved.

No part of this book may be reproduced in any form or by any electronic or mechanical means including information storage and retrieval systems, without permission in writing from the author. The only exception is by a reviewer, who may quote short excerpts in a review.

Chris Breen

Printed in the United Kingdom

First Printing: November 2011

Second Edition April 2012

Version 2.0

INTRODUCTION

Chris Breen is a Registered Nurse who served with the RAMC, a Paramedic and Clinical Tutor with additional qualifications in Trauma and Remote Medicine. He has had a long term interest in emergency medicine and is the Medical Advisor for a Preparedness group and runs courses in Survival Medicine.

Craig Ellis is a Medical doctor who trained as a Specialist Emergency Physician. He has a special interest in austere medicine and medical practice during prolonged disasters. He has both worked and taught austere medical practice.

The contents of this book are derived from a number of articles which have been published online and the syllabus of Course they run.

Its aim is to provide key information on Clinical Assessment and Diagnosis in an understandable way, suitable for both beginners and Experienced practitioners.

In addition to detailed medical and trauma assessments, explanations of common diseases and conditions at provided with signs and symptoms. Red flag indicators for each body system and individual conditions are also detailed.

To support this chapters are included on Pharmacology, Nutrition, Child Birth, Triage, Dermatology, Ophthalmology, Ear Nose and Throat (ENT). In our changing world information on gunshot injuries and CBRN threats are also covered.

However reading a book is never a substitute for proper training and experience. Anyone seriously interested in using this knowledge should seek additional training with a reputable training organisation to the desired skill level. The authors take no responsibility for the use of the information contained.

Chapter 1 Examination of Patients

In order to diagnose an illness or ascertain the extent of an injury a history and full patient examination should be made.

History taking and examination is just practice. It isn't difficult, the trick is to know what is abnormal. When you are first learning clinical examination you should practice examining people who are not ill; partners, children, and friends, as many as you can convince to let you do it. The purpose of this is to know what is normal. Once you achieve this it becomes much easier to recognise the abnormal.

Getting started (The 60 second assessment)

Before you touch or speak to the patient take a mental step back and look at the patient - an 'end of bed' assessment.

It doesn't matter if the presenting complaint is a sprained ankle or massive trauma, you should apply the same basic concept to every patient you see.

This initial survey can tell you a lot about them.

How do they appear? Are they pale, sweaty, shaking, do they appear anxious?

How are they sitting are they holding an injured or tender part of their body?

Do they appear to be struggling to breathe?

Can you hear any wheeze or rattle when they breathe?

Shake their hand. Does it feel cold? What is their capillary refill time?

Is there anything around that gives clues to the situation?

Don`t overlook the obvious ask the patient what's wrong, they might have experienced it before and know what the problem is and what needs to be done to resolve it.

In patient assessment the aim is for early identification of any potentially life threatening problems sometimes referred to as 'Red Flag indicators'. The extent of an illness or injury can be judged on a sliding scale usually defined as being between 'Well' and 'Very sick' or 'Big sick'. It is usually easier to say if a patient is at either end of the scale but more difficult to place where a patient is along the length of the scale.

This initial information helps you identify sick vs. not sick, but also what your ongoing assessment needs to be the trauma / critical ill primary and secondary survey approach or the more slow paced and system specific medical assessment.

Trauma Assessments

The full sequence below is primarily aimed at a seriously injured trauma patient, but elements of the assessment can be applied to any patient and apply just as equally to the initial assessment of a sick medical patient. The more stable the patient is the slower and more relaxed the history and examination can be.

Patient Position

Always consider the most appropriate patient position for examination. If the patient may have suffered serious traumatic injury before examination lay the casualty flat on their back. If collapsed and unconscious but without injury consider placing them in the recovery position. If conscious sit or lay as appropriate, they should be encouraged to adopt the most comfortable position. If shock is suspected then lay them down and raise legs, unless they are injured. If shocked and breathless, support head and shoulders but still raise legs if practical.

The patient also needs to be appropriately exposed. It's important to respect the patient's modesty, but not at the expense of being able to see exactly what is going on. If you don't uncover it you cannot see it. Modesty frequently causes sub-optimal assessment, so try and strike a balance.

An approach

First Aid students are taught the DRS ABC approach to casualty examination this will identify life threatening problems with the casualty and its equally applicable here. DRS ABC stands for;

- Danger
- Response
- Shout for or get Help
- Airway
- Breathing
- Circulation

If the patient is conscious and talking then it is safe to assume that they have a clear airway and an adequate breathing rate and pulse. But these observations still might not be normal due to illness and injury so still need to be assessed.

If a patient has a problem with their airway this needs attention before moving on. Without a patent airway both breathing and circulation are quickly compromised. Similarly a problem with breathing needs to be resolved before circulation is assessed.

The main aims of care in these circumstances can be described as follows;

To (P)reserve the casualty's condition

To (P)revent deterioration in the casualty's condition

To (P)romote Recovery

These are collectively known as the three P's

As discussed above, there are two basic type of examination firstly one for trauma patients who have had an accident or have been injured or are medically seriously unwell and secondly those who have a less serious medical problem. Many parts are common to the two types of assessment. When performing a medical assessment each body system needs to be assessed. Once you have a better knowledge of clinical assessment you can be more focused and just look at the systems you believe are effected (or the presenting problems), but while learning examine each system.

When providing more in depth care the DRS-ABC sequence is expanded to DRS-ABCDEFGHI, doing a full assessment of the casualty.

D- Danger:

Danger can come in many forms. It may be environmental, caused by adverse weather condition or the remoteness of a location. It may be manmade such as with traffic on a road or electricity in a building. Or it may be a tactical situation. Danger may come from a confused patient or an intoxicated or aggressive bystander.

Slippery or uneven ground can pose a danger to the rescuer, particularly if they rush to help an injured friend then become a casualty themselves. Also before kneeling next to the casualty check the ground next to them for sharp objects and bodily fluids.

As you approach the scene of an incident, you must be constantly aware of (and be continuously reassessing for) potential dangers, and be aware of the casualty and the area around them.

R- Response

After looking for any potential dangers before approaching a casualty, the first Vital Sign we measure is the Patients Level of

Response or Level of Consciousness (LOC). This can be measured simply as Conscious or Unconscious or using an extended scale such as the Glasgow Coma Scale (GCS) which is difficult to remember and for beginners can be confusing. A good compromise is to use the AVPU Scale.

A = Awake/ Alert

Alert and oriented to: Time, Date, Place and recent events

V= Responds to voice

Responds appropriately

Confused

Makes incomprehensible sounds (Grunts, groans, etc.)

P= Pain

Response in some way to a pain stimulus

U= Unresponsive

No Response

Anyone who is not Awake & Alert should have their level of consciousness (LOC) monitored and constantly reassessed.

Reason for unconsciousness

There are several common causes of unconsciousness which can be described using the acronym FISHSHAPED;

- Fainting,
- Intoxication,
- Stroke,
- Sepsis (infection),
- Heart attack,
- Shock,
- Heat imbalance,
- Anaphylaxis,
- Poisoning,
- Epilepsy and
- Diabetes or Dysrythmias (abnormal heart rhythms).

If you attend a patient who is unconscious without a clear history of cause consider all possibilities.

Use of Glasgow Coma Scale should be used to guide the management of head injured patients. The Glasgow Coma Scale is difficult to apply to children under 5 years of age. Although modifications exist, great care needs to be taken with its interpretation. It is especially useful to track changes in conscious state over time. At face value it is easy to use – but you must be literal in the interpretation of each component. Even health care workers commonly misapply it. (See Appendix 1)

S- Shout for help. This applies to normal situations where someone may be close by to assist you, fetch first aid or medical equipment or call for an ambulance.

Primary Assessment

A - Airway:

Secure the airway while taking precautions to stabilise the cervical spine if injury is suspected (see Spinal Immobilisation). Remember airway maintenance is always more important than spinal immobilisation but both should be achieved if possible.

If the casualty is conscious, they will have assumed a position where they can breathe comfortably. Any further interventions must not impair their capacity to breathe.

If the casualty is unconscious, log roll them onto their back and examine their airway. 'Look', 'Listen' and 'Feel' for movement of air.

By placing your left ear near the casualty's mouth you will feel the presence of the breath and will hear any sounds that the breathing produces. If air movement is partially obstructed then the amount of air you feel will be decreased and breathing noisy. Noise on breathing in (*Inspiration*) is indicative of a blockage in the upper respiratory system, whereas noise on breathing out (*Expiration*) indicates a lower blockage. The tongue partially blocking the windpipe may cause a 'snoring' sound or a 'gurgling' sound which would suggest liquid or semi-solid matter such as vomit in the windpipe.

The simplest method of opening the airway is by tilting the head and lifting the chin. This is achieved by pushing the forehead backwards with your left hand whilst supporting the back of the neck. Then place two fingers of your right hand under the tip of the jaw and lift the chin as this will move the tongue from the back of the throat and help clear the airway.

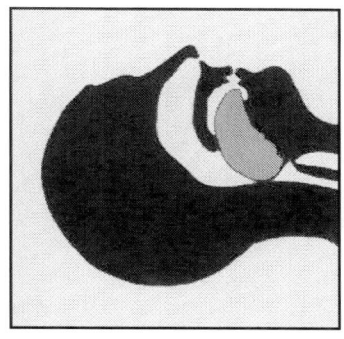
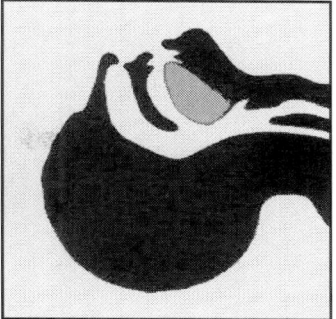

Briefly check mouth for obstructions either from the tongue or the presence of blood, vomit, oedema, loose teeth, dentures or other foreign matter. If you see any debris, sweep your fingers in the casualty's mouth to remove it. Do not sweep blindly as this may increase the obstruction by moving debris further down the airway.

If you have suction equipment or airway adjuncts they can now be used. However if the patent is maintaining their own airway it is often better to avoid unnecessary interventions as these can trigger the gag reflex and cause the patient to choke.

After any airway adjunct has been inserted check if it works by repeating the 'Look', 'Listen', 'Feel' procedure to detect breath sounds and movement.

While examining the airway, check for any smells on the breath such as Alcohol, Cannabis, Pear drops which indicate the presence of Ketones in patients with High blood sugar (hyperglycaemia), Solvents; etc.

A patient who is unable to talk or is hoarse may have swelling, damage or a blockage which could compromise the airway.

B - Breathing:

The assessment of breathing includes providing oxygen and ventilation support if required do not move beyond the breathing stage until this if required is provided.

The acronym RIPPAS can be used to remember the steps needed to fully assess breathing. These are detailed in the section on chest examination.

    Rate of Respiration

    Inspection for damage or defect in chest wall.

    Palpate (feel for injury)

    Percuss (tap for resonance)

Auscultation (listen for air movement)

Saturations of Oxygen and capnography

Once an airway is established; look down the body. If the windpipe is completely blocked but the casualty is still making a respiratory effort then you may still feel and see chest movements, so the presence of breath must be verified. If the blockage is in one of the branches of the windpipe leading into the lungs then chest movement may be uneven.

Observe for a maximum of 10 seconds, in that period you should see and or feel at least two breaths. If breathing is inadequate CPR must be started. This can be achieved by mouth-to-mouth ventilation with or without an airway adjunct or with a bag, valve, mask device (BVM)

RESPIRATION RATE

Is the breathing:

Normal

Normal breathing is regular, un-laboured, quiet and off moderate depth.

Deep

Excessively deep breathing

Shallow

Very small breaths

Laboured

Indicators of laboured breathing are; the patient is leaning forward with hand on knees (tripod Position), nasal flaring, inward movement of the muscles between and below the ribs as a result of reduced pressure in the chest (retractions), using the shoulder, neck and other muscles (accessory muscles) to expand the chest cavity and allow more airflow.

Normal respiration for Adults is *12 - 20 breaths/minute*

Abnormal 10-12 and 20-30 at rest

Serious <10 or >30

Normal Child range varies with age:

30-40 Resps/min newborn – 1 year Old

20-30 Resps/min 2 – 4 years Old

15-20 Resps/min 6 – 12 years Old

12-16 Resps/min at 14 Years Old

Remember: An increased respiration of an injured patient at rest may be the first sign of developing shock.

C - Circulation:

Determine pulse rate and blood pressure (see below). In conditions with serious blood loss, intravenous fluid replacement using saline or blood products is indicated. Only give fluids in the absence of a radial pulse and control the volume given until a pulse is restored.

When giving saline limit it to 250ml Boluses up to a maximum of 2 litres, if the casualty still needs fluid after this blood should be given.

Control haemorrhaging with direct or indirect pressure; or application of a tourniquet. If circulation is not present; begin CPR or Defibrillation (See Clinical skills).

Capillary Refill Time (CRT)

The CRT is the time it takes blood to return to an area after it has become blanched. CRT can either be measured peripherally on a nail bed, hand or limb. It can also be measured centrally on the chest or forehead

Press on the area for five seconds; it will go pale, then release, if the skin takes more than two seconds to re-colour it indicates reduced circulation. This is an unreliable measure if the patient is cold or already has circulatory problems.

A deficit in the peripheral circulation indicates a circulation problem. A deficit in the central circulation is a serious sign and may be due to shock.

Tissue colour is a good indicator of the state of circulation if you check the inside of the mouth and the lips are pale then the problem is peripheral if the tongue is pale then the problem is central.

Pulse

A pulse needs to be obtained this is usually taken at the radial site in the wrist but can be taken at the neck (carotid pulse) or anywhere an artery crosses over a bone and is close to the skin's surface. Other sites are the groin (femoral), upper arm, between biceps and humerus (brachial pulse), head (temporal), top of foot (dorsalis pedis), back of knee (popliteal). When feeling for a pulse use two or three fingers as the increased surface area will make location easier.

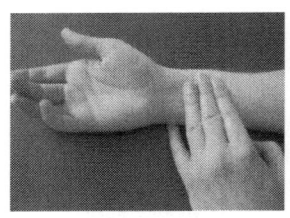 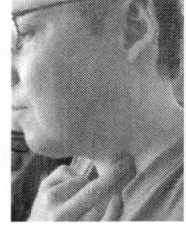 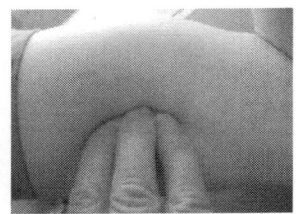

When assessing the Pulse the following should be taken into account:

HEART RATE Either count for 15 Seconds and multiply by 4 or for a full minute.

Average Adult	60-80 Beats/minute
14 Years	80-100 Beats/minute
6 Years - 12 Years	80-120 Beats/minute
2 Years - 4 Years	95-140 Beats/minute
New Born - 1 Year	110-160 Beats/minute

In Adults <60 is Bradycardia (slow pulse) >100 is Tachycardia (fast pulse)

RHYTHM

Regular

Regularly Irregular (With Extra Regular Beats)

Irregularly Irregular (with no discernable pattern, most often a rhythm called Atrial Fibrillation or AF)

QUALITY

Normal, strong and bounding, or weak and thread.

LOCATION

Location is important for three reasons:

Firstly by checking the pulse at the wrist (radial) and the pulse in the neck (carotid) you can roughly guess a blood pressure.

Radial pulse present = B/P $\geq$ 80 systolic

Femoral pulse Present = *B/P $\geq$ 70 systolic*

Carotid pulse present = *B/P $\geq$ 60 systolic*

Although the correlation is inexact, an absent radial pulse means patient is sick, an absent femoral and radial pulse means the patient is very sick.

Secondly, having unequal pulses in two arms may indicate a cardiac problem.

Thirdly, lack of pulses in a limb could indicate damage to the vessels from disease, direct or indirect trauma.

D – Deficits (Neurological): Level of Consciousness (LOC)

Assess the level of consciousness (LOC) by using AVPU (See Above) or GCS (see Appendix 1),

Check Pupils are Equal, Reactive to Light and Accommodating (PERLA).

Application of Glasgow Coma Score should be used to guide the management of head injured patients. However the Glasgow Coma Scale (See Appendix 1) is difficult to apply to a child under 5 years. Although modifications exist, great care needs to be taken with its interpretation.

Now move on to the secondary assessment

Secondary Assessment

E – Exposure / Search

In an unconscious or trauma patient remove clothing (Exposure) and look for additional wounds and any other unseen injuries (bleeding, bruising, burns or deformity). After an area is checked replace clothes or cover with a blanket to prevent heat loss. Check for medical alert bracelets, pendants or cards. Check if they are carrying any medication, a basic knowledge of common prescription medication will give you a good idea of a person's medical history providing of course the medication is theirs.

F – Fahrenheit

After exposing the casualty to check for further injury, care must be taken to preserve body heat (Fahrenheit) whilst performing any procedures required. If you have already started giving IV Fluids this will chill the body unless they have been pre-warmed.

G – Get a Set of Base Vital Signs

When assessing patients it is important to obtain a set of observations, sometimes known as vital signs, this is required for four main reasons;

- To aid identification of the underlying problem
- To gauge the severity of injury or illness
- To monitor the progress of the patient's condition
- To assess the effectiveness of treatment on the patient's condition

Vital signs include;

- Level of Consciousness (see above)
- Pulse (see above)
- Respiration Rate (see above)
- Blood Pressure (see under clinical skills)
- Temperature (see below)
- Capillary Refill Time (CRT) (see above)
- Skin Colour and Turgor (see below)
- Blood Glucose (see under clinical skills)
- Oxygen saturations (see under clinical skills)

TEMPERATURE

Normal Temperature range is 36.5 – 37.5 degrees Celsius.

Temperatures can be recorded with glass mercury, disposable paper (temp dot) or digital oral or tympanic (Ear) thermometer. Fever strips are also available to place on the forehead.

Four locations for placement are oral (under tongue), axilla (under armpit), tympanic (ear) or rectal (anus).

Thermometers should be left in place for 3 minutes. Axilla temperatures are generally one degree lower than oral ones.

SKIN COLOUR

Variation in skin colour can be indicate state of circulation and presence of disease;

PINK = Normal

PALE, WHITE, GREY = Can indicate *Shock*

FLUSHED (RED) = Carbon Monoxide, High Blood pressure, Fever

BLUE = Hypoxia (Decreased Oxygen)

YELLOW / JAUNDICE = Liver Injury / Failure, Hepatitis, Cirrhosis

Texture: Clammy, Wet or Dry
Temperature: Cold, Warm or Hot

Skin Turgor

Turgor or tenting is a measure of the elasticity of the skin. It can become reduced if the patient is dehydrated by around 10% or more. Dehydration is often caused by severe diarrhoea and/or vomiting or a decreased fluid intake. Infants and the elderly are most at risk especially those with a fever.

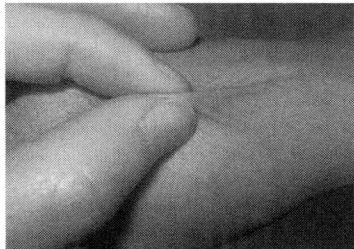

To assess lightly pinch some skin on the back of the hand, forearm or abdomen. Hold for a 5 seconds then release. Normally the skin would snap back to its normal position. If however the patient is dehydrated the skin returns slowly to normal or remains peaked.

H - History

If the patient is conscious ask them what happened, the events, signs and symptoms that led to their current condition. If not and if there were any witnesses to the incident or accident obtain as much information as possible from them. If they know the casualty asks about past incidents, medical history & any current medication or drug allergies. See Medical Assessment below.

Then perform a Head to Toe examination

H - Head-to-Toe Examination

Head to toe examinations are most commonly performed on patients who have been injured in a way that might cause multiple problems, such as falls and road accidents.

Each area of the body should be examined using the DCAPBTLS system looking for the presence of;

(D)eformity, (C)ontusion, (A)brasion, (P)uncture/Penetrating Injury, (B)urns, (T)enderness, (L)aceration & (S)welling

The areas are examined in order of importance; the area's most likely to kill or seriously disable the patient are examined first.

Additionally different areas have specific methods of examination;

Head

Examine the scalp for wounds. Look for blood, fluid or vomit in the mouth, blood or fluid in the ears. Observe for bruising behind the ear ("Battle sign") and bruising around the eyes ("racoon eyes") which may indicate a fracture of the base of the skull.

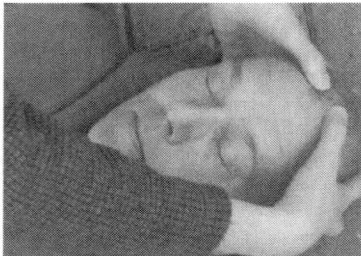

Yellow tinged blood or fluid coming from the nose or ears indicates the presence of cerebral spinal fluid CSF. This fluid encases the brain and its presence in blood indicates a skull fracture.

Whist examining the head recheck the pupil reactions. Look in the eyes and check for redness or a puffy appearance, is there blood or pus present? Are the eyes yellow suggesting the patient is jaundiced.

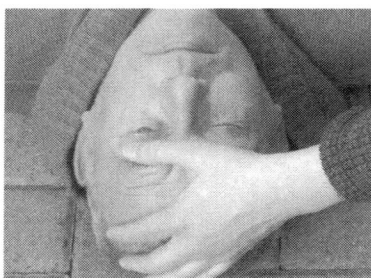

Wounds to the head, face, mouth or neck may suggest possible cervical spine injury.

Check central capillary refill on forehead.

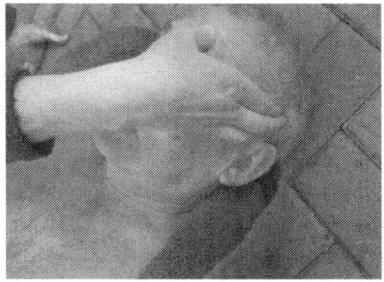

Airway compromise from facial injuries is potentially lethal due to haemorrhage, swelling and debris. Immediate stabilisation of the airway is imperative. Airway patency should be re-evaluated throughout care and transport.

Neck

Distended neck veins may result from a tension pneumothorax (Punctured Lung) or cardiac tamponade (Punctured Heart). Tracheal deviation may indicate a tension pneumothorax although this is a late sign and the patient would be seriously ill at this stage.

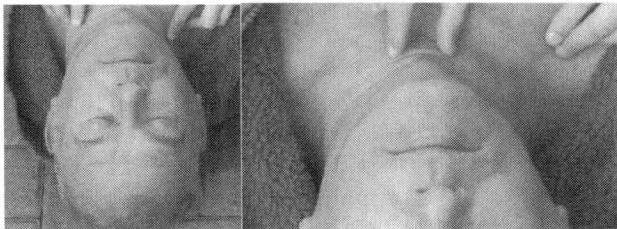

Crumpling cellophane sensation under the skin of the neck may indicate a pneumothorax with subcutaneous emphysema (Air in tissue).

Neck wounds require aggressive airway management due to the potential for rapid deterioration. Intubation should be attempted immediately in an unconscious patient if increasing neck swelling may compromise patient's airway.

Torso

Trunk wounds may consist of damage either to the chest or abdominal cavity.

Chest

Examine the chest using DCAPBTLS see above. Observe for equal and symmetrical chest rise. Place thumbs on breast bone (sternum) and fan fingers out along each side of ribs. Use firm pressure to check for deformities in the chest wall by moving hands down sternum and ribs. When the patient exhales place thumbs tip to tip on their sternum, now as they inhale your thumbs should move apart equally. This will give you an indication of the symmetry and depth of breathing.

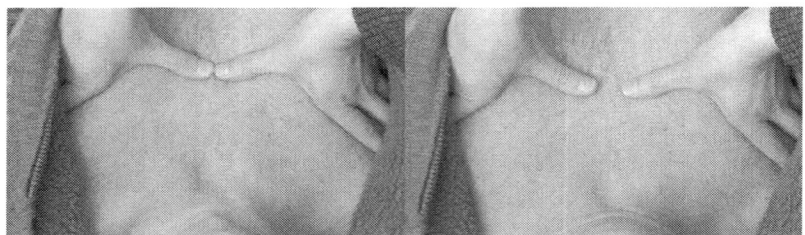

Using a stethoscope listen to the chest for breath sounds (Auscultation). Start at the front (Anterior) of Chest and listen from side to side then move from top to bottom avoid the areas covered by bones

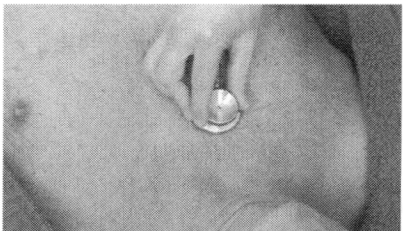

Compare one side to the other looking for differences. Note the location and quality of the sounds you hear.

In a trauma assessment you are primarily concerned with the presence or absence, rate and depth of breathing and noises that indicate a blockage to the airways. You may also hear other sounds these are detailed under respiratory assessment below.

Abdomen

Examine the chest using DCAPBTLS see above.

Feel the abdomen to check for tenderness, distension or rigidity which can indicate damage to organs and internal bleeding. For a more detailed abdominal examination see medical assessment below.

Pelvis

If the pelvis is fractured poor handling can cause significant blood loss. See trauma chapter for more details. Look for signs of incontinence this can indicate spinal damage or seizure activity.

Legs and Arms

Examine the legs first as these contain the larger bones and blood vessels from which patients can lose the most blood. Move on to collar bones, shoulders, arms and hands. When you reach the wrist check for a radial pulse and check peripheral capillary refill at fingers

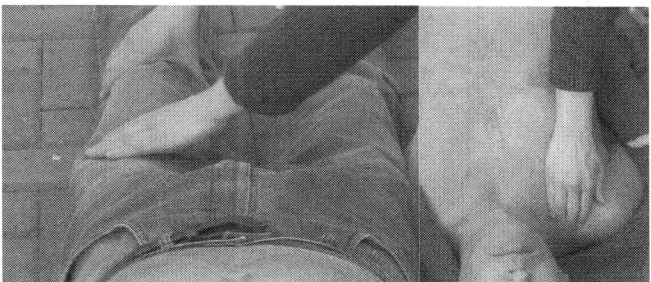

Evaluate extremities using DCAPBTLS.

Then check for Circulation, Sensation and Movement (CSM):

(C)irculation

Is the skin a normal 'Pink' Colour or are extremities pale or cyanosed? Can pulses be felt away (distal) from the site of the injury?

(S)ensation

Can the casualty feel you touching them, is the sensation the same on both sides of the body? If not this can be due to a neurological problem.

(M)ovement

Can the casualty move limbs, fingers and toes? Does pain restrict movement? If not do they have a fracture or muscular injury.

I – Invert ("it's not over until they are over")

Turn the casualty over using a log roll to examine their back. Feel along the spine for irregularities and tenderness.

Medical Assessments

The above assessment applies to trauma and critically ill medical resuscitations, the majority of non-trauma medical patients don't need the same rapid interventions and head to toe assessments. They can be slower and more focused. A set of vitals and a quick review of A,B,C,D needs to occur, but the exam can be guided by the history and more focused.

The art of questioning and obtaining a good history is the key to patient assessment and takes practice. An experienced practitioner will often come quickly to a working diagnosis after which the questioning will aim to confirm or exclude that diagnosis, they will often also have one or more differential diagnoses to work with.

Phrasing Questions

Always ask open questions or seek clarification rather than use closed questioning technique. It is well documented that when asking closed questions patients often agree with you even if they are not experiencing what you ask them about. This is because patients often feel that the questioner knows more about the condition than they do and if asked if they suffer a particular symptom feel they should have it so agree to please the questioner. It is better to ask "What sort of pain is it" rather than "Is it a crushing pain". After you have finished asking questions summarise the information and ask if your impression is correct and do they wish to change or expand on anything. Some patients are very verbose in response to open questioning, so on occasions a mixture may need to be used.

Before you finish the history taking ask if they have any other health concerns or recent health problems. It is well documented that patients often omit facts that they consider irrelevant to their currently presenting problem but may have a bearing on your differential diagnosis's.

Medical Model of Assessment and Documentation

This is the model for a professional assessment, for a simpler example see SAMPLE below.

- **Record Date and Time**

- **Referral from whom and Why referred**

- **Biographical Details; Patient Name, Address, Age and Sex**

- **Presenting Complaint (P/C)**
  If unconscious/confused document e.g. Poor historian and if history is taken from family

- **History of Presenting Complaint (HPC)**
  What happened why the patient sought help.

- **Previous Medical History (PMH)**
  Specifically ask about the following using the acronym as a memory aid MJ THREADS: M - myocardial infarction, J - jaundice, T - tuberculosis, H - hypertension & heart disease, R - rheumatic fever, E - epilepsy, A - asthma & bronchitis, D - diabetes, S - stroke

  Exclude diseases/conditions e.g. hysterectomy 5 years ago excludes pregnancy.

- **Surgical History (SHx)**
  Ask about any scars, exclude minor details but a previous removed gall bladder or appendix allows you to exclude inflammation of that relevant organ in the presence of abdominal pain.

- **Allergies, Sensitivities and previous side effects.**

- **Drug History (DH)**
  What doses, check compliance with taking medication, are they taking any over the counter medication, recreational drugs, herbal remedies etc. Ask about Inhalers, creams, and drops not just tablets. When was their medication last reviewed, should be within 6 months.

- **Family History (FHx)**
  Significant family medical history, Parents, siblings still living, if not what did they die from and at what age.

- **Social History (SHx)**
  Married status, lives with?, Occupation/school, contact with parents, Alcohol and smoking intake.

- **On Arrival (OA)**

  Appearance, position, obvious discomfort or guarding, colour, work of breathing, alertness.

- **On Examination (OE) - Review of Systems**
  Observations, Physical exam findings, Use Diagrams to illustrate problems/pain

  Systems Review
  - Head, Eyes, Ears, Nose, Throat (HEENT)
  - Respiratory (Resp)
  - Cardiovascular (CVS)
  - Gastrointestinal (GI)
  - Neurological (CNS)
  - Genital / Urinary (GU)
  - Musculoskeletal (Ortho)
  - Psychiatric (ψ)

- **Differential Diagnosis (DD or ΔΔ)**
  May be multiple possible diagnosis

- **Plan**
  Treatment including Drugs to be given (inc. Batch No. & Expiry date) Referral, Discharge, Self Care, Advice, Follow – up, safety netting.

SAMPLE History

A SAMPLE history is a structured way of recording a patient's history. It's not the only way, and perhaps not the best, but provides a good workable system for the lay person.

- Signs and Symptoms
- Allergies
- Medications
- Past Medical History
- Last (Eaten, Bowel Open, Urinated etc)
- Events leading up to current situation

Gathering this information, even in a first aid situation is useful to pass on to the emergency services in the event the patient becomes unconsciousness before they arrive as it gives them clues to the patient's condition and therefore treatment options.

Signs and Symptoms

A Sign is anything you can see, hear, smell or feel that is pertinent to the patient. Typical signs include bleeding, pale skin, deformity of a bone, noisy breathing, smell of alcohol or crepitus etc. A Symptom is anything the patient feels; hot, cold, tired, thirsty, nauseous etc.

Allergies

It is important to note any allergies or drug sensitivities such as Aspirin, Ibuprofen or Penicillin or any other reactions to substances such as latex or plasters as this may alter the treatment a patient receives.

Medication

A list of the patient's medication will give some clues to their medical history. It never ceases to amaze practitioners how many people claim to have very little wrong with them but are taking over a dozen different drugs. These people are either ignorant of why the medication was prescribed to them, trusting in what the doctors tell them, or are in oblivious about their multiple medical problems.

Past Medical History

A list of pertinent points of interest about the person's past medical history is important to record, the fact that a person has high blood pressure or diabetes is important, the fact they broke their wrist 20 years ago is less so.

Last (Eaten, Bowel Open, Urinated etc)

The recording of when they last ate or drank used to be recorded in case they needed an operation, obviously this depends on circumstance. It is more important with a diabetic patient or someone who is dehydrated. This can also be applied to other symptoms.

Events

The sequence of events that led up to a particular incident can give clues to the cause. For example, if a person is found to be unconscious it's important to know what happened prior to the event.

Did they hit their head or fall, did they complain of head or chest pain, have they been drinking and are intoxicated?

If the patient has pain or Dyspnoea then this can be assessed using either the OPQRSTA or SOCRATES formula.

OPQRSTA

(O)nset

When did the pain start, what were you doing or had been doing before it started.

(P) Provoke, Palliate or Prevent

Does anything bring the pain on (Provoke), lessen (Palliate) or Prevent it. Pain that is more intense when taking a deep breath is more likely to be caused by problem with the lungs or the muscles between the ribs (Intercostals). But a patient with a constant central chest pain is more likely to have a heart problem.

(Q)uality

What's the pain like is it sharp, dull, crushing or tight? Be causious with this as the patient's idea of what the pain feels like may not fit with a textbook answer. A person may describe both the discomfort caused by a heart attack and asthma as a heavy pain. But others could separately describe them as crushing and tight.

(R)adiation / (R)epeat

Does the pain go anywhere else, both chest and abdominal pain can often spread through to the back, arms, neck and shoulders. In the case of shortness of breath the 'R' for Radiation becomes Repeat i.e. has this happened before and what was the outcome.

(S)everity

How bad is the pain, is it at a constant level or does it come and go. A good measure is to use a Pain score, ask the patient to set a number against the pain "where zero is no pain and ten is the worst pain they have experienced" again this can be subjective but is a good measure to see if treatment is effective. Score the pain at the beginning and after each intervention that could relieve it.

T)ime

How long and how frequent is the pain.

(A)ssociated Symptoms

Such as nausea or a feeling of doom felt by people having a heart attack.

SOCRATES

(S)ite

Where is the Pain

(O)nset

When did the pain start, what were you doing or had been doing before it started.

(C)haracter

What's the pain like is it sharp, dull, crushing or tight? Be causious with this as the patient's idea of what the pain feels like may not fit with a textbook answer. A person may describe both the discomfort caused by a heart attack and asthma as a heavy pain. But others could separately describe them as crushing and tight.

(R)adiation

Does the pain go anywhere else, both chest and abdominal pain can often spread through to the back, arms, neck and shoulders. In the case of shortness of breath the 'R' for Radiation becomes Repeat i.e. has this happened before and what was the outcome.

(A)ssociated Symptoms

Such as nausea or a feeling of doom felt by people having a heart attack.

(T)ime,

How long and how frequent is the pain.

(E)xacerbating/relieving factors

Does anything bring the pain on (Exacerbating), lessen (relieving) or prevent it. Pain that is more intense when taking a deep breath is more likely to be caused by problem with the lungs or the muscles between the ribs (Intercostals). But a patient with a constant central chest pain is more likely to have a heart problem.

(S)everity

How bad is the pain, is it at a constant level or does it come and go. A good measure is to use a Pain score, ask the patient to set a number against the pain "where zero is no pain and ten is the worst pain they have experienced" again this can be subjective but is a good measure to see if treatment is effective. Score the pain at the beginning and after each intervention that could relieve it.

Body Systems

Once you have a clear idea of the patients symptoms and have identified the signs they are exhibiting you are on the first step to making a diagnosis from which you can plan your treatment. The body is divided into systems a disease process will affect one or more of these systems. There are 11 body systems these can be divided into 7 groups;

- Cardiovascular System
- Respiratory System
- Nervous System
- Digestive System
- Genitourinary System (Reproductive & Urinary)
- Endocrine, Lymphatic and Skin
- Musculoskeletal System

Each system has key symptoms that would indicate a problem with that system. Some symptoms such as nausea are present in a variety of illnesses across a range of systems. These should only be used to support a diagnosis. Temperature usually indicates an infection this is most commonly a respiratory problem, In the absence of other respiratory symptoms, consider other systems such as an abdominal problem.

Endocrine, Lymphatic and Skin

The endocrine system provides and distributes hormones needed by the body to regulate its functions. The Lymphatic system carries fluid to and from tissue spaces. Lymph nodes exist throughout the body, mainly in the torso, but also in the neck, armpit and groin. They filter and control the lymph in the intestinal fluid for germs. Then produce antibodies to fight the infection, the increased number of cells within the nodes causes them to swell up when you have an infection. It could be a simple throat infection or a cancer.

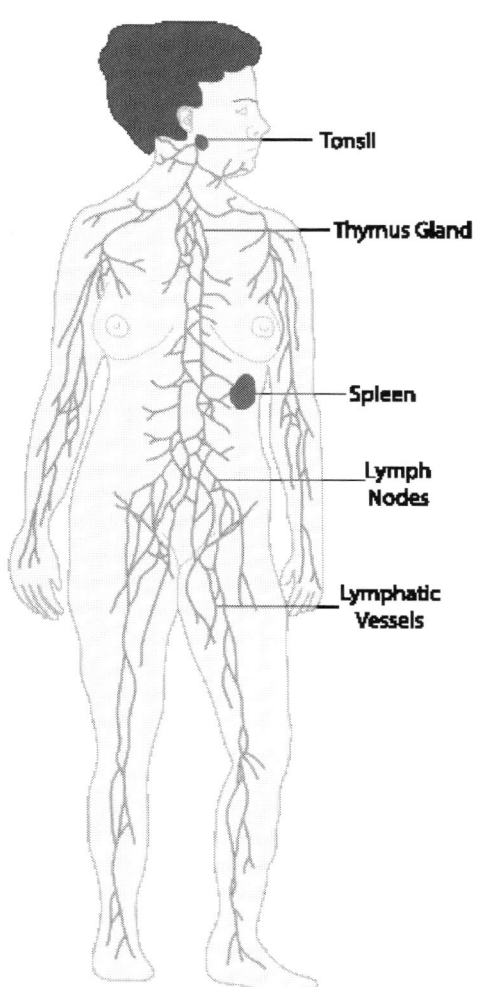

© TheEmirr

The skin main functions are to protects the body, give it shape, regulate temperature and absorb substances.

Symptoms
Heat or cold intolerance
Sweats, shivering and rigors
Rashes, itching and lumps

Musculoskeletal System

This system consists of the bones of the skeleton, muscles, joints, cartilage, tendons and ligaments. It supports the body, allows movement, provides stability and protects underlying organs.

Symptoms
Pain and/or stiffness in any bones, joints or muscles

Musculoskeletal Assessment

A musculoskeletal assessment is usually focussed to a particular joint where the patient is experiencing pain or discomfort. To minimise the discomfort for the patient always look before you feel and feel before you move the joint.

Questioning

When did the pain start?
Any injury or event before pain?
If injury, what was the mechanism?
Can you put weight on an injured lower limb?
Has it affected your strength?
What can't you do that you could before?
Does it affect a single or multiple joints?
Did it come on after an incident or was progression slow?
Any prior problems with the affected area?
Systemic symptoms, high temperature etc?

Examination

To perform an examination of the muscles, bones, and joints, use the following;

Inspection (Look)
Always compare each joint and muscle group on both sides.
Check each joint for asymmetry, deformity and wasting. Look for swelling, deformity, lesions and colour changes. Feel the joint, check to see if it's hot, if the joint is swollen this may be due to an excess build up of fluid (Effusion). A small amount of fluid is normal within a joint but some diseases cause this to increase. Check to see where the joint is most tender and visualise the underlying anatomy to identify the affected structure.

Palpation (Feel)
Feel each joint and muscle group in sequence

Manipulation (Move)
Lastly mobilise the joint this is to check it has a normal range of movement (ROM). The first movement is passive allowing the patient

to move the joint themselves, then actively with you moving the joint. Check the stability of the joint and supporting ligaments.

Isolate each axis when testing for normal range of movements i.e. hold the forearm when asking the patient to move wrist this will stop them using the elbow to help.

Putting it all together

A key concept to understand is of a differential diagnosis, a list of possibilities of diseases or injuries which explain the patient's problem.

History + examination findings + environment + circumstances = differential diagnosis.

You need to think of all the possibilities which could explain the problem, sometimes it is incredibly obvious, other times it can be extremely hard. Order your list from most to least likely. It should be based on the balance of probabilities of it being that disease. This is based on your experience, the patient's previous experience (they might have had it before) and the situation / environment you are in.

Once you have your list think: "What more information do I need to differentiate the possibilities on my list?" Ask more questions, examine some more or do some simple tests.

Look up the most likely diagnoses in a reference book, read about each and think – "does this explain the presentation?"

You need to make a plan. It will not always be the right one but you need at some point to make a decision.

Remember:
    Patients don't present like textbooks
    Is it a reasonable diagnosis = right age / right sex / right geography
    If you're not sure wait and reassess – 6 / 12 / 24 / 48 hours – depending on the problem

Chapter 2 Assessing Children and the Elderly

Recognition of the Sick Child

Early identification of seriously ill children is vital as they competence well then tend to crash. Therefore A rapid initial assessment and primary survey should be performed to identify life-threatening problems

General Impression

A useful 'door step' or 'end of bed' assessment tool is the Paediatric Assessment Triangle this can be undertaken as you approach the child. This is derived from (PEPP) Paediatric Education for Pre-hospital Professionals by AAP

Airway & Appearance (Open/Clear – Muscle Tone /Body Position)

What's Abnormal:

Abnormal or absent cry or speech.

Decreased response to parents or environmental stimuli.

Floppy or rigid muscle tone or not moving.

What's Normal:

Normal cry or speech.

Responds to parents or to environmental stimuli such as lights, keys, or toys.

Good muscle tone.

Moves extremities well.

Breathing, Work of (Visible movement / Respiratory Effort)

What's Abnormal:

Increased/excessive (nasal flaring, retractions or abdominal muscle use) or decreased/absent respiratory effort or noisy breathing.

What's Normal:

Breathing appears regular without excessive respiratory muscle effort or audible respiratory sounds.

Circulation to Skin (Colour / obvious bleeding

What's Abnormal:

Cyanosis, mottling, paleness/pallor or obvious significant bleeding.

What's Normal:

Colour appears normal for racial group of child. No significant bleeding.

Initial Assessment
Airway & Appearance (Open/Clear – Mental Status)
- Look & listen for possible obstructions.
- Inspiratory stridor is indicative of upper airway obstruction.
- Wheezing indicates obstruction of the lower airways.
- Volume does not indicate severity.
- Do not attempt blind finger sweeps.
- Newborn & infants – neutral alignment.
- Avoid hyperextension in young children.

What's Abnormal:

Obstruction to airflow.

Gurgling, stridor or noisy breathing.

Verbal**, P**ain**, or U**nresponsive on AVPU scale.

What's Normal:

Airway clear and maintainable. **A**lert on AVPU scale.

Breathing (Effort / Sounds / Rate / Central Colour)

Assess the rate, effort and effectiveness of breathing

1. Assess the respiratory rate:

Age	Respiratory Rate
<1 year	30-40 breaths per minute
1-2 years	25-35 breaths per minute
2-5 years	25-30 breaths per minute
5-11 years	20-25 breaths per minute

Clinical Practice Guidelines 2006 (JRCALC)

2. Assess the amount of effort being used to breathe:
Are there any inspiratory or expiratory noises such as stridor, wheeze or grunting?

Can you see accessory muscles being used?

Is sternal recession evident?

Are the nostrils flared?

3. Assess the effectiveness of breathing:
Listen to breath sounds (auscultate) and measure the oxygen saturation levels to assess the effectiveness of breathing.

What's Abnormal:

Presence of retractions, nasal flaring, stridor, wheezes, grunting, gasping or gurgling.

Respiratory rate outside normal range. Central cyanosis.

What's Normal:

Easy, quiet respirations. Respiratory rate within normal range. No central cyanosis.

Circulation (Pulse Rate & Strength / Extremity Color & Temperature / Capillary Refill / Blood Pressure)

1. Assess the heart rate:

Age	Heart Rate
<1 year	110-160 beats per minute
1-2 years	100-150 beats per minute
2-5 years	95-140 beats per minute
5-11 years	80-120 beats per minute

Clinical Practice Guidelines 2006 (JRCALC)

2. Assess the pulse volume – absent peripheral pulses and weak central pulses are signs of advanced shock.
   The presence of certain peripheral pulses can not be used to estimate systolic blood pressure in children.

3. Assess the capillary refill using the forehead, sole of foot or sternum.

4. Blood Pressure – should not be routinely measured in pre-hospital care because:

It varies with age

It is maintained until shock is very severe

Hypotension is a pre-terminal sign

Age	Lower Limit of Normal Systolic BP
<1 year	>60 or Strong Pulses
1-3 years	>70 or Strong Pulses
4-5 years	>75
6-12 years	>80
13-18 years	>90

What's Abnormal:

Cyanosis, mottling, or pallor. Absent or weak peripheral or central pulses; Pulse or systolic BP outside normal range; Capillary refill > 2 sec with other abnormal findings.

What's Normal:

Colour normal. Capillary refill at palms, soles, forehead or central body ≤ 2 sec. Strong peripheral and central pulses with regular rhythm.

Fluid Loss (Hypovolaemic) Shock in Children

Signs	<25% Blood Loss	25-40% Blood Loss	>40% Blood Loss
Heart Rate	Increased	Increased	Increased or Reduced
Systolic BP	Normal	Normal or Reduced	Reduced ++
Pulse Volume	Normal or Reduced	Reduced	Reduced ++
Cap Refill	Normal or Increased	Increased	Increased
Resp Rate	Increased	Increased	Sighing
Skin Temp	Cool	Cold	Cold
Skin Colour	Pale	Mottled	White/Grey
Mental State	Mild agitation	Drowsy	Reacts to pain only

Remember: A child with >25% shock needs blood & urgent hospital care

Disability

1. Assess levels of consciousness – AVPU (Modified GCS during secondary survey)

Glasgow Coma Scale for Children <4 Years

Glasgow coma scale (<4 years)	
Response	Score
Eye Opening	
Spontaneously	4
To verbal stimuli	3
To pain	2
No response to pain	1
Best Motor Response	
Spontaneous or obeys verbal command	6
Localises to pain or withdraws to touch	5
Withdrawn from pain	4
Abnormal flexion to pain	3
Abnormal extension to pain	2
No response to pain	1
Best Verbal Response	
Alert, babbles, coos, words to usual ability	5
Less than usual words, spontaneous irritable cry	4
Less than usual words spontaneous cry	3
Moans to pain	2
No response to pain	1

2. Observe the child's posture

- Floppy (hypotonic) – if new onset, assume child is seriously ill until proven otherwise

- Stiff (hypertonic) or back arching – if new onset, regard as a sign of cerebral upset

- Decerebrate or decorticate posturing – indicates serious cerebral abnormality

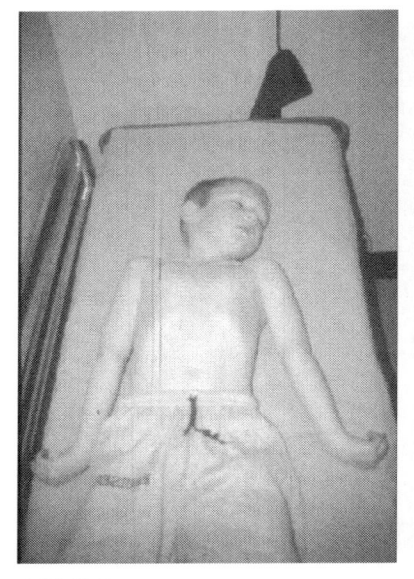

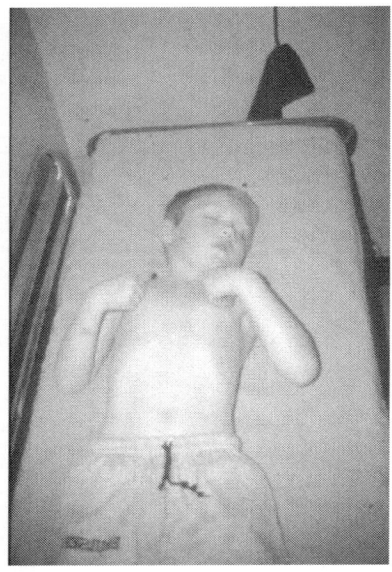

©EMAS

Decerebrate Rigidity **Decorticate Rigidity**

3. Assess the pupils

- Pupils should be equal, normal size and react briskly to light

4. Measure the blood glucose level

   Any child presenting with significant difficulties involving:

- Airway
- Breathing
- Circulation
- Disability

Must be treated as time Critical

Ongoing Assessment

Use structure of initial assessment for any ongoing assessments

CUPS Method of classifying Sick Children

Critical	**Absent airway, breathing or circulation**
	(cardiac or respiratory arrest or severe traumatic injury)
Unstable	**Compromised airway, breathing or circulation**
	(Unresponsive, respiratory distress, active bleeding, shock, active seizure, significant injury, shock, near-drowning, etc.)
Potentially Unstable	**Normal airway, breathing & circulation but significant mechanism of injury or illness**
	(Post-seizure, minor fractures, infant < 3mo with fever, etc.)
Stable	**Normal airway, breathing & circulation**
	No significant mechanism of injury or illness
	(small lacerations or abrasions, infant ≥ 3mo with fever)

Specific Conditions in Children

Febrile Convulsions

A febrile convulsion, also known as a fever fit or febrile seizure, is a convulsion associated with a significant rise in body temperature. They most commonly occur in children between the ages of 6 months to 6 years and are twice as common in boys as in girls

The child is unable to regulate its own body temperature due to an immature hypothalamus. As body temperature rises rapidly during an episode of infection, usually >39°C most children will experience a brief full body seizure that is tonic-clonic in nature usually lasting 1-2 minutes. But can last up to 15minutes, a simple febrile convulsion should not reoccur with 24 hours. However a complex febrile convulsion can occur and is characterized by longer duration, recurrence, or focus on only part of the body.

34% of all children between the ages of 3 months and 5 years will have a febrile convulsion and 1:3 risk further convulsions. There is evidence that indicates a higher risk of further seizures if the first seizure occurs before the age of 1 year. However, only 1% of children will go on to develop epilepsy.

Croup

This is a breathing problem most commonly seen in children between 6 months and 5–6 years of age that is caused by an infection of the upper airway causing swelling inside the throat which in turn causes the classic "barking" seal like cough. Other symptoms are a grating upper airway sound (Stridor), hoarseness, difficulty in breathing, fever, rhinitis, drooling and sternal recessions. Symptoms vary in intensity and can be worse at night. Normally treated by GP but in rare cases can be very serious.

Normal Stages of Human Development (Birth to 5 Years)

The flowing information is derived from the Child Development Institute: Parenting Today

It is important to keep in mind that the time frames presented are averages and some children may achieve various developmental milestones earlier or later than the average but still be within the normal range.

Birth to 1 month

Feeds: 5-8 per day, Sleep: 20 hrs per day
Sensory Capacities: makes basic distinctions in vision, hearing, smelling, tasting, touch, temperature, and perception of pain.

Emotional: Generalized Tension

Social: Helpless, Asocial, Fed by mother

2 to 3 months

Sensory Capacities: colour perception, visual exploration, and oral exploration.
Sounds: cries, coos, grunts
Motor Ability: control of eye muscles, lifts head when on stomach.

Emotional: Delight, Distress, Smiles at a Face

Social: Visually fixates at a face, smiles at a face, may be soothed by rocking.

4 to 6 months

Sensory Capacities: localizes sounds
Sounds: babbling makes most vowels and about half of the consonants
Feedings: 3-5 per day
Motor Ability: control of head and arm movements, purposive grasping, rolls over.

Emotional: Enjoys being cuddled

Social: Recognizes his mother. Infant distinguishes between familiar persons and strangers, no longer smiles indiscriminately. Expects feeding, dressing, and bathing.

7 to 9 months

Motor Ability: control of trunk and hands, sits without support, crawls about.

Emotional: Specific emotional attachment to mother, protests separation from mother.

Enjoys games such as "peek-a-boo"

10 to 12 months

Motor Ability: control of legs and feet, stands, creeps, apposition of thumb and fore-finger.
Language: says one or two words, imitates sounds, and responds to simple commands.
Feedings: 3 meals, 2 snacks. Sleep: 12 hours, 2 naps

Emotional: Anger, Affection, Fear of strangers, Curiosity, exploration

Social: Responsive to own name. Wave bye-bye. Plays pat-a-cake, understands "no-no!" Gives and takes objects.

1 to 1 ½ years

Motor Ability: creeps up stairs, walks (10-20 min), and makes lines on paper with crayon.

Emotional: Dependent Behaviour, Very upset when separated from mother, Fear of Bath

Social: Obeys limited commands, repeats a few words, Interested in his mirror image, feeds himself.

1 ½ to 2 years

Motor Ability: runs, kicks a ball, and builds 6 cube tower (2yrs) Capable of bowel and bladder control.
Language: vocabulary of more than 200 words. Sleep: 12 hours at night, 1-2 hr nap

Emotional: Temper tantrums (1-3yrs), Resentment of new baby.

Social: Does opposite of what he is told (18 months).

2 to 3 years
Motor Ability: jumps off a step, rides a tricycle, uses crayons, builds a 9-10 cube tower.
Language: starts to use short sentences controls and explores world with language, stuttering may appear briefly.

Emotional: Fear of separation, Negativistic (2 ½ yrs), Violent emotions, anger, Differentiates facial expressions of anger, sorrow, and joy. Sense of humour (Plays tricks)

Social: Talks, uses "I" "me" you" Copies parents' actions. Dependent, clinging, possessive about toys, enjoys playing alongside another child, negativism (2 ½ yrs), resists parental demands, gives orders.

3 to 4 years
Motor Ability: Stands on one leg, jumps up and down, draws a circle and a cross (4 yrs) Self-sufficient in many routines of home life.

Emotional: Affectionate toward parents, Pleasure in genital manipulation, Romantic attachment to parent of opposite sex (3 to 5 yrs), Jealousy of same-sex parent. Imaginary fears of dark, injury, etc. (3 to 5 years).

Social: Likes to share, uses "we" Cooperative play with other children, nursery school. Imitates parents. Beginning of identification with same-sex parent, practices sex-role activities. Intense curiosity & interest in other children's bodies. Imaginary friend.

4 to 5 years

Motor ability: mature motor control, skips, broad jumps, dresses himself, copies a square and a triangle.
Language: talks clearly, uses adult speech sounds, has mastered basic grammar.

Emotional: Responsibility and guild, Feels pride in accomplishment

Social: Prefers to play with other children, becomes competitive prefers sex-appropriate activities.

Baby check

Information adapted from
http://www.nicutools.org/MediCalcs/BabyCheck.php3

Baby Check can help you assess the severity of illness in babies in the first six months of life and measure improvement or worsening of condition.

It's not a substitute for clinical judgment or common sense and assesses signs and symptoms of generalized illness. Some conditions, such as injury, a convulsion or an abscess, where the baby is not systemically ill, may get a low score but still need medical assessment or treatment

	Signs and Symptoms		Score
1	Unusual cry	E. g. high itched, weak, moaning or painful	2
2	Fluids taken in previous 24 hours	Less than normal	2
		Half normal	4
		Very little	9
3	Vomiting	Vomiting at least half of feed in the three previous feeds	4
4	Vomiting bile	Any green bile vomit	13
5	Wet nappies (urine output)	Less urine than normal	3
6	Blood in nappy	Large amount of blood in nappy	11
7	Drowsiness	Occasionally drowsy	3
		Drowsy most of the time	5
8	Floppiness	Baby seems more floppy than usual	4
9	Watching	Baby less watchful than normal	2
10	Awareness	Baby responding less than normally to the surroundings	2
11	Breathing Difficulties	Minimal recession visible	4
		Obvious recession visible	15
		Normal Respiratory rate 25-35 ≥ 40 = tachyponea	

12	Looking Pale	Baby more pale than normal or has been pale in last 24 hours	3
13	Wheezing	Baby has wheezy breathing sounds	2
14	Blue Nails	Apparent blue nails	3
15	Circulation	Baby's toes are white, or stay white for 3 seconds after squeezing	3
		Normal heart rate 110 – 150bpm ≥ 160 = tachycardia	3
16	Rash	Rash over body, or raw weeping area > 5 x 5 cms	4
17	Hernia	Obvious bulge in scrotum or groin	13
18	Temperature	Greater than 38.3 c (tempadot)	4
19	Crying during checks	Baby has cried during checks (more than a grizzle)	4

Total scores

0-7	Baby is only a little unwell, medical attention in not necessary
8-12	Baby is not seriously unwell; parents would be advised to seek advice from a health professional
13-19	Baby is ill, parents would be advised to contact a doctor
>20	Baby is seriously ill, parents would be advised to seek immediate medical attention

Paediatric Trauma Score (PTS)

	+2	+1	-1
Weight	>20 Kg (44lbs)	10-20 Kg (22-44lbs)	<10 Kg (22 lbs)
Airway	Patent	Maintainable	Non maintainable
Systolic BP	>90 Radial	50-90 Carotid	<50 Non palpable
CNS	Awake	Responsive	Unresponsive
Fracture	None	Closed or ?	Multiple or open
Wounds	None	Minor	Major, Penetrating or >10% Burns

9-12 Minor Trauma

6-8 Potentially Life Threatening

0-5 Life Threatening

<0 Usually Fatal

Assessing the Elderly patient

A person becomes elderly at the age of 65 however as this is based on retirement age, in countries such as India this becomes irrelevant and a person is considered an Elder or Elderly at around 50. At 85 a person is termed the oldest old. The current average life expectancy for males is 77.4 years and 81.6 years for women also the number of people living to 100 years in the UK has tripled since 1985 reaching 11,600 in 2009. Whatever term is used it is an inevitable part of aging that the body will start deteriorating and eventually fail leading towards death.

Each body system changes as we get older;

The Respiratory System (Lungs and Airways)

The airways contain cilia that are tiny hairs that move backwards and forwards and push dust and foreign bodies out towards the nose or down the throat, but in the elderly patient this movement is decreased so choking may occur.

As people age the number of alveoli where gaseous exchange of oxygen and carbon dioxide between inspired air and the blood decrease. The lungs lose their elasticity and lung volume is decreased. Changes in the density of bones often cause curvature of the spine called kyphosis and weakening of the muscles of the diaphragm and between the ribs decrease the maximum amount of air that is breathed in and out

As less air is breathed out this leaves some in the lungs which hampers gaseous exchange and increases the amount of carbon dioxide in the blood. Cells in the body called Chemoreceptor's control the amount of oxygen in the blood these become less sensitive in an elderly patient hence an oxygen saturation reading of 93% to 95% may be normal. In a younger person a level of 96%+ is considered normal. Chronic obstructive heart disease (COPD) can be caused by smoking or underlying lung diseases, it usually affect patient from 35 years of age and death usually occurs 10 years after onset of breathlessness.

The Cardiovascular System (Heart and Blood Vessels)

A build up of fatty deposits (atherosclerosis) in the blood vessels together with the loss of elasticity will make the vessels more rigid which increases systolic blood pressure. As cardiac function declines with age, there is a decrease in blood volume, pulse and the amount of blood pumped with each heartbeat (stroke volume).

There are natural sensors in the blood vessels called baroreceptors these measure the pressure of blood in the vessels and send signals to the brain when the body needs to adjust the pressure when moving. In the elderly these become less sensitive so systolic blood pressure can suddenly drop when moving from a sitting to a standing position this can cause fainting, but a drop of less than 20 mmHg could be normal for the patient. As part of the aging process the number of cells that control the electrical signals in the heart decrease by up to 90% by the age of 75, there is also a loss of the fibres that channel electrical impulses through the heart. This causes irregular heart rhythms (Arrhythmias) such as atrial fibrillation (AF). Coronary heart disease is a failure of the hearts circulation to supply adequate oxygen to the cardiac muscle and surrounding tissue a failure of this system leads to heart attacks and angina.

Nervous System

The weight of the brain shrinks 10 to 20% by 80 years of age and losses between 5 to 50% of brain cells (neurons) more in patients with dementia. The junctions between neurons, motor and sensory networks become slower and less responsive.

The shrinking brain stretches the blood vessels from its surface to the inside of the skull this can lead to haemorrhage. Nerves in the skin deteriorate which results in less pain being felt from injuries.

Skin

The skin becomes thinner, more wrinkled, drier, loses elasticity and become more fragile as we age. Fat layers below the skin becomes thinner and outer skin loosens

In older skin uncontrolled bleeding produces large bruises (Haematoma) underneath the skin.

Temperature

In the elderly the core body temperature drops, so a temperature of between 35-36 degrees C may be normal and explains why older people feel colder. It also means that an older person with a temperature of 37.1 C has a more virulent infection than a younger person due to the difference in normal core temperatures.

Kidneys, Liver and Digestive system

Kidneys reduce in size and there ability to filter the blood can reduce by up to 50% by the age of 90. The liver shrinks and its blood flow decreases. Changes in the stomach and intestines reduce nutritional intake and metabolism. Taste bud sensitivity and the production of saliva declines as well as gastric acid. Older people develop a degree of glucose intolerance which can lead to diabetes and is often overlooked until it becomes a more serious problem it can be diagnosed by taking a blood sample after fasting overnight, a raised blood sugar is an indication of diabetes.

Musculoskeletal

Muscle fibres become smaller and fewer, ligaments and cartilage of the joints lose their elasticity, muscle mass decreases and is replaced by fat and bone density reduces. Osteoporosis is common in the elderly affecting around 50% of women and 20% of men, the bones fracture more easily, falls can result in fractured hips which have a high related death rate of 30% within a year following the fracture.

Cancer

Cancer cells in the body grow and reproduce in an uncontrollable way. It can spread to other areas of the body and this is called metastasis. The damaged cells invade nearby healthy cells and destroy them hastening the process. With the benefit of modern medicines, radiotherapy and chemotherapy cancers are often curable without these the death rate is high. One in three people will have some form of cancer during their lives, half of these occur in the over 55s.

Trauma Section

Revised Trauma Score (RTS)

GCS	Systolic BP	Resps	Points
15-13	>89	10-29	4
12-9	76-89	>29	3
8-6	50-75	6-9	2
5-4	1-49	1-5	1
3	0	0	0

Chapter 3 Fractures & Spinal Trauma

When assessing any casualty with a traumatic injury, some important points should be kept in mind;

- Is it a fracture or dislocation?
- Does it involve nerves or blood vessels?
- Is the patient shocked?
- Does it involve any internal organs?

It is important to eliminate potentially life-threatening or complicated injuries before treating as a simple strain or sprain.

When examining the patient always **look** first, then **feel** for deformity before finally **moving** limbs or joints. If your initial observation or tactile examination reveal a significant problem do not the move limb as this will inflict unnecessary discomfort and pain.

When performing an assessment of limbs, remove clothing and evaluate extremities using the pneumonic CSM;

(C)irculation

Is the skin a normal 'Pink' Colour or are extremities pale or cyanosed showing poor circulation. Can pulses be felt away (distal) to the site of the injury. Is capillary refill normal. Do they feel colder than the same limb on the other side.

(S)ensation

Can the casualty feel you touching them? is the sensation the same on both sides and are they able to distinguish between sharp and dull stimulus.

(M)ovement

Can the casualty move limbs, fingers and toes normally in a full range of motion. If pain restricts movement don't force patient to move beyond comfortable limits.

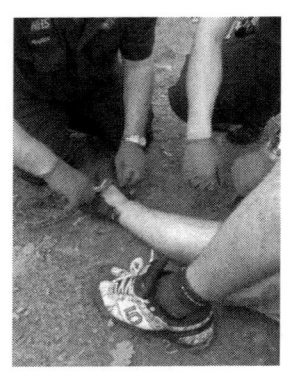

Observe for signs of shock, be aware that multiple injuries may co-exist such as a fracture with dislocation of a joint, internal injuries and/or soft tissue damage.

Referred Pain

In the absence of a clear history of injury the pain the patient feels in a limb or joint, may be 'Referred Pain' this arises when the brain is confused over where the pain stimuli is coming from. E.g. nerves relating to the heart join the spinal cord at T1, T2 level this is the same area that supplies the left arm, which is why people having heart attacks sometimes complain of pain or a heavy sensation in their left arm. A pain in the shoulder with no history of injury result from a more serious underlying problem, such as pneumonia, punctured lung, aneurism, ruptured spleen or ectopic pregnancy. In injury it is also more common in children where hip injuries may present with complaints of knee or ankle pain. In order to accurately identify what is injured always examine the joint and bone above and below the joint where pain is.

Fractures

Some fractures are obvious and involve deformity of a limb or bones coming through the skin, unfortunately most are not. In the absence of x-ray facilities any injury that could be a fracture should be treated as such until proved otherwise.

Fractures are either caused by acute injury, overuse and stress or disease processes such as osteoporosis if there isn't a suitable history the injury is unlikely to be a fracture.

If don't know if it is a fracture or not, immobilise it for 72 hours then reassess it – if there is still severe pain and loss of function it makes a fracture much more likely than a sprain or contusion.

Fractures can be diagnosed by any or all of the following;
- Pain at the site of injury,
- Loss of movement or function,
- Swelling or bruising,
- Crepitus (grating of bones)
- Deformity including shortening, bending or twisting of a limb.

Pain and tenderness caused by fractures appear at the site of injury and around the circumference of the bone. Pain on one side only is more likely to be bruising and a fracture.

Types and sub types of fractures.

Closed Fractures

Closed fractures occur where the bone breaks but is not exposed to the air through a break in the skin. In multiple trauma the skin may be broken but if the fractured bone is nor exposed the fracture is still classed as being closed.

Open Fractures

If the fracture is open part of the bone may protrude through the skin this adds the risk of bleeding and wound infection to that of the fracture. If underlying blood vessels and nerves are affected the fracture is termed complicated.

Stable/Unstable Fractures

One further distinction is that of stable and unstable fracture. Stable fractures occur when the bones are either not completely broken or when the ends are impacted and don`t move. Unstable fractures move independently and can cause additional injuries if not splinted securely.

Hairline Fractures

Hairline or stress fractures occur when trauma damages the bone but there is insufficient force to break the bone.

Greenstick Fractures

Occurs in children where the bone splinters on the opposite side of the bone to which the force is applied. This can appear to make the bone bend with obvious deformities.

Simple Fractures

Simple fractures occur when the bone is broken but the two parts remain touching the break can be relatively transverse (less than 30 degrees) at an oblique angle (Greater than 30 degrees) or in a spiral. Without X-Ray it would be difficult to tell them apart other than the fact that transverse fractures tend to heal quicker and are more stable.

Comminuted Fractures

There are many different types of comminuted fractures but most involve the bone fragmenting into multiple pieces. These types of fractures require surgical intervention to repair and involve the use of screws and plates to rebuild shattered bones, some may also require external fixation.

Avulsion fractures

Produced by muscle contraction or stretching of ligaments. These cause pieces of bone to break off where the muscle connects to the bone.

Displacement of fractures

If the bones have moved away from their normal positioning then the fracture is said to be displaced and unless it is repositioned it will either heal with a deformity or not heal at all.

There are different types of displacement which can exist on their own or in combination.

Lateral – Displaced to side of other part of bone

Posterior - Displaced behind other part of bone

Angled - Displaced at angle to other part of bone

Rotated - Displaced at rotation to other part of bone

How Bone Heal

Damaged bones can replace themselves completely given time. When a bone is fractured a blood clot forms at the site of the injury. The body then sends all the materials needed for bone replacement to the injury site and this replaces the clot. In well aligned bones a soft callus joins the bone fragments together and stabilises them. If the bone fragments are not aligned or separated union of the pieces can still take place but the join is often distorted and prone to further damage. This bridging phase takes 3 to 4 weeks. Over the next few months consolidation occurs and the soft callus is replaced by a hard bony callus although it may take up to 2 years before the bone remodels itself to its original shape.

Blood Loss with Fractures

The most serious fractures are those of 'Long Bones' damage to these bones can produce massive blood loss. Blood is lost through three mechanisms;

- Damage to large blood vessels
- Leakage from Bone Marrow
- Bleeding from muscles

The average adult has 5-6 litres of blood in their bodies, a more accurate measure is;

- 70ml/Kg Adult
- 80ml/Kg Child
- 100ml/Kg Infant

Typical long bone injuries have the following blood losses;

- Humerus 500ml-750ml
- Tibia 500ml-1000ml
- Femur 1000ml-2000ml
- Closed Pelvic Fracture 2000ml-3000ml
- Open Book Pelvic Fracture 4000ml

A 40% Blood loss is classed to be Life Threatening. If you have a normal total volume of 5000ml (5L) 40% is only 2000ml (2L) which can easily be lost in Long bone fractures.

There are two main aims in the treatment of fractures. To ensure ends of bones at point of fracture meet without deformity and to restore full function of the affected part.

The first step in treating any fracture is to determine if the bone has been displaced this can be determined by careful examination of the affected area and comparison to the opposite side of the body. A shortened limb on affected side would suggest a lateral or posterior dislocation. A limb moving in an unnatural way could indicate an angular displacement. A hand or foot pointing in the wrong direction suggests a rotational displacement.

Ottawa Rules for Fractures of the Ankle

The presence of a fracture is more likely in patients with any pain in the area around the bones that protrude either side of the ankle (malleolus) and 6cm up the fibular (malleolar zone) and the inability to walk four weight bearing steps immediately after the accident and upon later examination.

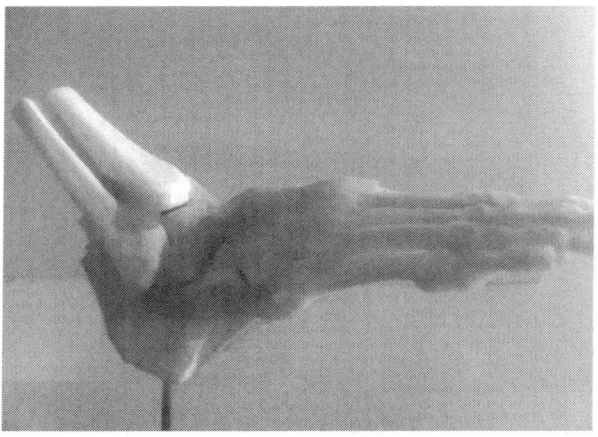

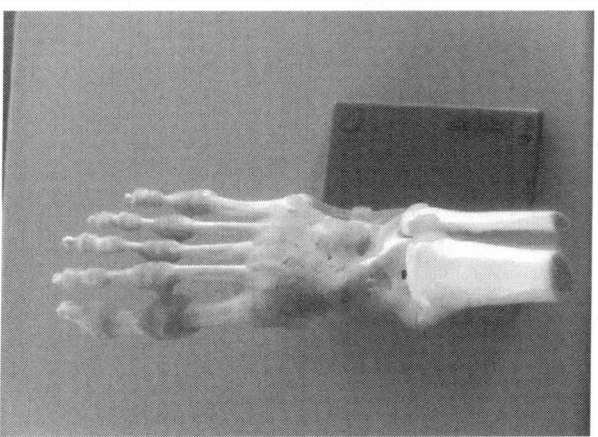

Ottawa Rules for Fractures of the Foot

The presence of a fracture is more likely in patients with foot injuries with any pain in the top of the foot (mid foot zone) and any of the following:

- Tenderness at Navicular bone just below the malleolus (see above).

- Tenderness at base of the little toe (5th metatarsal) remembering the bones of the toes extend much further back into the foot than the portion where they divide and articulate.

- Inability to walk four weight bearing steps immediately after the accident and in upon later examination

Ottawa Rules for Fractures of the knee

The presence of a fracture is more likely in patients with knee injuries with any of the following:

- Over 55 years of age
- Tenderness at the head of the fibula
- isolated tenderness of the kneecap
- inability to bend knee to 90 degrees
- inability to walk four weight bearing steps immediately after the accident and upon later examination.

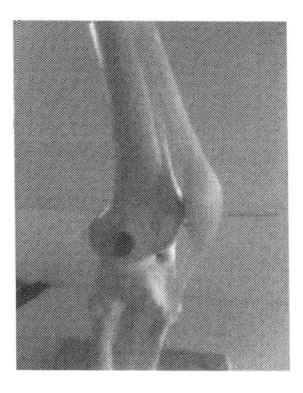

Upper Leg (Femur)

A lot of force is needed to fracture the femur, and femoral fractures are often associated with other serious complications. The strong muscles in your thigh will cause fractured bone ends to overlap and damage surrounding tissue and blood vessels leading to serious bleeding. A femoral fracture can be identified by;

- Shortening of the limb
- Swelling
- Pain
- Signs of shock

If the femoral artery is damaged death from internal bleeding can be rapid. In order to minimize bleeding traction should be applied. But this is contra-indicated if there is damage to either;

- Pelvis
- Knee
- Top of Femur

Hip

Damage to the ball or socket of the hip joint is very painful and usually requires surgical repair. It is often diagnosed by an obvious shortening of the effected limb and an external rotation of the foot.

Pelvis

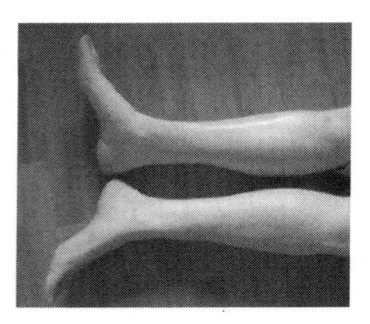

Fractured pelvis should be suspected with any high velocity injury such as falls or RTCs. If the pelvis is entirely broken the patient feet will both be externally rotated this is known as an Anterior-posterior or open book fracture.

The main complication of a pelvic fracture is major blood loss as mentioned above there are major blood vessels passing through the pelvis to supply circulation to the lower extremities. Other problems can occur if splinters of bone penetrate abdominal organs.

Due to the forces needed to fracture a Pelvis the patient often has other serious injuries.

- 50% Serious Head Injury
- 50% Long Bone Fracture
- 20% Serious Chest Injury

There are different types of Pelvic Fractures;

- 60-70% Lateral Fractures
- 15-20% Open Book Fractures
- 5-15% Vertical Fractures

The most common type is a Lateral Fracture mostly caused by side impacts these rarely require operation and heal with bed rest. The other two share a 6% mortality rate and are often associated with severe bleeding.

© Sebastian Kaulitzki | Dreamstime.com

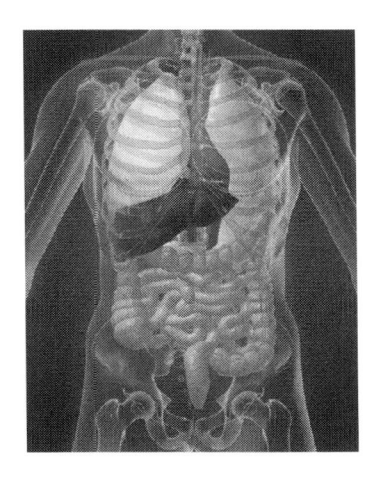

Ribs

Fractures to the ribs themselves usually heal without further intervention and should take around 4 weeks. The only real issue is pain and complications from not coughing or deep breathing because of the pain (infection).

Fractures to ribs can interfere in ventilation of the chest. If multiple adjacent ribs are broken in more than one place a 'flail segment' is created. The segment moves independently from the rest of the chest wall causing pain and impeding respiration. Pieces of ribs can penetrate the lungs causing a heamothorax (Blood in the pleural cavity) or a pneumothorax (Air in the pleural cavity). See section on chest injuries for more details.

Spinal Damage

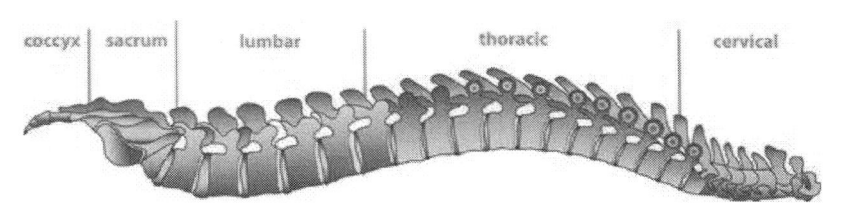

© Maryna Melnyk | Dreamstime.com

The spine is divided into five sections the cervical, thoracic, lumbar, sacrum and coccyx. Most spinal injuries occur in the cervical spine. Mainly as stresses are placed upon it as the head is shaken due to sudden acceleration or deceleration forces. These may be applied during traumatic injuries such as RTCs, blows and falls from heights.

The cervical spine is made up of seven cervical vertebrae separated by inter-vertebral disks and joined by ligaments. They are referred to as C1 to C7 starting from the base of the skull through to the top of the thoracic spine. Damage to C1 or C2 is often fatal if the spine is compromised as the nerves joining the spine at this level control breathing.

A set of rules to eliminate serious injuries to the C Spine is called 'clearing the C Spine'

If the following apply

- Fully alert (GCS 15) see Appendix 1
- Not intoxicated
- No distracting painful injury
- No neurological signs or symptoms such as 'tingling'
- No tenderness in the midline of the neck

And if any of the following are relevant;
- Neck pain is present but has a delayed onset
- Has walked unaided since injury
- Neck injury followed a rear end shunt

If the spine has been 'cleared' then immobilisation may not be necessary. However poor spinal management can have devastating effect on a casualties life and recovery if in any doubt about the presence of a spinal injury immobilise the casualty particularly in the following circumstances.

- Fallen >1m
- Diving accidents
- RTC>60mph
- In rollover RTCs or ejected from vehicle
- Pedestrian or Motorcyclist in RTC
- Patient over 65

Any casualty that is unconscious or has a head injury should be considered to have a cervical spinal injury until proven otherwise. These casualties should be immobilized.

Spinal Shock

The quality of treatment and immobilisation a casualty get immediately after an injury and for the next 8 hours has a significant effect on recovery of function. Poor management can worsen injuries, although the initial injury is usually the mechanism that causes the most damage.

After the initial injury the spinal cord swells. Treatment to reduce inflammation of the cord helps to prevent further nerve damage

Some patients recover with immobilization alone. The patient requires a semi-rigid collar and prolonged immobilisation lying still with minimal neck movement. The patient needs two months complete bed rest for this method.

The effects of the injury depend on the level at which the injury occurs. But often effects sensation and movement below that level and related organs. However some function can return in the first few weeks after an injury. So it is impossible to predict the final outcome for any patient at the time of injury.

Depending on the level of the injury initial disability will include the following. If the injury is at C8 for example the patient will also loose function of systems below

C4 and C5	Diaphragm (Breathing)
C5	Shoulder and Elbow Muscles
C6	Bending the Wrist
C7	Straightening the elbow.
C8	Bends the fingers
T1	Spreads the fingers
T1 –T12	Chest wall & abdominal muscles.
L2	Bends the hip
L3	Straightens the knee
L4	Pulls the foot up
L5	Wiggles the toes
S1	Pulls the foot down
S3,4 and 5	Bladder, bowel, anal, genitalia other pelvic muscles

Helmet Removal

If attending a motorcyclist with a full face helmet this should only be removed if you can see or suspect a head injury, if the patient is having airway or breathing difficulties or if they are unconscious. To do this safely requires two people.

The first person stabilises the patients head by holding either side of the helmet.

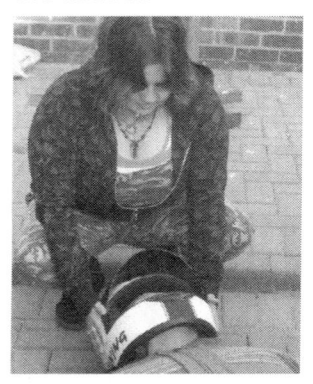

The second person places the thumb and first finger of one hand on the patients cheeks under the helmet and the other hand under the patients neck to support the head.

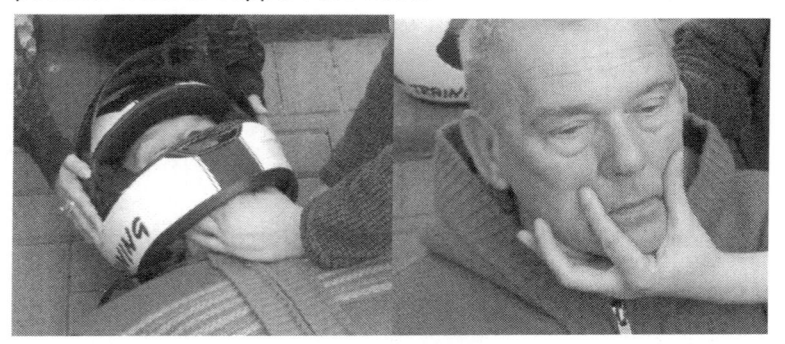

The right hand photo shows finger position without the helmet.

To remove helmet the first person, rocks it back and forth to clear the nose and the back of the skull.

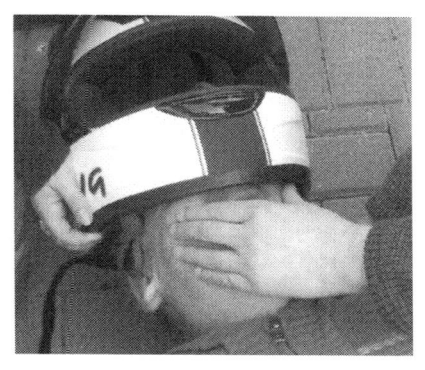

Once the helmet starts to be removed the second person can slide their hand up to support the weight of the head and reposition it in a neutral position.

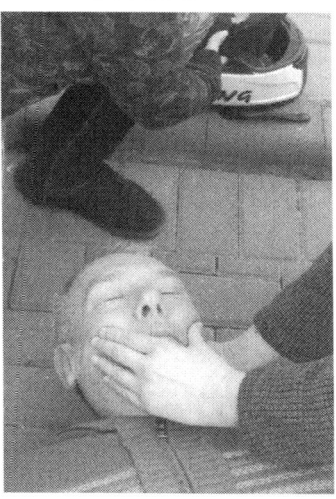

Chapter 4 Dislocations

When force is applied to a joint the first thing to occur is a mild sprain and the ligaments are strained, as progressively more force is applied a severe strain occurs and if the force continues the joint dislocates.

Jaw

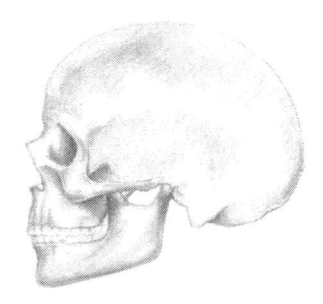

© Ciska76 | Dreamstime.com

Jaw (Mandible) dislocation is the displacement of the mandible from the rest of the skull, dislocations can be caused by traumatic and non-traumatic means. The point at which the two join is the temporomandibular joint (TMJ).

The jaw can dislocate in any direction, but moving forward (Anterior) dislocations are the most common, Backward (Posterior) dislocations can be caused by a direct blow.

Patients have pain and are unable to open or close mouth, you should check for damage to the mouth and the stability of the jaw for fractures. Other symptoms include a misaligned bite, difficulty speaking, dribbling, jaw may be sticking out.

Shoulder

Shoulders are the most common joint that becomes dislocated and the easiest to rectify.

When examining the patient the normal round symmetry of the shoulder looks squared off, they will hold arm in the most comfortable position and resist any attempts to move it due to pain. Check for underlying fractures and nerve and blood vessel damage. If any exist it significantly increases the risks of reducing the dislocation.

Elbow

The elbow is a sturdy joint and takes a considerable force to dislocate. Due to this a significant amount of elbow dislocations also have associated fractures. The elbow can be displaced to the front (Anterior) or more often the back (Posterior).

Finger

The two joints in each finger are called interphalangeal (IP) joints. The area where the finger joins the hand it is called the metacarpophalangeal (MCP) joint. The most common dislocation is of the proximal interphalangeal (PIP) which is the nearer joint to the body of the hand. It can dislocate to the front, back or side.

Hip

Hip dislocations can be to the back (Posterior) commonly caused by impacts in road accidents, to the front (Anterior) caused by falls or to the side (Lateral) usually associated with a fracture.

In all dislocations the patient is in severe pain, has severely limited movement in the limb. There is also a possibility of nerve or blood vessel damage. Damage to the femoral artery can cause fatal internal bleeding.

© Caroline Jackson

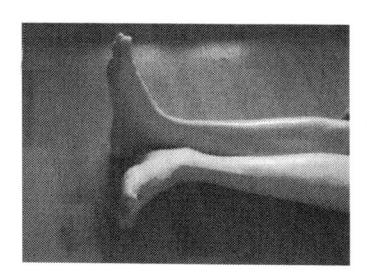

If it is a posterior dislocation the leg will be internally rotated towards the centre of the body whereas in an anterior dislocation the leg is externally rotated. In patients with total hip joint replacement dislocations are not uncommon but not usually associated with significant injuries in the same way traumatic dislocations are.

Knee

Knee dislocations are usually accompanied by extensive soft tissue damage, this will make reducing the dislocation easier as there will be less muscle mass working against you. There is a real risk of vascular injury and they may need to be re-manipulated to ensure a good circulation.

Kneecap (Patella)

When dislocated the kneecap usually moves to the outside and the deformity is obvious when compared with the other leg. The patient will keep their knee flexed in the most comfortable position.

Chapter 5 Wounds and Burns

Types of Bleeding

There are several type of blood vessels in the body, the three well known ones are Capillaries, Veins and Arteries.

Capillaries

These are the smallest vessels and supply a vast network of blood to the skin and organs. If a person is struck and a bruise appears this is actually the result of capillary damage releasing blood under the skin, if you graze your skin then any blood revealed is due to damages capillaries and tends to ooze out. Capillary bleeding is very unlikely to pose a significant bleeding risk however it does open the body up to infection so all grazes etc should be covered.

Veins

Veins are used to take de-oxygenated blood away from the tissues. The blood in them is said to be a darker red as there is less oxygen in it than arterial blood. If a vein is damaged the blood runs out steadily. venous bleeding is life threatening if not treated particularly if internal or in an unconscious casualty that cannot care for themselves.

Arteries

Arteries carry oxygenated blood from the heart to the tissues. Blood from arteries is forced out with each beat of the heart, hence the faster the heart rate the quicker the patient losses blood. Arterial bleeding is the most life-threatening but can be managed using proper techniques.

Principles of Wound Management

Most wounds in otherwise healthy individuals heal by themselves or with little intervention other than initial cleaning and having a dressing applied to protect them from further damage and infection.

When a wound is deep or complicated by other factors a regime needs to be implemented to manage the healing process. The management plan needs to consist of the following;

- To assess, plan, implement and evaluate care with consideration for the whole person not just the wound.

- To promote the natural healing process by maintaining a warm, moist and non-toxic environment.
- To use treatments that are safe, simple, non irritant and non-allergenic
- To use dressings that do not traumatize new tissues on removal and minimize frequency of changes

Physiology of Wound Healing

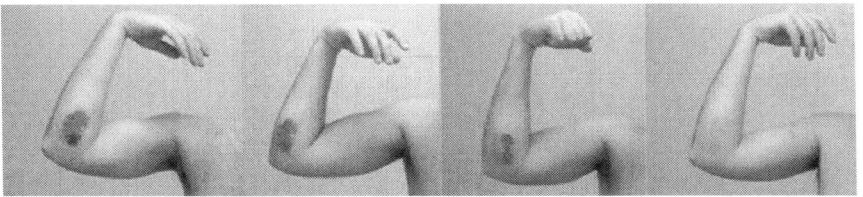

© Fedor Kondratenko Dreamtime.com

Wound healing is the term generally used to describe the mechanism through which the body repairs or replaces damaged tissue. An understanding of the healing process is essential if wounds are to be properly assessed and their management planned. Although the following headings are described separately, they often do overlap, particularly in chronic wounds.

This process can be described as progressing through three phases;
- Inflammatory Phase
- Proliferative Phase
- Maturation Phase

Wound healing varies considerably according to a number of factors which are discussed later. It is important to realize that although the surface of a wound may heal in days it might take months for the underlying tissue to heal properly.

The Inflammatory Phase (2-7 Days)

The first phase of healing is generally called inflammatory, because this is the most visible occurrence after injury. When tissue is damaged, blood vessels are injured and bleed into the space created. This blood then coagulates to form a fibrin clot, the injured blood vessels repair themselves, and the bleeding stops. The damaged tissue then secretes histamine, which has a number of effects, but principally acts to cause capillaries to constrict. During the next few hours, there is increasing tissue swelling and engorgement of surrounding blood vessels. This increased blood supply accounts for the inflamed appearance of; redness, warmth, swelling and pain. Anything which prolongs this inflammatory phase can delay healing, e.g. infection or physical damage caused during dressing changes.

The Proliferative Phase (8-24 Days)

During this phase, different types of cells arrive at the wound site to defend against bacteria, remove dead tissue and begin the repair process. In this phase the cells produce new strands of collagen which is the main constituent of skin, tendons, ligaments and scar tissue. The peak rate of production of collagen in a wound healing by primary intention is between the fifth and seventh day. It is therefore important to take Vitamin C at this stage as the body is unable to store it.

The longer the initial inflammation phase due to damage or infection the more likely scar tissue will be formed. As the proliferative phase proceeds further, there is a rapid increase in the tensile strength of the wound and the number of capillaries begin to decrease towards normal levels. Inflammation also decreases but the wound may remain red, raised and itchy.

The Maturation Phase (24 Days – 2 Year)

During this phase there is a progressive decrease in the blood supply to the scar tissue. The collagen fibres inside the wound move around to make the repair stronger. The dusky red appearance of tissue changes to pale white scar tissue. The strength of the wound, having increased rapidly in the first three weeks of healing will have regained only 50% of the normal tensile strength of a skin wound within the first six weeks, with the amount of collagen in the scar continuing to increase for several months. As it then gradually reduces more, so the scar flattens and softens. The tension within the wound causes the collagen to orientate itself at right angles to the wound margins in a three-dimensional "lacing" effect.

Epithelialisation

In addition to these four overlapping phases a further process Epithelialisation needs to be considered when the wound has been healing by secondary intention.(see below) This process takes place before maturation in such wounds. Following injury, epithelial cells at the edge of the wound migrate over the wound surface. These cells can only migrate over live tissue, and, therefore, if debris, blood clots or scar tissue are present, they have to migrate below causing scabs to form. The best epithelialisation occurs in moist wound environment.

Wounds heal either by *Primary or Secondary* intention

Healing by Primary Intention

Healing by primary intention can occur when the wound edges are either adjacent as In the case of an incision or brought together and closed with sutures, clips, glue or some other form of wound closure. The wound goes through the healing stages described above, but the minimal amounts of blood and exudates will have formed a natural barrier at the wound surface after forty-eight hours. Such a wound can be exposed after this time: a dressing should not be removed unless absolutely necessary within the first two days.

Healing by Secondary Intention

Healing by secondary intention takes place when there has been tissue loss (often extensive) and there may be debris and exudates to be cleared from the wound. Granulation tissue will form the base and sides of the wound, increasing in thickness slowly filling the wound.

Factors which affect wound healing

The human body is able in favourable conditions to heal most wounds without any outside intervention. However a number of factors may contribute to wound break-down and influence wound healing.

Gender

Males shed bacteria more actively and have a higher chance of infection and subsequently reduced healing rate than females.

Infection

Infection of a wound occurs when the germs are sufficiently virulent to overcome the body's resistance bacteria can affect the production of collagen and delay epithelialisation.

Haematoma

A build-up of blood within the tissues appears to have a toxic effect on the tissues as well as acting as a focus for infection. Also the pressures created can restrict blood supply and cause tissue damage.

Temperature of Wound

The best temperature for wound healing has been shown to be 37 degrees Celsius. Certainly extremes of heat and cold can show significant tissue damage. Hence, you should use warmed saline for irrigation/cleansing; and avoid removing dressings unnecessarily.

Nutritional Status

It is important to realize that malnourishment will slow healing: in particular the reduction of collagen synthesis as a result of protein deficiency. Deficiencies in Ascorbic Acid (Vitamin C, which contributes to collagen formation), zinc (probably through its effects on the enzyme systems involved in protein metabolism) and iron (through its effect on haemoglobin levels) have all been cited as factors affecting the rate of tissue healing. So it is worth stocking these supplements for medicinal use if none other.

Drugs

Although it is not usually possible to stop taking them if you have other problems it should be noted that the following drugs may have an adverse effect on wound healing;

Indomethacin (an *Anti-inflammatory*), Aspirin, Cytotoxic Drugs and Steroids

Embedded Object in Wound

The presence of an embedded object in a wound can act as a focus for infection in addition to the problem of provoking an immune reaction.

Good Blood Supply

A wound is dependent on the blood for a supply of nutrients and cellular material vital for wound healing. Well supplied areas such as the face usually heal quickly whilst extremities of the limbs receive a poorer supply.

Smoking

Studies have demonstrated that blood flow to peripheral vessels is reduced by the inhalation of nicotine. Some research also points to direct tissue damage and inhibition of the healing process.

Illness

Anaemia may in itself delay healing due to the supply of oxygen to the wound being reduced. A Circulatory disease will, in limiting the flow of blood, have a detrimental effect on the rate of healing. Other diseases that affect healing are Diabetes, Jaundice and increased Urea levels (Uraemia). Respiratory and Cardiac Disease`s will reduces oxygen to tissues and thus delay healing.

Patient`s Age

Ageing results in reduced skin elasticity and metabolic rate; there may be some muscle wastage (Atrophy). With increasing age, the inflammatory and repair mechanisms operate less vigorously and cells, therefore, are replaced more slowly. General blood supply may also be impaired.

Age of the Wound

It is probable that the older the wound when appropriate intervention commences, the slower healing will be, so treat early.

Surgical Technique

Rough handling, can damage tissue and provide a focus for infection. Poor suturing technique can also influence wound healing since applied too tightly they can cut through a wound edge, whilst incorrectly inserted they can damage weakened tissue. Remember that sutures are foreign bodies and although sterile can both; evoke an immune response or drag contamination though a wound.

Types of Wounds

Contusion

These are blunt, non penetrating injuries, that crush or damage small blood vessels and result in bleeding into the local area. Erythema (or redness) results from the dilation of the capillaries; Ecchymosis (or the bruise itself) results from blood leaking from small blood vessels and losing its oxygen. A hematoma is a palpable lump from where the blood has leaked out of vessels and pools in the tissues. The patient can lose a significant amount of blood before swelling is evident.

There is normally no specific treatment it is just painful and simple analgesia is enough. Usually there is not enough blood loss to be significant from a volume point of view, c\occasional if extensive bruising can be a problem due to blood loss but this isn't common.

A large haematoma has the potential to get infected, this presents as increasing pain / fever / swelling. The treatment is antibiotics initially and if not quickly setting may need incision and drainage.

Lacerations

A laceration is a straight cut to the skin, often superficial but may involve deeper structures. The main aim of managing these wounds is to close the skin.

You need to understand that there are many structures you cannot fix or are beyond your experience in a remote clinic environment, but you still need to consider and try and identify what deep structures are injured.

For deep lacerations Providone iodine sprayed into the wound before closing protects against infection. A low-adherent absorbent dressing such as polyurethane foam is ideal with pressure bandaging added if there is much discharge after suturing.

Discharge is usually light and within forty-eight hours, a natural barrier against pathogenic invasion will have been formed and the wound can, if required, safely be exposed at this point. Continued cleaning of such wounds will be unnecessary unless there are signs of breakdown or infection

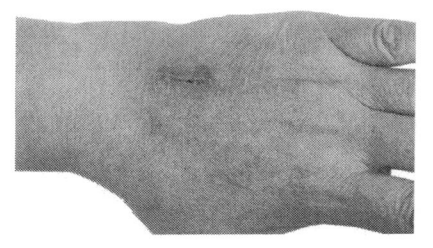

© Birgit Reitz-hofmann - Dreamtime.com

Crush Injuries

When dealing with Crushed fingers and toes you may need to fix an underlying fracture.

Often blood collects under the nail and is very painful, this is easily relieved by heating a paperclip and using it to melt a hole in he nail letting out the blood. If there is loss of a lot of tissue they should be dealt with as open wounds. A low-adherent absorbent dressing such as polyurethane foam or an alginate sheet should be used.

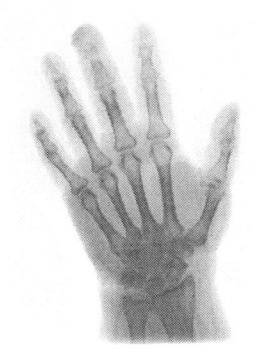

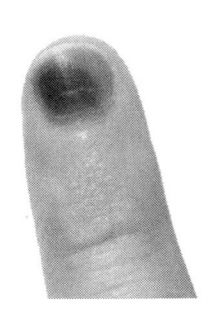

© Tallik Dreamstime.com   © Marcin Pawinski Dreamstime.com

Deep Penetrating Wounds

Penetrating wounds consist of a narrow but deeply penetrating tract; they may contain infection buried deep in the wound. These are caused by knives, low velocity bullets and other penetrating objects. Closing the wound is not an option as it will trap the infection. These wounds need to be opened more under anaesthetic to be cleaned properly. For penetrating injuries involving the trunk see chapters on abdominal and chest injuries. Following cleaning and depending on the size of the hole, either a biodegradable alginate ribbon or a hydrogel with ribbon gauze, loosely packed, are recommended.

Abrasions

Abrasions, although apparently superficial are usually very painful, and commonly have dirt and grit in the wound. They must be thoroughly cleaned and the dressing used must prevent further contamination and absorb discharge. Following thorough cleansing, a semi permeable film dressing can be used for low discharge wounds whilst a polyurethane foam or hydrocolloid sheet is recommended for a wound with high discharge. For high risk wounds use an antiseptic-impregnated dressing.

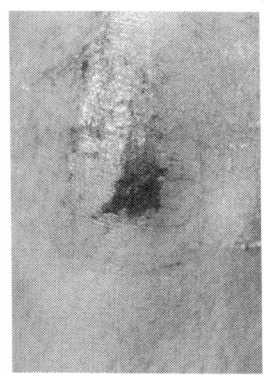

© Szefei| Dreamstime.com

Bites

Bite injuries produce a confined ragged wound with a high risk of infection – that is especially true for human bites. Thorough cleaning is essential. Bite wound should not be closed a short course (5 days) of antibiotics is usually advisable (e.g. Flucloxacillin, Augmentin or Cephradine)

De-gloving Injuries

De-gloving wounds cause layers of tissue to be torn away exposing deep tissues and may cause extensive damage to skin, fat muscle and bone. Such injuries will need thorough cleaning and possible skin grafting.

Use of Antibiotics

Most wounds will contain some bacteria, and chronic wounds may be heavily contaminated if there is debris or dead (necrotic) tissue. If you don't have the benefit of a Laboratory tests you need to use antibiotics where contamination is likely or signs of infection are present.

If infection exists then appropriate antibiotics should be started. Oral antibiotics will also be used following bite injuries. The only indication for the use of topical antibiotic is for an infected / malodorous wound when topical Metronidazole may be used.

The decision to close

Another question you need to ask is, is closing the wound the best option? In many outdoor medicine circles and novices working in austere environments, a big deal is made of the ability to suture but the reality is many wounds can live without it !

Is it clean?: Can you clean the wound? Never ever close a dirty wound. Infection is almost certain to result.

Can I close the layers appropriately?: What will happen if you don't close the wound? Are you just closing it for cosmetic reasons or is it big and gapping and needs to really be closed?

How long ago did it happen?: Closing old wounds > 8-12 hrs significantly increases the risk of infection. For old wounds, delayed primary closure should be used. For hands and feet and feet you have a little less time, 4-6 hours and for the head and face you have slightly longer 12-24 hrs

Long-term Wound Management

Older wounds need to be considered slightly differently if there are any they are slow to heal or are being allowed to heal by tertiary or delayed primary closure.

Necrotic Wounds

Necrotic tissue is dead tissue found in or around a wound. It is usually recognizable by its black or yellowish-brown colour. The first aim of managing such a wound is to remove the necrotic tissue without damaging the underlying or surrounding tissues.

Sloughy Wound

Slough is formed when dead cells accumulate in the exudates of a wound. Slough tends to be yellow in colour but care must be taken not to misinterpret slough either for, occasionally, epithelial tissue, or for the pus produced when an infection is present: the other signs and symptoms present which are likely to co-exist in an infected wound are outlined below. Further, some dressings may interact with the wound to produce fluids, which can be mistaken for slough or pus.

Granulating Wounds

Granulation tissue is recognised by its red 'healthy' appearance, as new blood vessels are formed and grow into the wound area. However, healthy granulating tissue, being well supplied with blood, bleeds easily and the avoidance of trauma and the promotion of granulation by providing a clean moist environment, are the aims of management at this stage, care must be taken however, not to assume a red wound equals a healthy wound. Infected wounds can also have a deep red coloration to them and the presence of any of the other signs of infection mentioned above must be taken seriously.

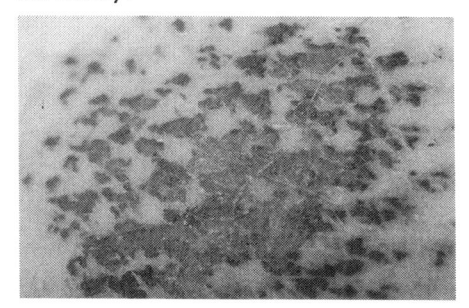

Granulation tissue

© Spe Dreamtime.com

Infected Wounds

Infected wounds often contain pus (frequently yellow in colour) and are likely to show signs of tissue destruction and delayed healing. There is likely to be some or all of the following signs and symptoms present: High temperature, heat and swelling around wound edge, inflammation, Cellulitis, offensive odour and greenish slough. Management must be aimed at treating the infection with antibiotics such as Flucloxacillin and/or providing the optimum environment for the body defence to overcome the invading infection.

Malodorous Wounds

Malodorous wounds have an offensive odour often arises when wound healing is complicated by anaerobic bacterial infection. Such wounds are often discharging exudates, lesions, as well as infected pressure sores and leg ulcers. Management of such wounds will often be dominated by the need to promote the patient's quality of life: care may, therefore on occasion be unconventional and aimed at symptom control rather than active treatment.

Epithelialising Wounds

Epithelial tissue begins to develop when a wound is filled with granulation tissue to the level of the surrounding skin. The colour of this type of wound can vary from pinkish through to yellowish and may require careful assessment to distinguish the epithelial tissue from slough. Fragile epithelial tissue develops best under moist conditions when cells can migrate readily across the surface of the wound: although the avoidance of trauma during dressing changes is an equally important requirement of management regime.

Sinus or Fistula

Almost any type of wound could be complicated by a sinus or fistula. The presence of pus might alert one to the possibility of a sinus within a wound, the pus being discharged into the wound cavity from the abscess beyond: whilst the presence of body fluid e.g. faecal fluid, urine, bile discharging either into a wound cavity or via a suture line suggests the presence of a fistula.

A sinus is often difficult to heal as the cavity beyond often contains foreign material e.g. suture material. The management of such a wound ideally requires that any foreign material is removed. The sinus must be opened sufficiently wide to allow any exudates to drain or it should be opened out (often surgically) and allowed to heal by granulation from below. The exudates from a draining sinus should be absorbed and a means of ensuring that its opening cannot heal must be adopted but a tight pack will act as a bung and prevent the first requirement of sinus management -the free drainage of exudates.

A fistula may develop as a result of a disease process or due to breakdown of a surgical repair. Fistulae often close spontaneously or (further) surgery may be required. In the interim such wounds are usually managed symptomatically with care of the skin to prevent abrasions (Excoriation) from being a major consideration.

Treatment of Burns

Burns are fourth major cause of trauma related deaths, burns can be classified into three types;
- Superficial (First Degree)
- Partial thickness (Second Degree)
- Full thickness (Third Degree)

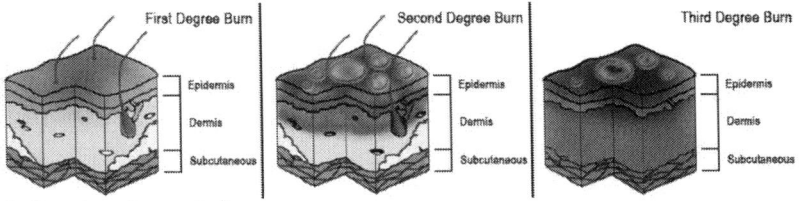

© Persian Poet Gal

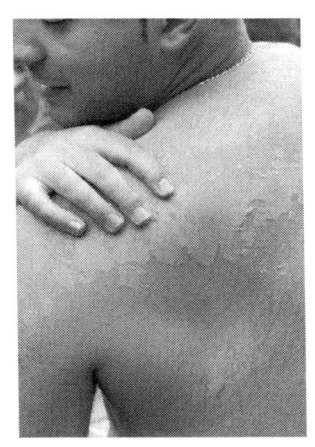

© Arenacreative | Dreamstime.com

Superficial burns only affect the top layer of skin, they are denoted by reddening and swelling of skin and tenderness.

Partial thickness burns affect the epidermis causing reddening and rawness. Blisters are formed from plasma released from tissues.

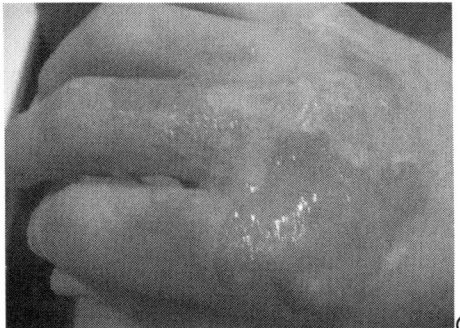

© Alcedema

Full thickness burns affect multiple layers of skin and can affect nerves, blood vessels and underlying muscles.

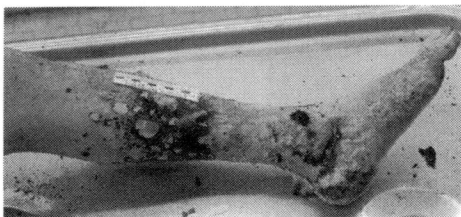

© Goga312

A casualty who is trapped in a burning structure or vehicle can experience a number of problems apart from tissue loss. As always our priority is to **maintain (A)irway, (B)reathing and (C)irculation**.

Burns cause progressive cell death as temperatures rise above 45°C, instantaneously above 60°C, heat is also conducted into surrounding tissues, causing further injuries.

Burns cause fluid loss from cells this may happen over several hours and is relative to the area burned see below.

Injuries of over 15% of the body surface (10% in children) cause sufficient loss of fluid that the patient will require additional fluids to be administered to prevent shock developing.

Early cooling of a burn will reduce the local inflammatory response. Injuries above 25-30% of the body surface cause Systemic Inflammatory Response Syndrome (SIRS). This continues to develop for several hours after the burn.

The clinical signs of SIRS can be delayed. Toxins released from the burn wound further stimulate the SIRS. In the healthy, excessive i.v. fluid administration can be compensated for by an increased urine output. In the burn victim, too much fluid results in excessive oedema.

Smoke Inhalation

This is a serious problem and affects the body in different ways;

Burns to the airway are caused by hot gases from flame, smoke and steam. Usually affecting the upper airway which can swell causing an obstruction. The patient may appear initially ok but as the swelling can occur up to 36 hours later and develops slowly they must be observed carefully. The lining of the airway may become ulcerated leading to secondary infection.

If the gasses are toxic and are deeply inhaled into the lungs they dissolve, leading to chemical injury which can lead to pulmonary failure, this may take hours or days to become apparent.

Absorption of toxic gases through the lungs into the blood leads to blood poisoning.

The two leading causes of death are due to carbon monoxide and cyanide poisoning. Carbon monoxide replaces molecules of oxygen carried in blood it also causes cells to function abnormally.

The patient will experience fatigue, nausea and confusion this can lead to a decrease in brain function and eventually death in severe cases.

It's important therefore to assess their respirations for adequacy and depth.

Calculating the % burnt

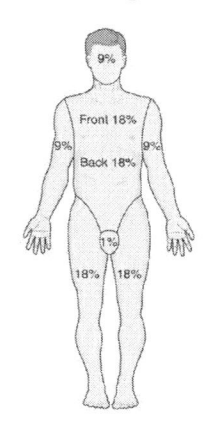

The Rule of 9s.

Head [9%]

Chest and Abdomen [18%]

Back[18%]

Each arm [9%

Each leg [18%]

Genitals[1%]

© Legger| Dreamstime.com

Don't count areas of first degree burn only in estimating the total burnt area for purposes of these calculations. Initial fluid requirement should be based on 20ml/kg weight of the patient up to 2 litres. Fluid required in the first 24 hours is often underestimated and is based on;

4ml x patient weight in kg x BSA burned.

With half the total being given in the first 8 hours.

Thus a 80kg man with 40% burns would initially need 1.6 litres of fluid, another 4.8 litres in the first 8hrs and a further 6.4 litres in the next 16 hours. For a total of 12.8 litres in the first 24hrs. If the patient is unconscious all of this would need to be given IV.

Significant or critical burns are gauged as full thickness covering 10%+ of BSA or partial thickness of 30%+ of BSA or burns affecting the hands, feet, face, airway or genitalia. Probable mortality is calculated as the patient's age + BSA burnt as a percentage. Bizarrely one of the killers in burn victims is hypothermia, where blood plasma that seeps into burnt areas is evaporated leading to rapid heat loss and severe hypothermia.

Chapter 6 Head, Chest and Abdominal Trauma

Head Injuries

A head injury often causes nothing more than a bruise, lump or headache. There are however several serious conditions which need to be excluded;

Concussion

Concussion is where the brain, which is suspended in Cerebral Spinal Fluid (CSF) shakes within the skull hitting its inside surface, the casualty may briefly lose consciousness and become confused. There may be a brief loss of memory, followed by nausea, dizziness and headache from a few hours to a few days. Recovery is usually complete.

Compression

Compression is usually caused by an injury due to either a skull fracture or laceration to the brain where it has hit the inside of the skull due to sudden deceleration. Compression can be caused by bleeding inside the skull which holds a fixed volume of material or by swelling of brain tissue caused by trauma or infection. Pressure on brain tissue causes patients to display symptoms below as well as increasing disability.

In severe cases the brain can become herniated as it is pushed down into the opening where the spinal column joins the brain. This has the potential to be fatal.

Management

Any patient with a head injury who has a significant mechanism of injury, say from a Road Traffic Collision (RTC), fall or blow also has the potential for a spinal injury.

Assess level of consciousness using the Glasgow coma scale (see appendix 1)

A physical examination of the casualty should be performed. Look for blood with straw coloured fluid from the nose and ear this is cerebral spinal fluid (CSF) and is indicative of a basal skull fracture. Other signs are panda eyes, which are black circles of bruising around one or both eyes and battle sign which is bruising behind the ear.

Check pupil reactions by shining a light directly into the casualties eyes, preferably in dim light. Note the size of each pupil in millimetres, some pen torches have a gauge on the side showing pupils sizes.

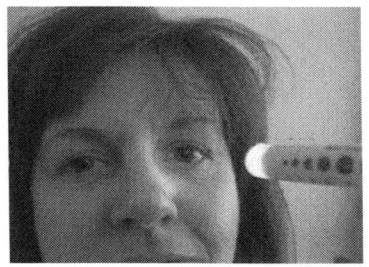

The pupil should go smaller (constrict) in reaction to the light, note if a reaction takes place, if it is brisk or sluggish and if both eyes react the same. A difference in pupil sizes or reaction speed is often a clue to an underlying head injury. Check to see if they can follow the light from side to side and if their vision is blurred.

However don't become fixated with pupils; 10% of the population have asymmetrical pupils (some quite dramatically) and pupil asymmetry is only meaningful if there is other evidence of serious head injury.

Check the casualty can remember what happens (amnesia) a loss of less than a minute is rarely serious. Whereas a loss of greater than 30 minutes usually indicates a serious injury.

Note any history of unconsciousness although not a definite guide less than two minutes is associated with concussion whereas longer periods with compression indicates bleeding or swelling off the brain

- Further checks can include;
- Hearing in both ears
- If they can move all limbs, have normal sensation and no numbness or pins & needles
- Finally check to see if they can stand and walk without staggering

Even if the patient passes all the tests they should still be monitored for possible deterioration as initial injury may cause swelling of brain tissue or slow bleeding into the brain. Signs they should be alert for are;

- Increased drowsiness
- Increased headache
- Confusion
- More than one episode of vomiting
- Weakness in Limb
- Facial Droop or Speech difficulties
- Dizziness, loss of balance
- Blurred vision
- Difficulty breathing
- Convulsions or Absences

Chest Wounds

There are several different chest injuries.

Fractures of the chest wall have been previously covered.

Remaining injuries either effect;

- Lungs
- Diaphragm
- Trachea
- Heart
- Major Blood Vessels
- Oesophagus

Lungs

There are a number of lung injuries that can result from trauma;

Pulmonary contusion

Pulmonary contusion is bruising of the lungs causing bleeding into the Alveoli. This decreases gaseous exchange and lowers oxygen level in blood. Support patient with IV fluids (if shocked) and oxygen if available. Excessive fluid therapy may causes more complications,

Simple Pneumothorax

A simple Pneumothorax is caused by trauma or can happen spontaneously. Degree of compromise to breathing depends on size of Pneumothorax. Small tears will heal themselves, monitor in case it becomes a tension Pneumothorax and treat symptomatically.

Open Pneumothorax

An open Pneumothorax is known as a 'sucking chest wound' caused by penetrating trauma which will allow air to enter the chest cavity from outside. Bubbling of blood in the wound may be seen on expiration. Air may be present in the surrounding tissue (Subcutaneous emphysema) which feels like "bubble wrap".

Tension Pneumothorax

A Tension Pneumothorax occurs when air enters the pleura but cannot escape, as pressure builds up it collapses the lung on the affected side, as it progresses it can also affect the heart and other lung. Potential signs include; diminished or absent breath sound, unilateral chest movement, fast breathing, lowering blood pressure, distended neck veins and cyanosis. If you see the trachea has moved away from the midline towards the unaffected side this is a very serious problem.

Haemothorax

A Haemothorax is bleeding into the chest cavity will present with both breathing and circulation problems. Which will both require support.

Diaphragm

This is a sheet of muscle that stretches across the bottom of the chest and is an essential part of respiration. It can be damaged by blunt or penetrating trauma or by pressure changes during an explosion. If it tears, abdominal organs may become herniated through the tear which will interfere with respiration and may damage the organs.

Trachea

Damage to the trachea will affect breathing. Monitor respiration rate, oxygen saturation, movement of chest, listen for unequal or absent breath sounds.

Heart

Two conditions affect the heart during trauma;

Myocardial Contusions

Which is bruising of the heart muscle, this shows the same signs as a heart attack and can cause cardiogenic shock it should be treated in the same way with careful monitoring of patient vital signs particularly blood pressure and oxygen saturations. It presents as central chest pain following a history of chest trauma.

Cardiac Tamponade

Which is bleeding inside the sac surrounding the heart. As the blood builds up it compresses the ventricles of the heart and rapidly affects the heart function. It presents with three symptoms known collectively as Becks triad; a low blood pressure, muffled heart sounds and distended neck veins. Patients are often also breathless and confused.

Major Blood Vessels

Vessels can be damaged by blunt or penetrating trauma, explosion or deceleration injuries. If the aorta is completely severed death is rapid, if it is damaged but not severed a third of casualties die in first 24 hours and half within 48 hours. Aortic dissection is characterised by sudden onset ripping chest pain. Pain is often said to go through to back or into neck or jaw. Blood pressure is often low.

Oesophagus

In traumatic injuries the Oesophagus can be damaged by penetrating trauma. The main problem with this is that it allows gastric content to enter the chest cavity which can lead to pneumonia and sepsis.

Small tears may heal themselves, larger ones require surgery and are rapidly fatal.

Abdominal Injuries

The abdomen contains many organs and is separated from the thoracic cavity by the diaphragm. If the injury occurs before inspiration then the diaphragm will be high in the chest, at around nipple level. If the chest is fully expanded then the diaphragm will be flattened. This has to be considered when evaluating injuries. Three types of structure exist in the abdomen;

- Solid Organs
- Hollow Organs
- Vascular Structures

Solid organs include the Liver, Kidney, Pancreas and Spleen these tend to be very vascular and damage causes serious bleeding. Hollow organs such as Intestines, Stomach, Bladder and Gallbladder these rupture when damaged causing their contents to spill into the abdomen, leading to severe infection. The third group of structures include the Aorta, Femoral Artery and Vena Cava, if these are damaged it usually causes life threatening bleeding. If the diaphragm ruptures then abdominal content will enter the thoracic cavity become herniated and interfere with breathing.

Damage to the abdomen may be caused by blunt, penetrating, shearing, deceleration and blast injuries.

Chapter 7 Road Traffic Collisions (RTCs)

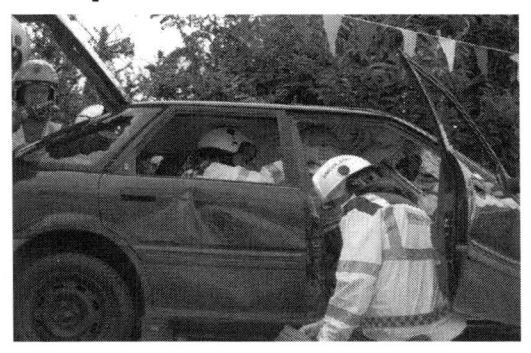

The focus of this chapter is dealing with a RTC, while this is mostly applicable to urban areas with active Emergency Medicine Systems. Equally though a RTC can occur anywhere cars and trucks are on the road, in the third world or after a catastrophe.

Your ability to treat casualties at an accident is both limited by your expertise and equipment that is available.

A few general principles apply to most road traffic collisions. If you stop at an accident do so behind the incident blocking the road. Park your vehicle 'defensively' at an angle rather than straight in the road so that if traffic behind you fails to spot the accident and unfortunately hits your vehicle it will not be pushed into the accident causing further injury to the casualties or yourself.

Assess the scene for possible hazards such as fire, fuel spills and hazardous loads. Only approach the scene if it is safe to do so. If it is dark and you have one wear a Hi-viz vest or coat.

Call the police and ambulance if it is possible to do so.

If you are not alone send another person to set up a warning triangle between 100-200 meters behind your vehicle and if it is dark break some snap light on the road. Both should be carried in your vehicle together with an adequate first aid kit.

If possible approach any vehicle occupants from the front, call out to them, say you are there to help and tell them not to move. If they do have a spinal injury the last thing you want them to do is look over their shoulder to see who is approaching behind them. The emergency services bang the bonnet of the car to focused the casualties attention forward whilst talking to them.

If the car doors are locked or jammed you may need to gain entry by smashing a window, a rescue hammer is good for this and usually comes with a seatbelt cutter as well. A thick pair of gloves is essential too.

Ensure you minimise further danger. ALL engines to be switched off, and do not allow people to smoke nearby.

Check that casualties are breathing, if not you need to get them out of the car as quickly as possible to perform CPR, it is very difficult to do this when someone is in a vehicle and should only be attempted in situ if they are trapped.

If the casualty is conscious and has suffered any type of head injury or was hit from any side with force, always consider the possibility of a spinal injury and try and encourage them to stay in the car if it is safe to do so.

If possible get them or help them to sit upright and support their head/neck from behind in a neutral position, do not flex the neck if you can help it. You may need to kneel on the backseat of their car to do this effectively, always explain why you are doing things to the casualty as it helps reassure them and calm the situation.

If they are unconscious but breathing insert an oral or nasal airway (if you have them) and open their airway using the Jaw Thrust method if you are trained to do so.

If the occupants are conscious check that they are all accounted for, there have been many cases where unrestrained children and adults have been ejected from vehicles into ditches or over hedges and not immediately been found and babies and small children that were on passengers laps and have been thrown into the foot well. Occupants may have been injured wandered away from the accident then collapsed.

If there are casualties on the road who are not conscious try to get someone to stay with them to monitor their breathing but do not move them unless you have too. If you do not have enough people, try and get them into the recovery position whilst supporting their neck as best as you can to stop it moving about. Treat any bleeding and support any fractures before moving them.

The decision as to whether to remove someone from a vehicle can sometimes be difficult to make particularly if you do not have the equipment or personnel to move them safely.

If they are not breathing or are in imminent danger then they need to come out quickly. If you think their condition is deteriorating such as changes in breathing rate, pulse or level of consciousness you should try and get them out in a controlled manner supporting their spine, airway and any injuries they have sustained. If you do have to move them place them on their back in a neutral position and do not leave them. Other dangers may come from traffic or environmental factors where in your judgement leaving them where they are is more dangerous than moving them. In these situations you need to use common sense.

A Neutral position keeps the head upright and in line with the spine like a soldier standing to attention and prevents further aggravation to any possible injury sustained in the RTC.

Chapter 8 Joints, Muscles, Tendons and Ligaments

General Examination of Injuries

History Taking

- Note any history of Trauma or musculoskeletal disease
- Check on Medication that has adverse effects on the Musculoskeletal system i.e. Statins, ACE-inhibitors, Anticonvulsants, Diuretics, Aspirin
- Family History – Consider conditions with inheritable traits i.e. Osteoarthritis, Rheumatoid arthritis, Osteoporosis.
- Social History – Occupation (Repetitive Strain Injury, Vibration white finger, Fatigue fractures)
- Dietary History – Calcium intake / supplements

Questioning the patient

- Pain – Character, Onset, Site
- Stiffness – Joints involved, when is it worse, is it related to rest or activity
- Locking – Mechanical block
- Swelling – Joint affected, onset is it constant or intermittent, Temp, colour
- Deformity – Time frame, Associated symptoms, Acute / Chronic
- Weakness – Localized / Generalized
- Sensory disturbance – Extent of disturbance
- Loss of Function – New or old, Compensatory mechanisms in place
- What is the functional limitation
- Symptoms within a single region or affecting multiple joints
- Acute or slowly progressive
- If injury, what was the mechanism
- Prior problems with the affected area
- Systemic symptoms

Examination

General Inspection
- Appearance, ability to balance and walk if lower limb injury

Assessment
- Inspection (Look)
- Palpation (Feel)
- Manipulation (Move)
- Special Tests & Function

- Patient loosely dressed or with the joint fully exposed
- ALWAYS begin each joint exam with inspection for asymmetry, deformity, atrophy
- ALWAYS compare each joint and muscle group bilaterally
- Palpate each joint and muscle group in sequence
- Isolate each axis when testing Range of Movements (ROM)

Sprain

A sprain is an injury to ligaments which are strong tissues which support joints and attach bones together. They can be injured, by being stretched during a sudden pull.

Grades of Ligament Injuries

Grade I: Partial tear of a ligament without joint instability.

- Mild tenderness and swelling
  Slight or no functional loss (i.e., patient is able to bear weight and move with minimal pain)
- No joint instability

Grade II: Incomplete tear of a ligament, with moderate functional impairment but without causing joint instability.

- Moderate pain and swelling
  Mild to moderate bruising
  Tenderness over involved structures
- Some loss of motion and function (i.e., patient has pain with weight-bearing and walking)
- Mild to moderate instability of joint

Grade III: Complete tear and loss of integrity of a ligament with instability of the joint.

- Severe swelling
- Severe bruising

- Loss of function and motion (i.e., patient is unable to bear weight or move)
- Full joint instability

A damaged ligament causes swelling, inflammation, pain and bruising around the affected joint.

Strain

A strain is stretching or tearing of muscle fibres. Caused by muscle stretching or sudden contraction.

First degree strain

A mild strain affecting a few muscle fibres which are stretched or torn. The injured muscle is tender and painful, but has normal strength.

Second degree strain

A moderate strain with a greater number of injured fibres. There is more severe muscle pain, tenderness, mild swelling, some loss of strength, and a bruise may develop.

Third degree strain

This strain tears the muscle completely with a complete loss of function.

Musculoskeletal Red Flags

- Osteoporosis
- Absent distal pulses
- Systemically unwell patients
- Heat around joints
- Significant mobility impairment
- Suspicion of pathological injuries
- Locking or joints giving way
- Abnormal neurological assessment
- Falls Risk
- Injury not compatible with history
- OTTOWA rules? (see below)

Arthritis

Any inflammation of a joint is known as arthritis. There are different types of arthritis. The three most common are Rheumatoid arthritis, Osteoarthritis and Gout. Arthritis can also occur following some viral and bacterial infections and are usually self limiting.

Rheumatoid arthritis

This is a common form of arthritis affecting about 1% of the population, three quarter of sufferers being women. In these people the body makes antibodies that attack the synovium causing inflammation, this can damage the joint, cartilage and adjacent bones. It is progressive, disfiguring and quite disabling for some people.

It can affect a few or many joints. Most often small joints are affected such as fingers, wrists, ankles and knees, although any joint can be affected. Rheumatoid arthritis is a chronic disease, the severity and time between episodes is different for each patient.

Symptoms include;

- Painful, stiff joints
- Small, painless lumps appear over joints
- Deformity of the joints.
- Tiredness and weight loss
- Fever

In rare cases the inflammation can occur in the lungs or heart this can be serious.

Osteoarthritis

Osteoarthritis is the most common type of arthritis, it causes inflammation of tissues around the joints. It causes damage to cartilage and bony growths appear on the edge of the joints. It mostly occurs in the knees and hips although almost any joint can be affected. It mostly affects women over 50, but also affects men and can occur at any age. It is one of the most common reasons for hip and knee joint replacement.

Symptoms include:

- Pain, stiffness and difficulty moving joints
- Tender joints
- Joints slightly larger or more 'knobbly'
- Grating or crackling in joints
- limited range of movement
- Weakness and muscle wasting

Gout

Gout is a common type of arthritis affecting mainly men between 40 and 60, usually affects the joint of the big toe but can affect any joint. The affected joint swells and is painful, it is caused by a build-up of uric acid in blood that forms crystals. Eating too much red meat, seafood and drinking beer and being overweight worsens the condition. Diabetes and Hypertension also have an effect.

Neck Pain

A set of rules to eliminate serious injuries to the C Spine is called 'clearing the C Spine'

If the following apply

- Fully Alert (GCS 15)
- Not Intoxicated
- No Distracting Painful Injury
- No Neurological signs or Symptoms such as 'Tingling'
- No tenderness in the Midline of the neck
- Not complaining of Spinal Pain
- No tenderness or deformity of vertebra

And if any of the following are relevant;

- Neck Pain is present but has a delayed onset
- Has walked unaided since injury
- Neck injury followed a rear end shunt

See section on trauma for more detail regarding the dangers of spinal injuries.

Once the above has been eliminated ask the patient to perform a range of movements (ROM) as below, if they are unable to do so immobilise their neck.

- Flex =chin to chest
- Extend, = Look up
- Rotate. = look left and right
- Lateral bend = ear to shoulder (Both Sides)

Whiplash

When the head and neck are suddenly and forcefully whipped forward and back, mechanical forces place excessive stress on the cervical spine. This is known as an acute neck sprain or whiplash injury. It strains the muscles and ligaments of the neck beyond their normal range of motion. There is often pain and stiffness in the side of neck or shoulders for the first few days following a whiplash injury.

Wryneck (Torticollis)

Causes the head to be tilted to one side. It has many precipitation factors such as a birth defect, muscle spasm, trauma, nerve damage or may just happen without apparent cause. The muscles affected are usually those supplied by the spinal accessory nerve.

Back Pain

Back Pain can be acute (less than three months old) or chronic where the pain develops gradually over time, lasts more than 3 weeks, and causes long-term problems.

The pain is usually centred around your lumbar region sometimes referred to as the small of your back this region holds your upper body weight plus any weight you are lifting or carrying, it is under a continuous pressure, especially when you're are bending, twisting and lifting. Between 80-90% of the population will experience one or more episodes of lower back pain during their lives, most will be of unknown cause (idiopathic).

Pain may come from the muscles in your back or from your spine;

Latissimus dorsi: these form the largest muscle in the back, stretching from the middle of the lower back to behind the armpits.

Trapezius: sits above your latissimus and forms a trapezoid shape along your neck, shoulders, and the middle of your back.

Rhomboids: The rhomboids stretch from your spine to your shoulder blades.

Erector spinae: The erector spinae stabilize your back.

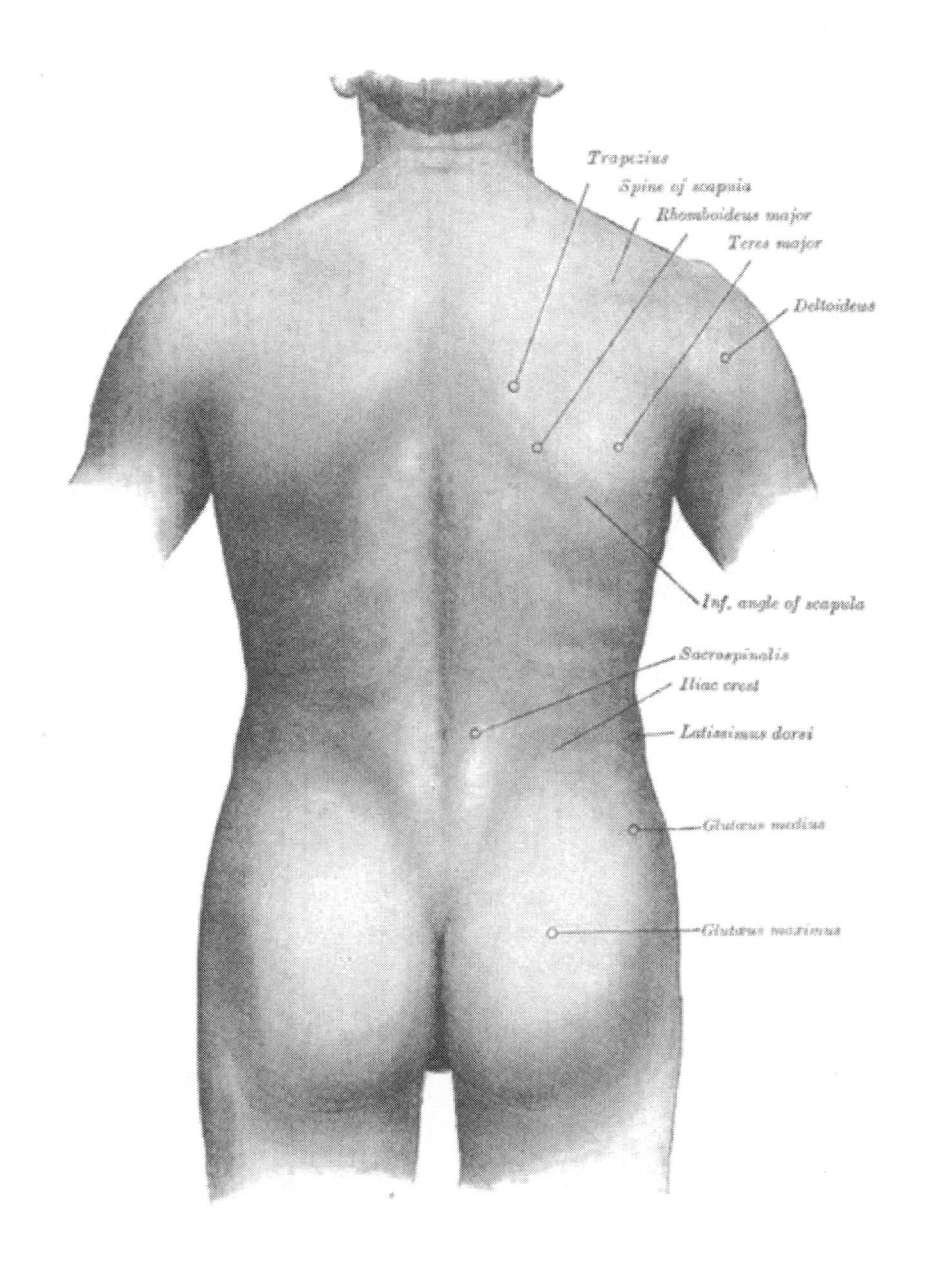

Intra Veritable Discs

Disc conditions and injuries such as degenerative disc disease and herniated discs are among the most common type of problems causing back pain or neck pain.

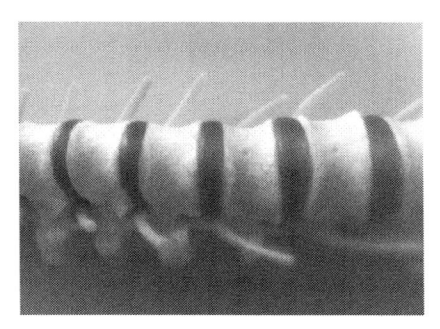

Sciatica - This is an umbrella term to describe pain, weakness, numbness, or tingling in the leg. It is caused by injury to or compression of the sciatic nerve.

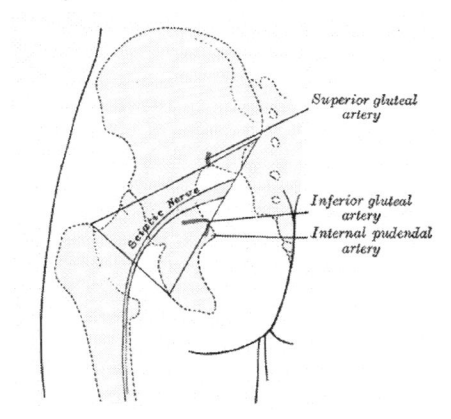

Sciatic Nerve stretch test – Lay patient on back and have them raise their leg to 90 degrees, straight up in air. Now bend foot at ankle so toes are pointing downwards. If this causes pain shooting at the back of the thigh this is an indication of Sciatic nerve tension.

Treatment is aimed at maximising mobility and independence. In some cases, no treatment is required and recovery is spontaneous.

Red Flags

There are a variety of serious pathologies that can cause low back pain. These should be ruled out by questioning or examination

Fracture;

- Age >70 years
- Significant trauma (Major in young / minor in elderly)
- Prolonged use of Corticosteroids
- History of Osteoporosis
- Altered sensation from trunk down

- Clinical diagnosis of a fracture

Cancer;
- Age under 20 or over 55
- Unexplained weight Loss (>4.5kg in 6 months)
- Previous history of cancer
- Pain that doesn't improve when lying down/resting
- Insidious onset
- Systemically unwell
- Constant, progressive, non mechanical pain
- Altered sensation from trunk down
- Clinical diagnosis of Cancer

Infections;
- Systemically Unwell
- Constant, progressive, non mechanical pain
- Recent bacterial infection e.g., UTI or Skin Infection
- Intravenous Drug Use
- Immune suppression from steroid, transplant or HIV
- Altered sensation from trunk down
- Clinical diagnosis of Infection

Cauda equine syndrome;
- Acute onset of Urinary retention or overflow incontinence
- Lose of anal spincter tone or fecaal incontinence
- numbness between buttocks and genitalia (Saddle anesthesia)
- Widespread >1 Nerve root or progressive motor weakness in the leg or gait disturbances
- Clinical diagnosis of Cauda equina syndrome

Inflammatory Disorder;
- Gradual onset before after 40 years
- Pain that doesn't improve when lying down/resting
- Insidious onset

- Systemically unwell (e.g. fever, chills)
- Constant, progressive, non mechanical pain
- Morning backpain >30 mins
- Peripheral joint involvement
- Limitation of joint movement in all directions
- Iritis, skin rashes(psoriasis), colitis, urethral discharge
- Family history of arthritis or osteoporosis
- Pain improves with exercise
- Clinical diagnosis of inflammatory disorder

Abdominal involvement
- Any possibility of pregnancy:
- Associated abdominal pain or vomiting :
- Worrying medical history for abdomen or back:

Knee Assessment

Make sure that both knees are fully exposed.

Inspection
- Is there any evidence of bowing or knock-kneed deformity
- Any scars present
- Does the knee appear red or swollen
- Any rashes present

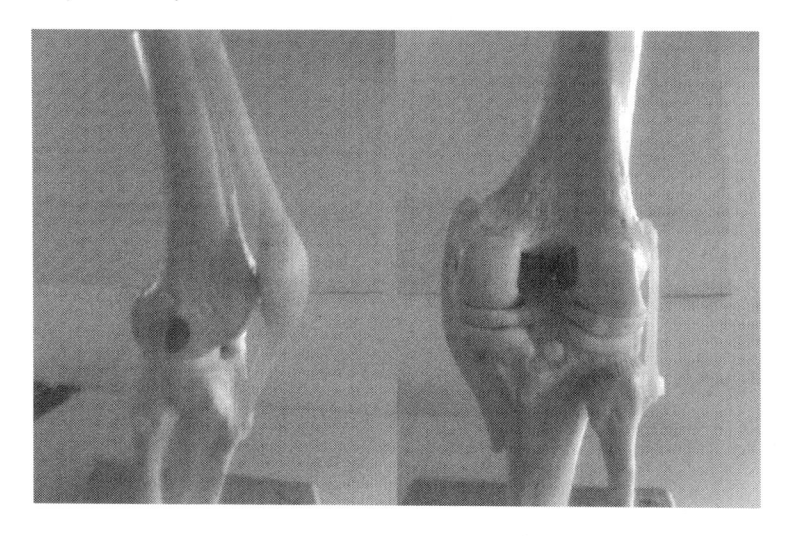

Assess for an effusion (Water on the knee) - Bulge test

- Using your thumb and index finger - milk down any fluid from above the knee. Keep this hand in this position
- Now with the other hand stroke the inside of the knee to empty the medial compartment of fluid then stroke the outside.
- Observe the medial side of the knee for any bulging? This may indicate an effusion (water)

Movement

The normal range of motion of the knee is from: 0 degrees *(Extension)* to approx 135 degrees *(Flexion)*

Active movement

Ask the patient to fully bend *(flex)* then straighten *(extend)* their knee. Always compare the range of movement with the other knee. Is there any reduced range of movement?

Passive movement

Place one hand on the patient's knee and then with the other hand flex *(bend)* the knee as far as possible & then extend the knee. With the hand that is placed over the knee do you feel a 'grinding' sensation? Such a grinding sensation (crepitus) is usually indicative of degenerative knee disease.

Lateral Collateral Ligament test

Cradle the patient's lower leg between your arm and body. The knee should be flexed to 30 degrees. Now with your other hand apply pressure to the knee joint and move leg towards the centre line. Compare to uninjured side excessive movement indicates ligament damage.

Anterior Cruciate Ligament test

Have your patient lay on their back with knee bent and foot flat. Sit on foot in order to stabilise lower leg. With the patient's hamstring muscles relaxed, wrap your fingers around the back of the knee, keeping your thumbs in front of the kneecap. Now pull forward. In a relaxed normal patient there is usually a small degree of movement. Compared injured and uninjured side for differences.

Posterior cruciate ligament test

Repeat as above but instead of pulling - push the patients lower leg.

Excessive movement in either plane may be indicative of cruciate ligament injury.

Apley's grind test

Place the patient face down and bend their knee to 90 degrees. Using your hand to stabilize their lower leg, grip the patient's heel with your other hand. Now gently push down while rotating the ankle back and forth.

A grinding sensation or pain may be indicative of menisci damage, the meniscus being C shaped discs of cartilage which separate the bones in the knee joint.

Serious internal derangement and fractures

Serious damage to structures inside the knee or a small fracture are more likely if any of the following are present. These are usually a trigger for an x-ray and often an MRI scan:

- age 55 or over
- isolated tenderness of the Kneecap(patella)
- tenderness at the head of the fibula
- inability to flex knee to 90 degrees
- inability to weight bear both immediately and in later on examination (4 steps - unable to transfer weight twice onto each lower limb regardless of limping).

Anterior Cruciate Ligament (ACL) Rupture

The anterior cruciate ligament, or ACL, is one of four major knee ligaments. The ACL is critical to knee stability, and people who injure their ACL often complain of symptoms of their knee giving-out from under them. Most often ACL tears occur when turning / twisting whilst running or landing from a jump. The knee gives-out and sometimes a popping sound is heard when the ACL is torn. Women are known to have a higher risk of sustaining this injury.

Ankle Assessment

Mechanism

Inversion

Ankle twisted inwards.
Consider lateral ligament injury or a fracture to base of 5th metatarsal (outside of foot).

Eversion

Ankle twisted outwards.
Consider deltoid ligament injury, navicular injury (Small bone at top of foot)

Inversion / eversion / forced dorsiflexion (toes towards shin)
Consider anterior tibiofibular ligament or navicular injury.

- The patient may hear an audible snap. This does not often correlate with the presence of a fracture. It is an unreliable sign.
- An ankle should be fully assessed at all times to ensure that you do not miss anything

Inspection

- Look for Swelling and/or deformity

Palpation: (feel)

- Ankle joint
- Malleoli (Boney prominence either side of foot)
- Oedema (Fluid under skin)

Check Range Of Movement:

- Foot can be moved up and down at the ankle (dorsiflexion and plantarflexion)
- Subtalar joint Inward/Outward (eversion / inversion)
- Subtarsal joints Inward/Outward (eversion / inversion)
- Hold heel; twist midfoot
- Toes can move freely (Metatarsophalangeal heads)

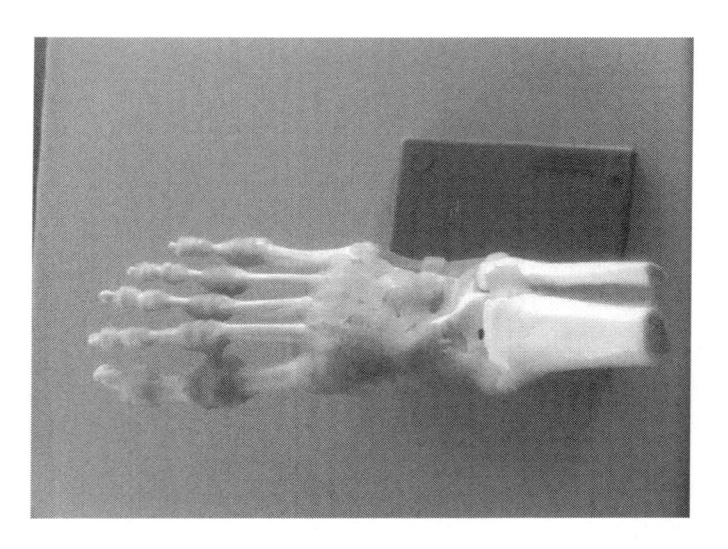

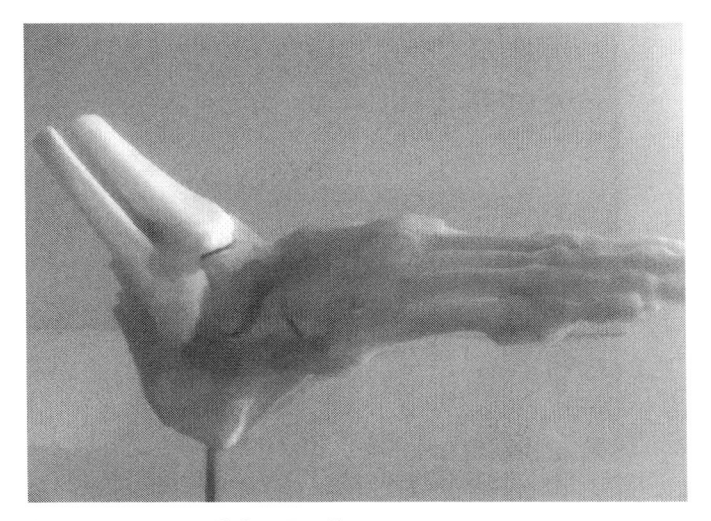

Ottawa Ankle Rules

As with other injuries it can be difficult to distinguish a small fracture from a strain without an x-ray and ultimately time will tell, but application of the Ottawa ankle rules can increase the chance of a fracture. Patients with malleolar or mid-foot zone pain and *any* of these findings are said to be Ottawa ankle rules positive and the more strongly positive, the more likely a fracture:

Bone tenderness along the distal 6 cm of the Anterior or posterior edge of the fibula or tip of the lateral malleolus.

Bone tenderness at the base of the fifth metatarsal.

Bone tenderness at the navicular bone.

Calf Muscle Rupture

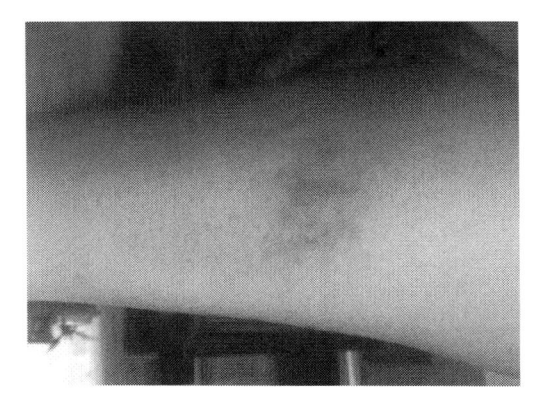

A common cause of calf pain is a pulled or torn calf muscle. It occurs when part of the muscles of the lower leg (gastrocnemius or soleus) are stretched beyond their ability to withstand the tension. This stretching can result in small microtears to the muscle fibers or, in a severe injury, a complete rupture of the muscle fibers.

It can feel like you've just been hit in the back of the leg and an audible "pop" is sometimes heard. There will be sudden, sharp pain in the back of the lower leg, or pain, swelling and even bruising over the calf muscle. Most calf injuries will make it difficult to tolerate weight on injured side and make it very difficult to stand on the toes.

Calf strains may be minor or very severe. In an austere situation accurate grading is academic as the treatment is the same – the length of time to recovery will differentiate the grade. The main issue is ensure the injury is not actually an Achilles tendon rupture.

Calf strains may be minor or very severe and are typically graded as follows:

Grade 1 Calf Strain:

The muscle is stretched causing some small micro tears in the muscle fibres. Full recovery in approx 2 weeks.

Grade 2 Calf Strain :

There is partial tearing of muscle fibres. Full recovery in approx 5-8 weeks.

Grade 3 Calf Strain:

This is the most severe calf strain with a complete tearing or rupture of muscle fibres in the lower leg. Full recovery in 3-4 months and, in some instances, surgery may be needed.

Ruptured Achilles Tendon

The Achilles joins the gastronomies (calf) and the soleus muscles of the leg to the heel of the foot. Tendons are strong, but not flexible so they can only move so far before they get inflamed and tear or rupture.

Causes of Achilles Tendon Rupture

Ruptures can be caused as a complication of Achilles tendonitis, an imbalance in strength in front and back leg muscles or more commonly when overstretched during exercise.

If the toes of the foot move towards the shin as the foot flexes at the ankle while the lower leg moves forward and the calf muscles contract, a rupture may occur. A classic sign of an Achilles tendon rupture is the feeling of being hit in that area. There is sometimes a "pop" sound. There may be little pain, but the person cannot lift up onto his toes while standing.

The Thomson test for a rupture is a good indicator, have the patient kneel on a surface with their foot over the edge. Then squeeze their calf muscle. If the foot does not move a ruptured Achilles tendon is likely.

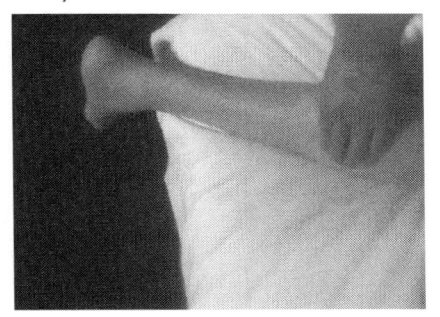

Medicine Section

Chapter 9 Allergic Reaction

A mild allergic reaction often causes no more symptoms than an itchy rash, this is not serious in itself, and may be treated with oral or topical antihistamines and cold showers / wet flannels. If difficulty in breathing or swallowing develops, and/or a sudden weakness regard these as serious symptoms requiring immediate treatment see below. Allergic diseases are on a spectrum with a mild rash at one end and life threatening anaphylaxis at the other.

Anaphylaxis
Anaphylaxis is caused by exposure to an antigen which triggers a cascading release of mediators (such as histamine). Causing the blood vessels to become leaky and inappropriately expanding (Dilation).

Anaphylaxis is potentially life threatening and requires prompt treatment to prevent deterioration and death. Its key features which differentiate it from an allergic reaction are;

- Airway swelling
- Airway constriction
- Low blood pressure
- Altered level of consciousness
- A sudden onset
- Wheeze and/or Stridor

It can be caused by insect stings, particularly wasp and bee stings. Certain foods such as eggs, fish, cow's milk protein, peanuts, nuts and drugs including blood products, vaccines, antibiotics and aspirin.

Chapter 10 Respiratory & Cardiac

Cardiovascular System

This System consists of the Heart and the blood vessels. Its purpose is to transport oxygen, water and nutrients to the cells and remove waste from them.

Symptoms
Cardiac chest pain
Tiredness and breathlessness on exertion
Fainting and dizziness
Ankle swelling in the absence of infection and injury
Breathlessness when lying down
Awaking breathless at night, Palpitations

Respiratory System

This system comprises the airways from the nose and mouth through the pharynx, larynx, trachea, bronchi to the lungs. It is supported by ribs, spine and sternum (Thoracic Cage) and the circulation to the lungs (Pulmonary). Its purpose is to provide ventilation of air to the lungs, exchange gases between air and blood and perfuse the lungs with blood.

Symptoms
Chest pain worsened by breathing (Pleuritic Pain)
Acute or chronic breathlessness
Hoarseness
Cough, sputum, blood in sputum (haemoptysis)
Wheeze

Cardiovascular and Respiratory Assessment

The heart and lungs both reside in the chest and their functions are so interlinked their assessments are also joined. There are a variety of signs, symptoms and tests which will aid a diagnosis but no single one will confirm it.

Questioning

Any pain present in chest?
What is the pain like? (Sharp or Crushing)
Is pain affected by breathing?
Do ankles ever swell?
Are you short of breath?
Are you breathless at night?
How much exercise before breathlessness occurs?

Do you ever feel faint or dizzy?
Do you have a cough?
Is it productive? What is the sputum like?
Do you ever wheeze?

Coughs

Cause:	**Character:**
Laryngitis	Cough with horse voice
Trachitis	Dry & very painful
Pleurisy	Sharp pain in chest wall
Post-nasal drip	Tickely
Asthma	Chronic, worse at night & after exercise
Oesophageal reflux	Dry & Nauseating
Epiglotitis	Barking
LVF	Productive and worse when laying flat

Sputum can be:
Bloody (Haemoptysis) indicating a Pulmonary Embolism or Tuberculosis
Is rusty coloured in pneumonia
Thick with coloured pus (Purulent)
Bacterial infections can produce yellow-greenish coloured sputum which often responds to antibiotic therapy. White, milky, or opaque sputum is often viral in nature and will not require antibiotic therapy.

Examination
Sit the patient up slightly reclined backwards, if they try to sit more upright or lean forward it can indicate they are repositioning themselves and using accessory muscles in the neck and shoulders to improve their breathing. For examination if possible, position patient sitting up on bed or couch at a 45 degree angle.

Before touching the patient observe their skin colour and moisture a flushed, sweaty patient may have a fever. A pale patient may be shocked. Blue tinged fingers, nose and lips (Cyanosis) indicates a serious circulation problem and is often a late sign of an ongoing problem. A reddened face (Mallar flush) may indicate a temperature or just a blush.

Listen to their breathing without a stethoscope. A wheeze on expiration may indicate asthma or COPD. A rattling on inspiration indicates a blockage or swelling in the throat (Stridor).

When questioning the patient are they able to talk in full sentences or do they need to pause between words for breath. Patients who are anxious often think they are short of breath but if they are well perfused and able to hold a conversation they are usually not.

Hands
Start your examination with the patient's fingers, look for;
Capillary Refill, Radial Pulse, nicotine staining
Clubbing, if you place the same finger of each hand nail to nail you should see a diamond shape at the base of the nails this is normal. If it's absent it's a symptom of chronic lung and heart disease, endocarditis, cirrhosis or bowel disease such as Chrons.

Clubbing

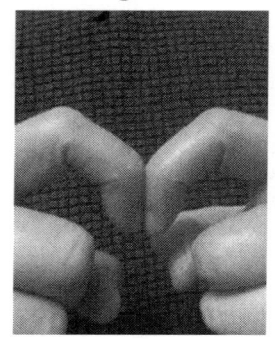

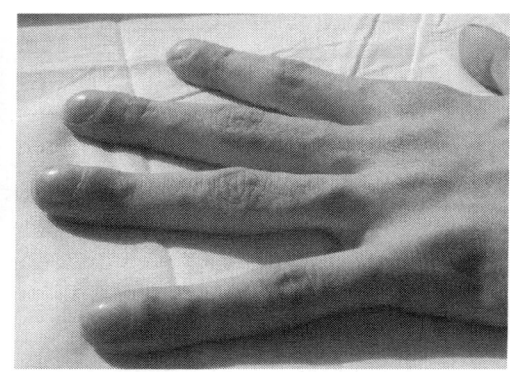

© Jerry Nick, M.D.

Also look at patient palm, the creases or lines should be tinged red or pink. Pale palmar creases are indicative of anaemia.

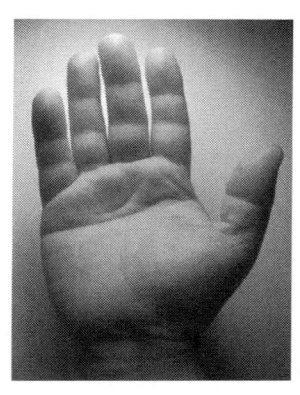

© WurdBendur

Palmar Erythema
This is characterised by red patchs on the patients palms. It has many causes chronic liver disease, portal hypertension, hepatitis, polycythemia, eczema, psoriasis, hand, foot and mouth disease, Rocky Mountain Spotted Fever, and Syphilis. It may also be a normal for the patient. It also occurs in around a third of cases of rheumatoid arthritis.

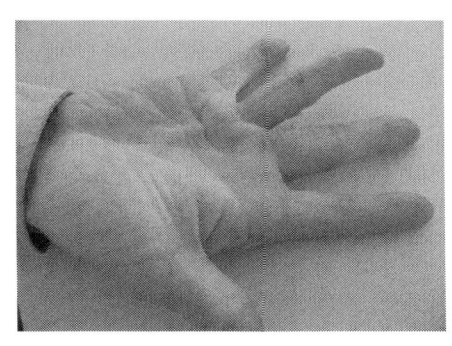

© Frank C. Müller

Dupuytren's contracture

This is a flexion contracture of the hand where the fingers bend towards the palm and cannot be fully straightened. It is an inherited connective tissue disorder. The ring finger and little finger are the fingers most commonly affected. The middle finger may be affected in advanced cases. (See photo above)

Arms

Check the arms for evidence of IV drug use and recent blood tests, Take a pulse at the brachial artery.

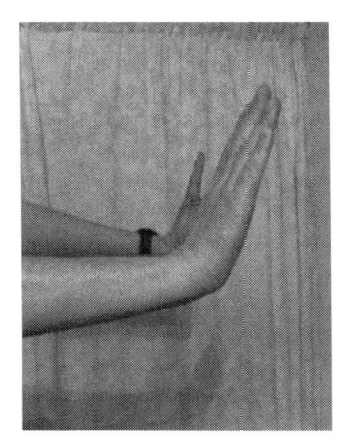

Ask the patient to hold out their arms in front of them for 30 seconds with the hands bent upwards at the wrist (Dorsiflexion) and fingers spread. If an abnormal "flapping" tremor occurs from the wrists this can be indicative of respiratory failure (COPD), Liver or Renal Failure.

Lymph nodes

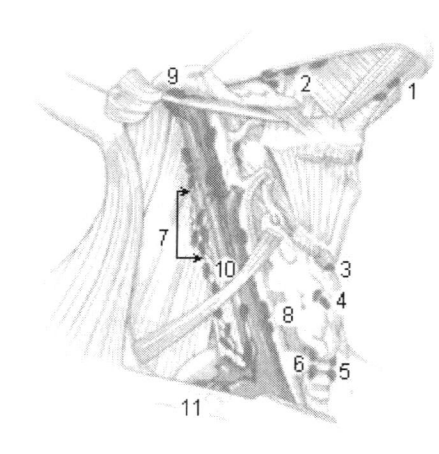

Deep Lymph Nodes
1. Submental
2. Submandibular (Submaxillary)

Anterior Cervical Lymph Nodes (Deep)
3. Prelaryngeal
4. Thyroid
5. Pretracheal
6. Paratracheal

Deep Cervical Lymph Nodes
7. Lateral jugular
8. Anterior jugular
9. Jugulodigastric

Inferior Deep Cervical Lymph Nodes
10. Juguloomohyoid
11. Supraclavicular

© Arcadian

Enlarged nodes may be visible on inspection or palpation. Normal nodes cannot be seen or felt. Feel in the armpits (axilla), above the collar bone (supraclavicular), in the neck and below the jaw (mandible). Infected nodes may also cause reddening of the surrounding tissue.

When evaluating lymph nodes the following should be considered;

Size:
< 1 cm normal.
Insignificant if < 2cm,
except in axilla then < 3cm.
In the supraclaviclar fossa > 1cm is significant (Virchow's)

Mobility
Mobile or fixed ("Matted" nodes are enlarged, fixed)

Consistency:
Soft (insignificant)
Rubbery (classically lymphoma) ,
Hard (classically malignancy & granulatous infection).

Tenderness:
Tender: inflammation *(infection)*
Non-tender (malignancy)

Warmth:
Suggests inflammation

small, movable, discrete, non-tender nodes often called "shotty"
Patients between 2-12 years old commonly present with insignificant lymph nodes in neck secondary to frequent viral infection

Virchow's Node

The left supraclavicular node (Virchow's node) drains lymph from most of the body via the thoracic duct which can be blocked by metastasis, possible diagnoses include lymphoma, intra-abdominal malignancies, breast cancer, and limb infections

An enlarged right supraclavicular lymph node drains thoracic malignancies such as lung and oesophageal cancer, as well as Hodgkin's lymphoma.

Neck
Ask the patient to turn their head to the side and examine the Jugular veins in neck they should be flat. If they are distended with blood it can indicate one of a number of conditions;
Cardiac Tamponade, Pericarditis, Pulmonary Embolism, Right Heart Failure, Cardiogenic or Obstructive Shock and Ventricular Tachycardia.

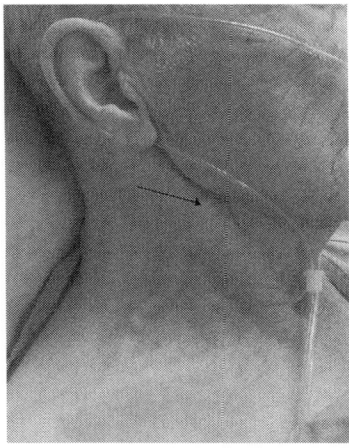

© James Heilman, MD

Check the trachea is in the midline, if deviating to one side it indicates a Tension Pneumothorax, this is usually a late sign and if detected the patient will be very unwell.

Eyes
Look for signs of anaemia or jaundice, yellowish nodules that appear around the eyes (Xanthelasma) and a grey opaque line which surrounds the eye (Corneal arcus) these indicates the presence of high cholesterol levels.

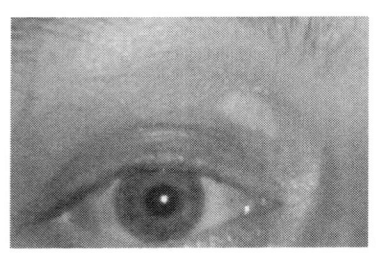

© Bobtheowl2

Mouth
A swollen, smooth and painful tongue can be caused by vitamin B deficiencies. A drier tongue can indicate dehydration and a pale or blue tinged tongue (Central Cyanosis).
If the corners of the mouth are inflamed and cracked it could be caused by a thiamine or vitamin B deficiency (Angulus stomatitis).

Chest
The examination of the chest is in 4 stages;
Inspection. Palpation, Auscultation and Percussion.

Inspection
Inspect the chest looking for scars, red spots with thin tentacle like lines radiating from them across the skin (Spider naevi). These can be normal but an excessive number can indicate chronic liver disease.

A rounded hyper inflated or barrel chest can indicate emphysema.
A pigeon chest with prominent sternum and costal cartilages signifies childhood asthma or rickets.

A funnel chest where the sternum and costal cartilages are depressed is also possible due a developmental defect.
Observe the normal breathing pattern and check for symmetry and normal expansion of both sides (bilateral). Look for skin being drawn in between ribs, above sternum and under rib cage (Retractions). This shows severe difficulty in breathing.

Look for bruises and wounds which can indicate underlying damage, observe breathing as in trauma assessment, uneven breathing can indicate damage to the chest wall or lungs.

Palpation
Feel the chest if it crunches like a crisp bag it indicates air trapped in the tissues (Surgical Emphysema) from a punctured lung. Feel the ribs from front to back for tenderness and deformity.

Place hands around chest starting at the top (upper lobes of lungs) and moving towards the lower lobes. Feel for symmetrical chest movement with respiration.

Auscultation
Using a stethoscope listen to the chest for breath sounds (Auscultation). Start at the Front (Anterior) of Chest and listen from side to side then move from top to bottom avoid the areas covered by bones. Listen at three levels at the front, under the armpit and lower at the sides then at three levels at the back.

Compare one side to the other looking for differences. Note the location and quality of the sounds you hear. Can you hear air moving quietly without additional sounds in each part of the chest? Silent areas can indicate damage or infection.

Lung Sounds	
Wet/ Crackles	These sounds are high pitched; they indicate the presence of infection. Mostly at the base of the lungs but sometimes throughout the lung field.
Stridor	Is an upper airway obstruction heard when breathing in.
Wheezes	Wheezes are heard in Asthma and similar diseases, in some cases they are audible without a stethoscope.
Bubbles	Bubbly sounds in the lungs are caused by fluid in the lungs in Cardiac failure
Rhonchi	These are often described as "snoring" or "gurgling" noises.
Silent	Collapse Lung or Pneumonia (Pus)
Crunching /Rub	Infection or Clot (Pulmonary Embolism)

Auscultation of Heart

Listen to the heart over the left side of chest. To discern all the individual heart sounds and abnormalities is well beyond the scope of this text. The normal sound is referred to as "Lub dub" and is followed by a pause then repeats. Any extra noises are abnormal. A rubbing sound may indicate inflammation of the hearts sac (Pericarditis). To hear the blood passing through the four valves listen at the following points.

Atrial	2nd Intercostal Space to Right edge of sternum
Pulmonary	2nd Intercostal Space to Left edge of sternum
Tricuspid	5th Intercostal Space to Left edge of sternum
Mitral	5th Intercostal Space mid axilla

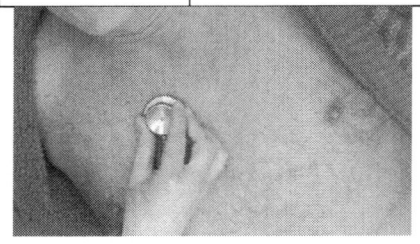

Percussion

Tap (Percuss) the chest, like all clinical skills practice this on well people before you have to do it on a potentially ill patient so you can tell what's normal and what's not. The correct method for this is to place the middle finger of one hand flat and firmly against the patient's chest and tap it with the end (not the pad) of the other middle finger, flicking the wrist to strike down.

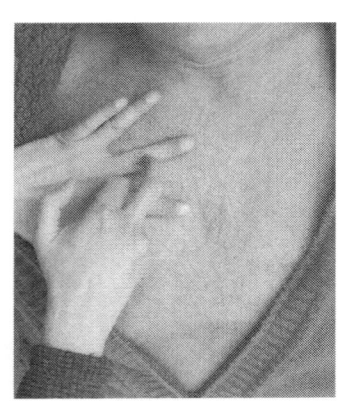

There are three tones;
Resonant (normal)
Hyper resonant (too much air, tension Pneumothorax)
Dull (Fluid or pus)

Base Line Observations
Record the Heart Rate, Blood Pressure, Respiratory rate, Oxygen Saturation, Temperature and Colour are all an indication of the state of perfusion which is the amount of blood reaching the tissues and organs. A pulse oximeter will measure the pulse for you but it is no substitute to feeling it yourself. This will tell you the depth, strength and regularity as well as the rate.

Cardiac and Respiratory Red flag Indicators
Red flag indicators if found usually indicate the patient needs further possibly life saving medical assessment and treatment beyond what is normally provided in the pre-hospital environment. If available this should be sought as soon as possible.

- Chest pain
- Increased shortness of breath
- Decreased level of consciousness or confusion
- Using accessory muscles to aid breathing
- Pale, sweaty appearance
- Pulse <60 or >100
- Respiration Rate >20
- Weight loss
- Unequal chest rise when breathing

Symptoms of Respiratory Illnesses

1. Asthma
2. Pneumonia
3. LVF
4. CCF
5. COPD
6. Hyperventilation
7. Anaemia

Information derived from Keith Hopcroft and Vincent forte (2008) Symptom Sorter 3rd Ed, Oxford: Radcliffe Publishing **(P=Possible)**

	1	2	3	4	5	6	7
Thick Phlegm	P	Y	N		Y	N	
Coarse Crackles	N	Y	N		Y	N	
Wheeze	Y	N	P		Y	N	
Fine Crackles	N	N	Y		P	N	
Reduced air entry	N	Y	N		N	N	
Worse lying down	N			Y	N		N
Ankle swell	N			Y	P		N
Cough	Y			Y	Y		N
Sputum++	P			Y	Y		N
Pallor	N			N	N		Y

Asthma

Asthma is a disease that affects the lower airways. It is usually triggered by an allergen although a viral respiratory infection, exercise or cold weather may precipitate it. It is part of the "atopy" (allergy) triad of eczema, hay fever and asthma. It manifests as an obstruction of the airways which is caused by a combination of swelling of mucosa and smooth muscle spasm of the small airway muscles causing them to contract and an increase in mucous production that blocks the narrowed airways. It is a common disease affecting over 10% of the population.

Signs and symptoms include shortness of breath (dyspnoea), increased respiration rate, productive cough and an audible wheeze. In children it may present as night-time (nocturnal) coughing.

Mild and moderate asthma presents with shortness of breath and chest tightness, plus sign of increased use of the chest wall muscles (the accessory muscles) to help with breathing and a slight reduction in sentence length and the presence of a wheeze when listening to the chest (Auscultation).

As it gets worse (severe to life threatening asthma) the patient will not be able to speak in full sentences, pulse may be >110/min, the respiratory rate >25/min, they may also start using the accessory muscles in the neck and shoulders. In life threatening asthma, no air movement and no wheeze can be heard when listening to the chest, the patient's extremities become blue-tinged (Cyanosed), their pulse rate drops (Bradycardia) and they become exhausted as breathing becomes more difficult.

Peak Flow Measurement

Peak flow is often used as a measure to further define the severity of an asthma attack. It relies on a patient being able to accurately undertake the measurement.

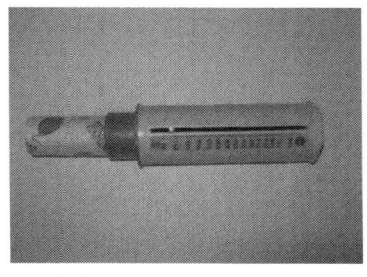

1/Zero the pointer on the scale
2/Breathe in as fully as possible.
3/Blow out as hard and fast as possible.
4/Repeat this sequence twice more.
5/The highest of the three readings is your peak flow.

A person having a serious asthma attack will struggle to blow into the Peak flow meter.

Although it is a good baseline measurement for treatment be aware of this.

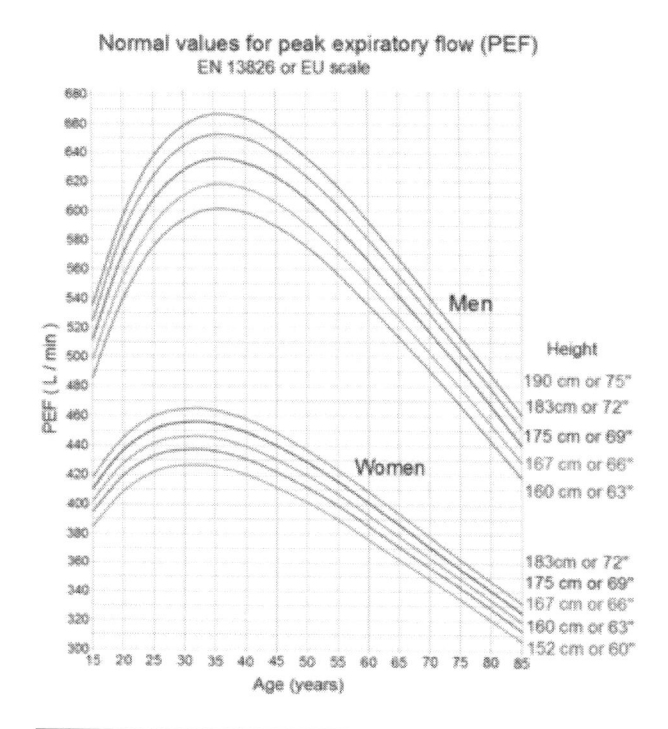

Nunn A, Gregg I (1989). "New regression equations for predicting peak expiratory flow in adults". *BMJ* 298 (6680): 1068–70.

Normal	80-100 % of Predicted Score
Mild Attack	51-79 % of Predicted Score
Severe Attack	33-50 % Predicted Score
Life Threatening	<33 % of Predicted Score

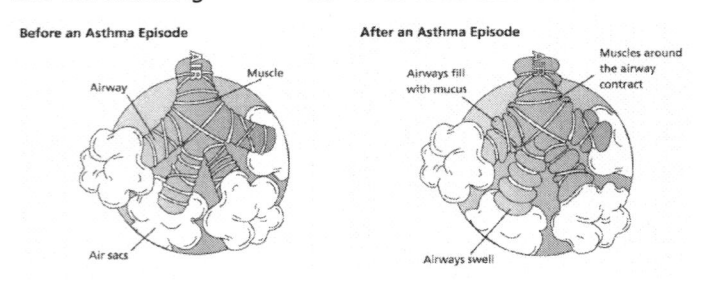

Pneumonia

Pneumonia is an infection in the lung tissue or bronchi, the distinction between acute bronchitis and pneumonia is academic without a chest x-ray and the treatment is broadly the same.

The cause can be broken down by age:

> Children
>> In infants and small children it can be Viral and/or Bacterial but it can be very difficult to tell which.
>>
>> In children less than 3 months it is almost certainly bacterial.
>>
>> Between 3 months and early adolescence it is usually viral, but it can be very hard to tell and if the patient is sick then treatment with antibiotics should probably occur, but is not essential for mild illness.
>>
>> In pre-teens and teenagers it can be caused by a cell without walls which is resistant to antibiotics (Mycoplasma) and/or a Bacterial infection.
>>
>> In older adults the cause is usually bacterial.

Secondary causes that can alter this are

> Aspiration of stomach contents or water when drowning, chemical irritation or bacteria from the mouth. These patients

will often get better without antibiotics and these should be reserved for those who have fevers or are critically ill.

Bacterial infection following a viral illness. This is discussed in more detail below, but the patient usually has a mild respiratory illness and other features of viral illness (runny nose, sore throat, sore joints, headache and/or unproductive cough) and are often getting better when they suddenly get much worse, this is usually a bacterial infection superimposed on viral infection.

Diagnosis

Often there is co-existing disease like asthma or chronic airways disease, but there will always be an element of chest infection.

Fever + productive cough = pneumonia

Fever + chest pain = pneumonia

Fever + shortness of breath = pneumonia

Common presenting features include shortness of breath, fever, cough (productive – green / grey / blood stained or unproductive), muscle aches, pleuritic chest pain, fast breathing rate / fast heart rate, reduced air-entry on effected side, dull to percussion, crackles on auscultation, increased work of breathing (In drawing and accessory muscle use) and if lips and tongue turn a congested blue colour (Cyanosis).

Heart failure

Is the inability of the heart to supply the body with sufficient oxygen. It can have many causes;

> Ischemic heart disease
> Enlargement of the heart
> Valve disease
> Diabetes
> High Blood Pressure (Hypertension)
> Obesity
> Smoking
> Drug effects
> Arrhythmias

And can be divided into Left or Right sided heart failure, although both with accompanying symptoms can co-exist.

Left ventricular failure (LVF)

This causes congestion of the veins within the lungs, thus the symptoms shown are manly respiratory despite the problem being cardiac. Symptoms include shortness of breath (dyspnoea) either on exertion or in advanced disease at rest. Patients often need to sleep upright, breathlessness being particularly pronounced when lying flat (orthopnea). This is accompanied by periods of severe breathlessness at night (paroxysmal nocturnal dyspnoea), wheezing, a 'bubbly' chest, dizziness, hypoxia and confusion.

Congestive Cardiac Failure

Right sided heart failure causes congestion of the capillaries in the body resulting in excess fluid leaking into the tissues called peripheral oedema. Either in the ankles of feet or in the scaral area if the patient is immobile. When fluid returns to the system at night it causes frequent nighttime urination (Nocturia). Fluid also accumulates in the abdomen (Ascites) and can cause liver enlargement, impairment and jaundice.

COPD

Chronic obstructive airway disease (COPD) covers a group of conditions including asthma (see above), emphysema and bronchitis.

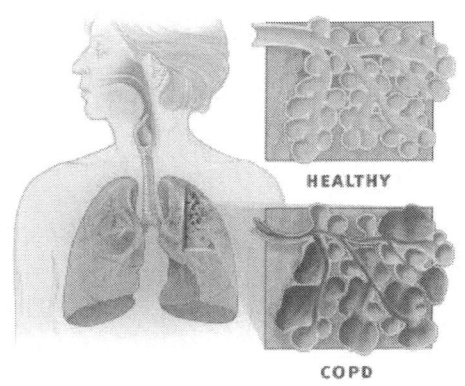

© Jtravers

Emphysema

In emphysema, the tissues that support the physical shape of the air sacs (alveoli) in the lungs fail upon exhalation usually due to a long time history of smoking. The main symptoms are shortness of breath (dyspnoea) and a change in the chest as it expands and becomes barrel shaped. Dyspnoea starts on exertion only but can progress so is present all the time to a lesser or greater degree, they use accessory muscles to breathe and will lean forward with arms extended or resting on something to help them breathe called the tripod position, cyanosis and their respiratory rate increases. The chest sounds hyper-resonant when listening (auscultation) and tapping (percussion). Patient with emphysema are referred to as "pink puffers" who has a pink complexion and dysponea.

Bronchitis

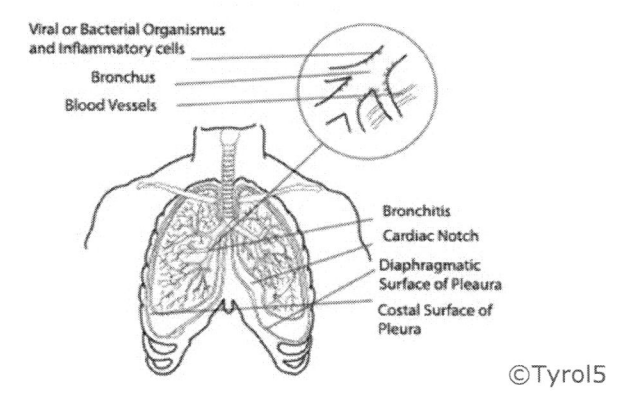

Bronchitis is inflammation of the mucous membranes of the bronchi, the airways that carry airflow from the wind pipe (trachea) into the lungs. Bronchitis can acute or chronic;

Acute bronchitis is characterised by the development of a cough, with or without the production of mucus (sputum) that is coughed up. Acute bronchitis often occurs with a viral illness.

In Chronic bronchitis the patient has a productive cough that lasts for three months or more per year for at least two years, caused by smoking, pollution or industrial irritants. They are sometimes called "Blue Bloaters" because of the bluish color of the skin and lips caused by cyanosis.

Hyperventilation

Breathing faster and or deeper than normal causing loss of carbon dioxide. It is usually caused by an anxiety episode but should not be dismissed as it can also be caused by some diseases and head injuries.

Symptoms such as numbness or tingling in the hands, feet and lips, dizziness, headache, chest pain, slurred speech, nervous laughter, and sometimes fainting. If the patient faints their breathing usually resets

Anaemia

Symptoms of Anemia

Red = In severe anemia

Eyes
- Yellowing

Skin
- Paleness
- Coldness
- Yellowing

Respiratory
- Shortness of breath

Muscular
- Weakness

Intestinal
- Changed stool color

Central
- Fatigue
- Dizziness
- Fainting

Blood vessels
- Low blood pressure

Heart
- Palpitations
- Rapid heart rate
- Chest pain
- Angina
- Heart attack

Spleen
- Enlargement

© Mikael Häggström

This is a decrease in number of red blood cells or a reducing of a normal quantity of hemoglobin in the blood.

In minor anaemia, patients will feel weak, tired and lose concentration. They can look pale (pallor) and become short of breath.

In more severe cases the heart rate will increase causing palpitations. Lack of oxygen to cardiac muscles can cause angina type pain and symptoms of heart failure (see above).

Less common symptoms may include swelling of limbs, heartburn, bruises, vomiting, sweating or blood in stools.

Avian / Bird Flu (H5N1)

Bird Flu (H5N1) is highly infectious amongst birds but is difficult for humans to catch or spread. It affects wild and domesticated birds. Since 2003 the World Health Organization (WHO) has confirmed over 400 cases of H5N1 in humans, there have been over 250 deaths.

The symptoms are similar to Swine Flu see below and can come on suddenly, but incubation is usually between 3 and 7 days and last for around a week. Those suspected of having Avian flu should be isolated for 7 to 10 days.

In serious cases, there can be rapid deterioration, with pneumonia and multiple organ failure, and this is generally fatal.

H1N1 — Easily spread, Rarely fatal

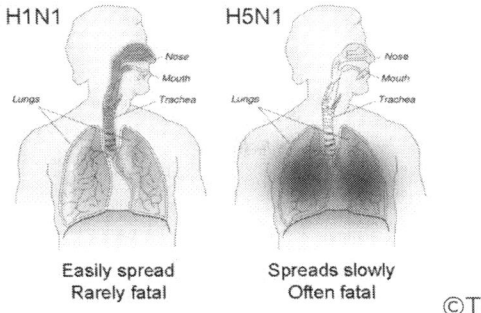

H5N1 — Spreads slowly, Often fatal

©TimVickers

Swine flu (H1N1)

Swine flu was first identified in Mexico in April 2009, it spread around the world and became a pandemic. By the spring of 2009 the number of cases declined. In August 2010 the World Health Organisation (WHO) declared the pandemic over, although new cases are still being reported in 2011.

Most cases were mild but some deaths occurred amongst patients who already had conditions such as diabetes which affected their immune or respiratory systems. The "at risk" group includes those over 65, pregnant patients and those with chronic health problems.

A vaccine is available which is currently included with the seasonal flu jab.

The following comments apply equally to an Influenza pandemic regardless of the classification it is given.

Symptoms of Avian and Swine flu include the following, however most are common to seasonal flu.

- Lethargy
- Fever 38C
- Aching muscles
- Headache
- Runny nose & sore throat
- Shortness of breath or cough
- Decreased appetite
- Diarrhoea and/or vomiting

Severe acute respiratory syndrome (SARS)

The infection is caused by the SARS corona virus (SARS CoV) is very serious and affects the lungs. Incubation is between 2 and 7 days.

Symptoms include;

- Temperature of 38°C +
- Lethargy
- headaches

- Fever and chills
- Muscle pain
- Loss of appetite
- Diarrhoea

Between 3 and 7 days after the onset of initial symptoms, it will affect breathing causing; a dry cough, difficulty breathing and a decrease in oxygen levels in the blood which if untreated is usually fatal. SARS is spread the same way as the flu virus through airborne infections and touching surfaces contaminated with droplets.

Acute respiratory distress syndrome (ARDS)

ARDS occurs when the lungs become seriously damaged through severe infection or injury. Causes include serious infections, such as pneumonia or blood poisoning (Sepsis) or injuries caused by such as near drowning, smoke inhalation, or severe chest trauma. Even with hospital treatment between a third and a half of patient die.

Symptoms include:

- Blue-coloured lips, fingers and toes (Cyanosis)
- Difficult, rapid, shallow breathing
- Increased heart rate
- Lethargy followed by confusion

Whooping Cough (Pertussis)

Whooping cough is an infection of the lining of the windpipe (trachea) and the bronchi leading to the lungs. Its highly infectious through droplets on surfaces and in the air from coughing and sneezing. Incidence have reduced significantly since the introduction of the childhood vaccine. It mainly affects infants and young children but can occur at any age. Incubation can be long 6-20 days before first symptoms appear.

- A mildly increased temperature (Pyrexia)
- Runny nose and sneezing
- Watering eyes
- Dry, irritating cough and sore throat

After 1 or 2 weeks more severe symptoms appear

- Main symptom is hacking cough with 'whoop' sound
- Cough is productive with thick phlegm
- Fatigue from strain of coughing
- Vomiting

Coughing comes in bouts roughly 12 to 16 per day. Complete recovery can take up to 3 months with frequency of bouts decreasing over that time.

Pneumothorax

A Pneumothorax is a collapsed lung. It can be caused as a consequence of trauma (see trauma section) or have a medical cause and can occur spontaneously. A typical candidate for a spontaneous pneumothorax is a tall, young male and is attributed to changes in growth.

The lungs are surrounded by the pleura which consists of two layers in between which is the pleural space. The Lungs are usually kept inflated by a vacuum (negative pressure) between the lung and the pleural space, the pressure in the pleural space is negative and sucks up the outside of the lung to keep it inflated, if you lose that negative pressure, you loose the mechanism to keep the lung inflated.

The patient usually presents with sudden onset shortness of breath and pleuritic chest pain. It can also be associated with strenuous effort.

The clinical findings include increased respiratory rate, reduced air entry and resonance to percussion. In hospital the diagnosis is usually made on the basis of a chest x-ray or CT scan. Usually if it is large enough to cause symptoms, it is clinically obvious without an x-ray.

Chest pain

This is a very common presenting complaint and is an absolute mine field. Trivial and life threatening can look exactly the same. The pain needs to be put in context:
- Trauma vs. not
- Age. Young vs. old
    Heart attacks are less common in young people
- Sex
- Type of pain
- Associated symptoms

Types of pain: There are broadly three types of pain:

- Pleuritic usually from an irritation of the lungs such as pneumonia, pulmonary embolism. Described as sharp, worse with inspiration and often pain is felt as a "catch".

- Visceral pain is more diffuse and harder to localise. Associated with damage or irritation of the heart, oesophagus or gut. Felt as a pressure, sweating and nausea and/or vomiting. It often radiates into the neck, arms and/or back.

- Musculoskeletal where the patient describes pain like a pulled muscle, worse with movement. Often the pain is sharp and well localised. There are some similarities to pleuritic pain.

Heart Pain

The heart is a pump. It requires oxygen to work. If it doesn't get enough oxygen it causes visceral pain.

The more activity the person does the more work for heart. The more work the more oxygen is required. Heart disease is the narrowing of blood vessels supplying the heart muscle caused by the build up of fatty deposits.

If the pain occurs during exercise and is relieved by rest its usually caused by Angina this can be stable occurs at same level of exercise or unstable occurs with progressively less exercise. Patients with very unstable angina are treated the same as a heart attack.

If the pain occurs at rest it is usually caused by an obstruction of blood flow, such as caused by a Heart Attack (Myocardial Infarction).

Heart Attack (Myocardial infarction) (MI)

If the blocked blood vessel is small and only supplies a small non vital area, the patient may recover without any treatment and only minimal effect. If however the blockage occurs towards the beginning of one of the main arteries supplying blood to the heart, it's more likely to cause significant damage. The larger the area of damaged heart the more likely it is to produce a lethal heart rhythm and for the patient to die. Most heart attacks occur between these two extremes. See below for a diagram of the heart showing the system of coronary circulation and plaque formation where a build up of cholesterol blocks (Occludes) the vessel.

The problem with heart disease is that a minority of patients present with the "classic" presentation of crushing central chest pain radiating to the neck and arm. The remainder may present with sharp musculoskeletal type pain or indigestion or even jaw or arm pain in isolation. Some patients will not experience any pain, which is more common amongst those that have diabetes due to degradation of nerves.

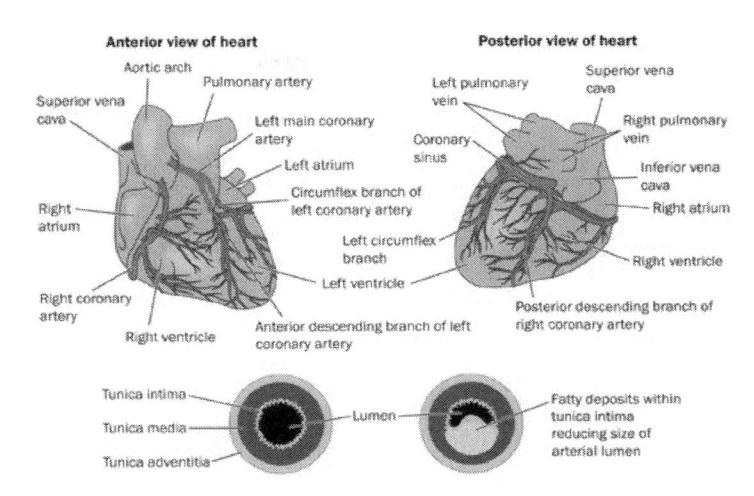

Depending on the intensity of pain and the nature of the damage to the heart, pulse and blood pressure may be raised or lowered and the pulse may become irregular. Oxygen saturations may also be decreased if the heart is struggling to pump blood around the body.

Other signs and symptoms can include nausea, vomiting, palpitations, shortness of breath and a feeling of dread. As you can see there is no such thing as a typical heart attack!

The diagnosis is usually made in hospital on the basis of an ECG recording and a blood test to measure changes in cardiac enzymes in the blood.

Indigestion
Indigestion is a very common problem and it can be tricky in that it can look similar to heart pain. It is characterized by burning pain behind the breast bone (Retrosternal pain), acid coming back into the mouth and may be related to certain types of food or meal times.

Deep Vein Thrombosis (DVT)

Deep vein thrombosis (DVT) are blood clots in deep veins particularly in the calf and the thigh, they affect around 0.1% of the population each year and are more prevalent in obese people and smokers. The main complication is that part of the clot may detach and travel to the lungs causing a pulmonary embolism.

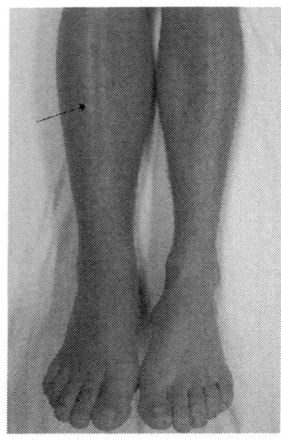

© James Heilman, MD

Symptoms include;

- Heavy aching Pain
- Swelling and or Redness
- Warm skin
- Tenderness particularly on the back of leg below knee

Clinical Feature	Score
Active cancer (treatment within last 6 months or palliative)	+1
Calf swelling >3 cm compared to other calf (measured 10 cm below tibial tuberosity)	+1
Collateral superficial veins (non-varicose)	+1
Pitting edema (confined to symptomatic leg)	+1
Previous documented DVT	+1
Swelling of entire leg	+1
Localized pain along distribution of deep venous system	+1
Paralysis, paresis, or recent cast immobilization of lower extremities	+1
Recently bedridden > 3 days, or major surgery requiring regional or general anesthetic in past 4 weeks	+1
Alternative diagnosis at least as likely	-2

Score of 2 or higher — deep vein thrombosis is likely.
Score of less than 2 — deep vein thrombosis is unlikely.

Scarvelis D, Wells P (2006). "Diagnosis and treatment of deep-vein thrombosis". *CMAJ* **175** (9): 1087–92.

Pulmonary Embolism (PE)

A pulmonary embolism is caused by a blood clot lodging in a blood vessel within the lung like a heart attack its effects depends on where the clot occurs, however any pulmonary embolism is a serious condition.

Risk factors for pulmonary embolism include a history of DVTs, use of contraception or long haul flights. Around 0.1% of the population develop DVTs and 10% of people with untreated DVTs develop pulmonary embolisms.

Most cases of pulmonary embolism develop when part, or all, of the blood clot travels in the blood stream from the deep veins in your leg to the lungs.

Symptoms are;

- Breathlessness that can come on gradually or suddenly
- Sharp pain which can be pin pointed
- Pain can increase on inspiration
- The patient is often tachycardic and may have coughed up blood

Clinical Feature	Score
Clinically Suspected DVT	+3
alternative diagnosis is less likely than PE	+3
tachycardia	+1.5
immobilization/surgery in previous four weeks	+1.5
history of DVT or PE	+1.5
haemopysis	+1
malignancy (treatment for within 6 months, palliative	+1

Score > 4 - PE likely.

Score 4 or less - PE unlikely.

Neff MJ (2003). "ACEP releases clinical policy on evaluation and management of pulmonary embolism". *American Family Physician* **68** (4): 759–60.

Angina

Angina is a disease where the coronary arteries have become narrowed due to the build up of cholesterol in the arteries supplying the heart with blood. The patient experiences pain as the heart muscle (myocardium) is starved of oxygen rich blood. There are two types of angina, stable and unstable.

In stable angina the patient generally knows what amount of exercise they can comfortably do without over exerting their heart. They are able to live their life within these boundaries. If they exceed their normal exercise tolerance they experience pain. This is relieved by using GTN spray or tablet which allows more blood to get to the heart muscle.

Varicose Veins

Varicose Veins affect around 30% of the population, more women than men and generally older or pregnant patients. They generally affect the legs but can occur in any vein. In most cases they don't cause any symptoms or problems although larger varicose veins can ache, cause reddening, tenderness, feel heavy or itchy. They affect the superficial veins which lie under the skin which can be seen and felt; these in turn feed into larger and deeper veins and back to the heart.

Varicose veins are enlarged (dilated), thickened and knobbly veins, often easily visible but sometimes hidden in overweight patients. The exact mechanism of development isn't fully understood but it is believed that they are caused by a weakness in the wall of the vessel causing the valves that stop blood draining backwards in the circulatory system to leak once this happens it causes extra pressure on the vein wall and more weakness in the valves.

Rare complications include; bleeding from trauma, Inflammation (thrombophlebitis), Swelling of the foot or lower leg, discolouration, eczema, skin ulcers or venous leg ulcers.

Venous Skin Ulcers

These can occur anywhere on the body but are most common just above the ankles, they present as a breakdown of skin revealing underlying tissue. Like varicose veins they mainly affect women and the elderly and occur in around 2% of the population. They can be painless or painful and if untreated break down surrounding tissue widening the affected area causing inflammation (dermatitis). Venous ulcers are formed when fluid leaks from enlarged veins into the tissue causing swelling, thickening and damage to the skin. The damaged skin may eventually break down to form an ulcer.

Thrombophlebitis

This is where blood clots develop in veins, usually of the legs. The condition may be inherited in people with a family history of blood clotting problem or as a side effects of varicose veins. It causes a painful, reddening and swelling varying from discomfort to a cramp-like pain. The pain is worsened when moving the foot at the ankle but subsides over a couple of weeks, leaving hard clots that can be felt. Ensure that this is Thrombophlebitis rather than a much more serious DVT (See above)

Peripheral vascular disease (Claudication)

Caused by hardening of the arteries (arteriosclerosis) fatty plaque building up and cause narrowing of the vessel, the walls of the vein also become less elastic resulting in decreased blood flow when muscles at work require more oxygen. This causes pain in the thighs or calf on exercising which is relieved by resting and as the condition worsens pain on resting too, risk factors include high cholesterol levels, Hypertension and Diabetes. This condition is often misdiagnosed and treated as muscular pains if in doubt refer on.

Chapter 11 Abdominal Assessment & illnesses

Digestive System

The Digestive system runs from the mouth to the anus, consisting of the mouth, oesophagus, stomach, intestines, liver, pancreas, gall bladder. Its purpose is to process food to make nutrients in food available to the body.

Symptoms
Abdominal pain
Indigestion
Last Time open Bowels, was it normal
Blood in vomit (haematemesis)
Blood in faeces (melaena)
Weight loss, loss of appetite
Jaundice, dark urine, pale faeces
Difficulty in swallowing (dysphagia)
Diarrhoea or constipation
Recent changes in bowel habits
Rectal bleeding or +/-mucus

Genitourinary System

This system consists of the kidneys, ureters, bladder and reproductive organs. The urinary system regulates the amount of fluid in the body and disposes of waste dissolved in urine. The kidney also produce some of the chemicals the body needs.

Symptoms
Loin or lower abdominal pain
Blood in urine (haematuria)
Unusual coloured urine
Urgency or incontinence
Painful urination (Dysuria)
Impotence or loss of libido
Urethral discharge
Menstruation problems
Labour, miscarriage
Painful sexual intercourse (Dyspareunia)
Vaginal bleeding or discharge (coloured or smelly)

Abdominal Assessment

This covers the Genitourinary and Digestive Systems.

Questioning

Looking at the symptoms above ask about;

Presence and location of pain?
Eating Habits?
Bowel Habits?
Colour, consistency of vomit?
Any fresh bright red or old blood dark red (coffee grounds) in vomit?
Colour and frequency of urination?
If female of child bearing age enquire if they may be pregnant?

In order to reach a diagnosis and understanding of the underlying anatomy of the abdomen is essential.

Two Pictures below used with kind permission of:
http://www.ambulancetechnicianstudy.co.uk

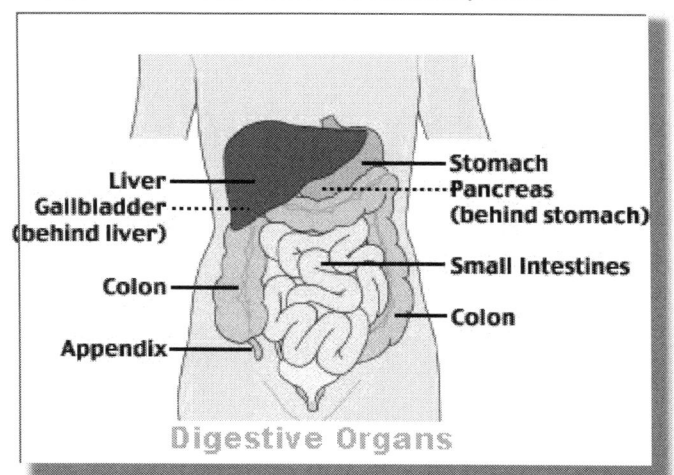

When describing the abdominal regions two systems are used the first divides the abdomen into nine regions as shown below centred around the navel called the umbilical region (see below), further the sides of the body are referred to as left or right regions. Pain may be in the right lumbar or left Iliac region. The denotation is based on the patients left and right rather than the practitioner looking at them. These names are difficult to remember so another system is commonly used dividing the abdomen into four sections centred on the Navel. The left and right Upper quadrants and the Left and Right lower quadrants. Abbreviated to LUQ, RUQ, LLQ, RLQ. These two systems can also be mixed as seen below.

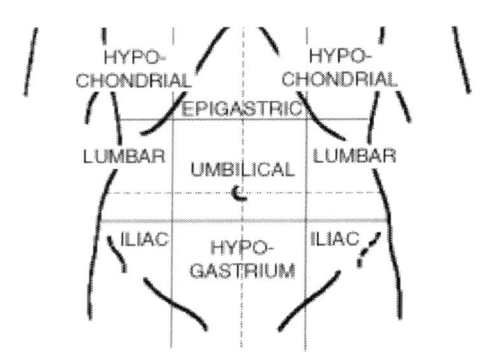

Anatomy and Diseases causing pain by Abdominal Region
In order to have an idea as to what might be causing symptoms it is important to know what organs and vessels lie in each quadrant.

Abdominal pain is a common problem and has dozens of causes. There are two primary sorts of pain;

- Visceral pain from the affected organ, patient's cannot clearly localise the pain.

- Peritoneal pain this is much more localised and reflects direct peritoneal irritation but occurs later in a disease.

Peritoneal pain come from the peritoneum which is a sack that surrounds the abdominal organs. The location of pain gives you help in identifying the problem, and this is why an knowledge of the anatomy is important.

RUQ

- Base of Right Lung,
- Right Lobe of Liver,
- Gallbladder,
- Head of Pancreas,
- Stomach: pylorus, duodenum,
- Right suprarenal gland,
- Right kidney,
- Right hepatic flexure,
- Ascending colon: Superior part,
- Transverse colon: right half

Typical conditions associated with RUQ are;
Cholecystitis, Duodenal ulcer, Hepatitis, Pyelonephritis
Appendicitis, Pneumonia.

LUQ

- Left Lobe of Liver,
- Spleen,
- Stomach,
- Jejunum and proximal ileum,
- Pancreas: body and tail,
- Left kidney,
- Left suprarenal gland,
- Left colic (splenic) flexure,
- Transverse colon: left half,
- Descending colon: superior half

Typical conditions associated with LUQ are;

Ruptured spleen, Gastric ulcer, Aortic aneurism, Perforated colon, Pyelonephritis, Pneumonia .

RLQ

- Caecum,
- Appendix,
- Most of ileum, ascending colon: inferior part,
- Right ovary,
- Right fallopian tube,
- Right ureter
- Right spermatic cord: abdominal part,
- Uterus (if enlarged),
- Urinary bladder (if very full)

Typical conditions associated with RLQ are;

Appendicitis, Pelvic inflammatory disease, ectopic pregnancy, Kidney stones, Strangulated hernia, Diverticulitis, Crohn's disease.

LLQ

- Sigmoid colon, descending colon: inferior part,
- Left ovary,
- Left Fallopian tube,
- Left ureter: abdominal part,
- Left spermatic cord: abdominal part,
- Uterus (if enlarged),
- Urinary bladder (if very full)

Typical conditions associated with LLQ are;

Constipated, Impacted Faeces, Pelvic inflammatory disease, Ectopic Pregnancy, Kidney Stones, Strangulated Hernia, Diverticulitis, Crohn's Disease, Ulcerative Colitis.

Central / Generalised abdominal pain
Any organ – visceral pain, Bowel

Epigastric
Indigestion, Pancreatitis, Myocardial infarction, Peptic Ulcer, Cholecystitis. (Liver, Stomach, Pancreas, Bowel)

Umbilical
Intestinal obstruction, Pancreatitis, Early sign off Appendicitis, Aortic Aneurism, Diverticulitis.

Suprapubic
Bladder, Uterus

Hypogastric
Urinary Tract Infarction (UTI)

Flanks
Aorta, Kidneys

Examination

Inspection

Ask the patient to empty their bladder then lie flat, exposing the abdomen, loosen belt and expose down to just above pubic hair line, with arms resting loosely at sides. Look at their face to determine if they are in pain or discomfort, observe their demeanour and look for a generalised jaundice.

Any abdominal examination should also include elements of respiratory / cardiac examination. Check hands, arms, face, eyes, mouth, neck, lymph Node and chest (See Respiratory/Cardiac chapter).

Examine the abdomen for signs of respiration, symmetry, pulsatile masses, visible peristalsis, stretch marks (striae) and engorged veins (caput medusa) caused by portal hypertension.

Scars

Look for previous abdominal surgery or scars. If they have had their appendix removed they will have a scar in the right lower quadrant of their abdomen.

Navel (Umbilicus)

Examine umbilicus if averted think fluid if inverted think fat.

Hernias'

Ask them to cough several times and observe, this may reveal the presence of a hernia. Getting them to place their chin on their chest can have the same effect.

Peristalsis

May be normally seen in very thin people, Increased peristaltic waves occur in Intestinal Obstruction.

Aortic Pulsations

Normal aortic pulsations can be seen in the Epigastrium, these are increased in aortic aneurysm. It can be palpated 2cm below the sternum slightly to the left of the mid-line, the aorta should be about 3cm in diameter. If an aneurysm is present pulsation may be increased on one side.

Gynaecomastia (and Small Testes)

is the abnormal development of large mammary glands in males resulting in breast enlargement. Caused by in low levels of free testosterone or the tissue responsiveness to them, may also be caused by an imbalance of an imbalance of estrogen.

Spider naevi

Found slightly beneath the skin surface, consisting of a central red spot and reddish extensions which radiate outwards like a legs or web. They are common and may be benign. However, greater than five spider naevi may be a sign of liver disease.

Inferior vena cava obstruction

The path of the vein can be seen bulging beneath the skinon the abdomen.

Look for;

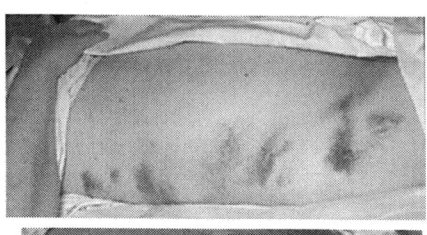

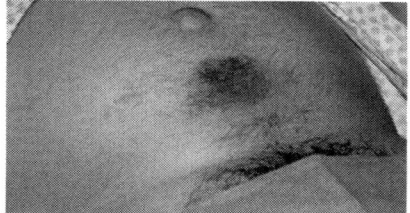

Bruising to the flank, called Grey Turners sign is an indicator of pancreatitis.

© Herbert L. Fred, MD and Hendrik A. van Dijk

Bruising around the umbilicus (navel) Cullen's sign is an indicator of pancreatitis or an ectopic pregnancy.

© Herbert L. Fred, MD and Hendrik A. van Dijk

Distension
Examine abdomen for signs of obvious distension, this can be summarised as the 7 'F's; Fluid – ascites / urine, Fat, Faeces, Flatus, Food, Foetus, Fibroids. Distension can also be caused by malignancy and phantom pregnancies.

Auscultation
Listen to the abdomen for bowel sounds using a stethoscope in each of the nine abdominal regions. Bowels sounds are normally heard 5-34 /minute but listen up to a maximum of two minutes before deciding they are missing. Absent bowel sounds is an indication of peritonitis or other serious abdominal problem. If bowel sounds are frequent with a high pitched tinkling quality this can indicate an obstructed bowel, these patients would also have a history of constipation. Sounds are transmitted throughout abdomen so listening at one point is sufficient.

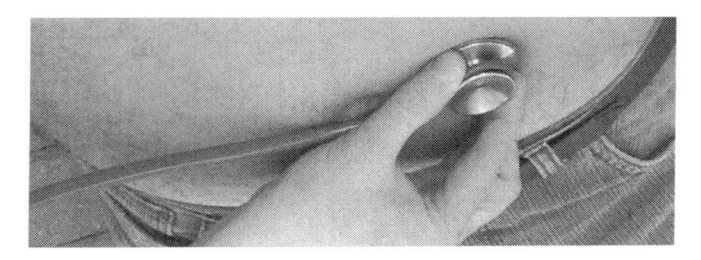

Bruits
Listen for a whooshing sound this can indicate a partial blockage (aneurysm) of the arteries.

Aortic Bruits
Listen 2cm below sternum left of Midline

Renal Bruits
Listen over the mesenteric arteries half way between the umbilicus and bottom of sternum 2cm away of Midline

Iliac Bruits
Listen over the Iliac arteries slightly below and either the umbilicus.

Femoral Bruits
Listen over inguinal ligament for femoral bruits

Friction Rubs
A grating sound can be rarely heard in the area overlying liver and spleen if heard be suspicious of a tumour of the liver of Splenic infarct.

Palpation

Feel (Palpate) the abdomen using the fingers of a flat hand don't dig or poke the surface as this will cause muscles to contract. If the patient is conscious and tells you they have pain in a certain area leave that part to last. They may be tender in other parts which are masked by more severe pain in one location. Note areas that are rigid, tender, where you feel resistance (Guarding) or cause pain when you press and then release (Rebound Tenderness).

Start by feeling the abdomen lightly, starting away from the pain and moving towards it. Feel for rigidity, distension, masses, tenderness and guarding across each of the abdominal regions. Then feel more deeply looking for enlarged organ (Organomegaly) normal sized organs are difficult to feel so identifying the edge of the liver, spleen or kidneys can indicate a problem. If the bladder is full it can also be felt. Feel for a pulsating mass in the Epigastric region this can indicate an aortic aneurism.

If you feel any hard areas note; size, shape consistency, mobility and if pulsation is present. It can indicate colonic carcinoma in any of the four quadrants however masses in the LLQ are frequently stool.

Murphy's sign

Push two fingers slowly into the abdomen over the gall bladder whilst the patient breathes in. If this is painful rather than just uncomfortable it indicates inflammation of the gall bladder (Cholecystitis).

McBurney's point

Press down in the right iliac fossa (McBurney's point) then releasing the pressure, if more pain is felt when you release the pressure (rebound tenderness), this indicates appendicitis.

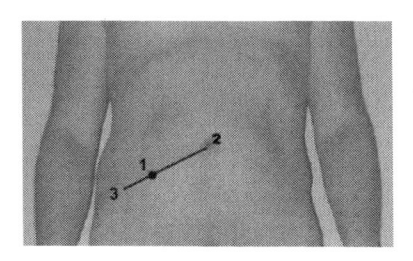

Location of McBurney's point (1), located two thirds the distance from the navel (2) to the anterior superior iliac spine (3).

© Steven Fruitsmaak

Rovsings sign

A further test for appendicitis or other peritoneal irritation is Rovsings sign where the abdomen is pushed from the left to the right this causes pain over the appendix if its inflamed.

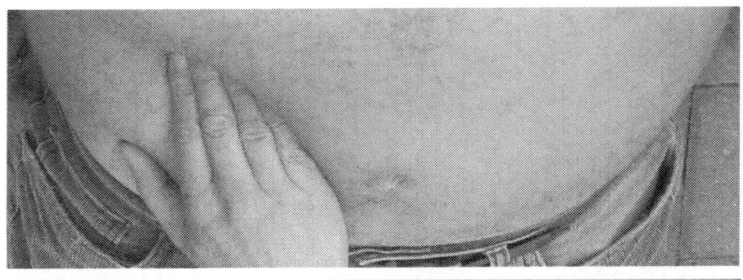

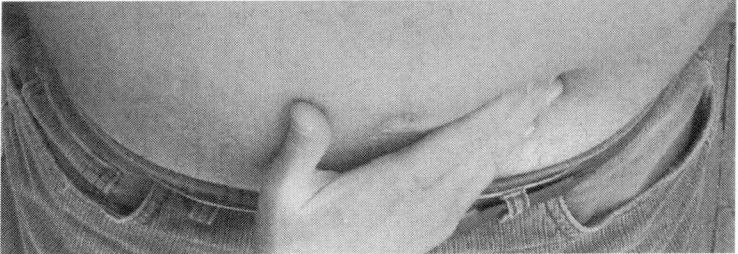

Psoas sign
Place hand on right knee and ask patient to raise thigh against your hand. Irritation of psoas muscle by inflamed appendix cause pain.

Obturator sign
Flex right thigh at hip with knee bent and rotate leg internally at the hip. This stretches the obturator muscle causing pain.

Percussion
Tapping (Percussion) of the abdomen can reveal if distension might be due to bowel gas (Flatus) or fluid (ascites), if a hyper resonance tone is heard it often indicates a gaseous distended abdomen. Enlargement of an organ can also be detected. When tapping over an organ the sound will be duller than over the lungs or bowel which is normally full of air. From this you should be able to identify the size of the organ and if it is enlarged. Abnormal dullness is heard over a distended bladder. If the whole of the abdomen in tender when percussed it indicates a generalised peritonitis which is very serious.

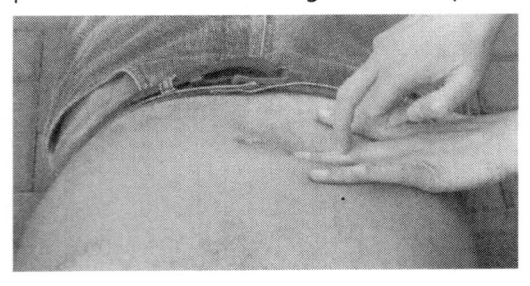

Ascites

This is free fluid in the peritoneal cavity often due to cirrhosis and severe liver disease, it can also more rarely indicate other serious medical problems such as heart failure and cancer. With the patient on their back Percuss from there umbilicus towards their flanks, on the top part of the abdomen it should be resonant, as you approach the flanks a dull sound will be heard if ascites is present. To confirm the dullness is fluid roll the patient onto their side and have them rest their for 2-3 minutes. If the area upmost is now resonant the cause is likely to be fluid which has drained downwards.

Splenic Percussion

The spleen needs to be significantly enlarge for it to be felt or percussed. Percuss down left lower anterior chest wall downward in rows (front to back) If normal it should be resonant throughout if dullness is heard then could be caused by an enlarged spleen.

Another test is to Percuss in lowest interspace left anterior axillary line continuously, asking the patient to breath deeply, it should be resonant throughout if dullness is on deep inspiration heard then could be caused by an enlarged spleen as it moves a lot during respiration. An enlarged spleen can be caused by Leukaemia, Lymphoma, Chronic liver disease, endocarditis, glandular fever or Chronic Malaria.

Bristol Stool Chart

Types 1 and 2 suggest constipation, with 3 and 4 being the "ideal stool" as they are the easiest to pass, and 5-7 tending towards diarrhoea. It was formally used as a measure of the time it takes matter to pass along the colon but this has since been disproved.

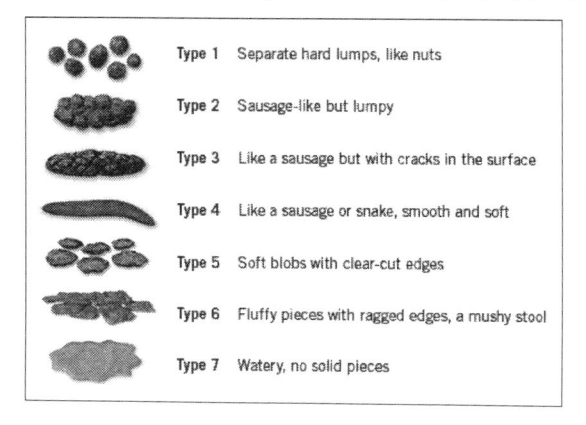

	Type 1	Separate hard lumps, like nuts
	Type 2	Sausage-like but lumpy
	Type 3	Like a sausage but with cracks in the surface
	Type 4	Like a sausage or snake, smooth and soft
	Type 5	Soft blobs with clear-cut edges
	Type 6	Fluffy pieces with ragged edges, a mushy stool
	Type 7	Watery, no solid pieces

Gastrointestinal Red flag Indicators

Red flag indicators if found usually indicate the patient needs further possibly life saving medical assessment and treatment beyond what is normally provided in the pre-hospital environment. If available this should be sought as soon as possible.

- Low blood pressure
- Decreased level of consciousness or confusion
- Signs of shock
- Generally unwell with high temperature
- Signs of dehydration
- Painful, rigid, guarded or tender abdomen
- Patient lying very still or writhing
- Absent or altered bowel sounds
- Associated testicular problem
- Blood in vomit or faeces
- Suspicion of medical cause for abdominal pain such as heart attack or lower lobe (lung) pneumonia

Differential diagnosis

It can be very difficult to tell exactly what may be happening with patients who are experiencing severe abdominal pain, without access to modern imaging. As discussed in the assessment chapter you need to work out what are the top 2 or 3 most likely diagnoses based on the history and clinical findings, and proceed from there with treatment.

Common Abdominal conditions causing Pain

1. Irritable Bowel Syndrome (IBS)
2. Constipation
3. Peptic Ulcer
4. Renal Colic
5. Biliary Colic
6. Appendicitis
7. Gastroenteritis
8. Urinary Tract Infection
9. Diverticulitis
10. Gallstones
11. GORD / Gastritis
12. Pregnancy

Symptoms of abdominal Illnesses (P=Possible)

Information in the table below is derived from Keith Hopcroft and Vincent forte (2008) Symptom Sorter 3rd Ed, Oxford: Radcliffe Publishing

	1	2	3	4	5	6	7	8	9	10	11	12
Variable swelling	Y	P										N
Diarrhoea	Y	P	N	N	N	P	Y	N	Y		N	N
Colicky	Y	Y	N	Y	Y	Y	N	N	Y			
Tenderness	N		Y	N	P	Y	P		Y			N
Fever		N	N	N	N	Y	P	Y			N	
High abdo Pain	P	P	Y					N	P			
Weight loss	N	N	P					P	N			
Rectal bleed	N	P	N					N	P			
Mucus PR	P											
Vomiting	N						P		P	P	N	
Chronic Pain	Y						N		P			
Constant Pain	N						N		Y			
Blood in stool	N						P		P			
Nocturnal Pain	N									P	P	
Relief antacids	N									N	Y	
Stress related	Y	N						N		N	P	
Radiates to back	N									P	N	
+ve Urinalysis		N						Y			N	
Related to eating		P						N			N	
D&V							Y					N
Increased bowel sounds							Y					

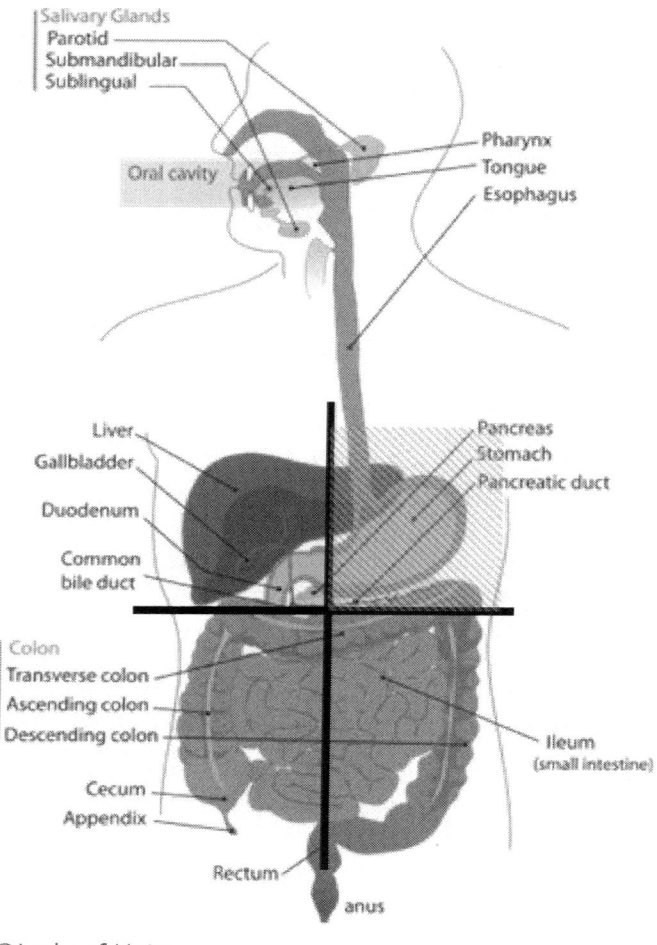

©Lady of Hats

Irritable Bowel Syndrome (IBS)

Irritable Bowel Syndrome affects 20% of the population at some point in their life, the cause is not fully understood but bouts are believed to be triggered by a number of causes including infections, nerves in the gut and intolerance to foods. But it often occurs in people with a normal digestive system which is free of disease and infection.

Common Symptoms include;

- Abdominal pain
- Bloating
- Diarrhoea and/or constipation
- Pellet or ribbon like fasces
- Mucous in faeces

Rare symptoms may include;

Nausea, headache, belching, loss of appetite, tiredness, backache, muscle pains, feeling quickly full after eating, indigestion and frequent and/or painful urination.

Constipation

Bowel habits vary enormously from person to person, and a change in habits and diet can provoke constipation. Definitions vary over exactly what constipation is – but infrequent hard stools twice or less a week are generally accepted as constipation. These motions often require straining to pass hard pellet like faeces. Sensations of pain and incomplete bowel movements can also occur

Constipation is normally attributed to either small, hard stools with normal muscle tone in the colon (colonic); or, normal stool with lack of muscle tone and failure to respond to the stimulus of faecal build up. As 'normal' bowel movements may occur anywhere from 3 to 20 times a week. The importance is in noting changes of an of individual bowel habits.

The causes include lack of dietary fibre, low fluid intake, immobility, slimming diets, and adverse drug effects such as the use of Codeine.

Paradoxically severe (longstanding) constipation may present with overflow diarrhoea and faecal incontinence.

Abdominal Examination - there may be (palpable faeces in lower and upper left quadrants of the abdomen or the examination may not reveal anything. A rectal examination may assist with diagnosis but it always requires a chaperone and is only usually performed by a Doctor.

Peptic Ulcer disease

This is an irritation or ulcers of the stomach or top part of the small bowel and is primarily due to excess acid production, but can also be caused by use of NSAID pain killing drugs and excess alcohol. Clinically it may present with burning Epigastric pain, relief with eating (usually), a comes and goes of varying severity.
Occasionally an ulcer can perforate through the wall of stomach, it presents with severe Epigastric pain and a rigid abdomen.

Biliary colic

This is pain caused by irritation of the tissue (viscera) surrounding the gall bladder caused by inflammation of the gall bladder (Cholecystitis) or gallstones.

The pain can be brought on by eating Fatty foods. Starting in the right upper quadrant, right flank, or the middle of the chest its steady, intense and starts quickly lasting from 30 minutes and to several hours. The pain may radiate to the back and shoulders, vomiting and diarrhea are possible.

Renal Colic

The pain from renal colic is caused by kidney stones passing through the urinary system. It comes in waves but can be constant and is often described as the worst pain the patient has ever experienced.

The kidneys process waste from the body and it is eliminated via urine. Sometimes the waste can form into crystals, these join together to form hard kidney stones. The problems occur when this stone tries to move from the kidney to the bladder. The ureters, connecting the two isn't designed for having stones move along it. Small stones <3-4 mm are washed out with urine, but bigger stones get stuck or move slowly.

The classic presentation is colicky pain, the patient may be writhing around the bed unable to sit still. The pain radiates from loin to groin as the stone moves, it may be associated with nausea and vomiting.

If you can test the urine (see clinical skills) it will reveal the presence of blood but no other indicators of infection.

Appendicitis

The appendix is believed to be the remains of an additional piece of intestine, which through evolution became redundant. It has also been suggested it has a role in the immune system. But no disability has been noted in the routine surgical removal of it.

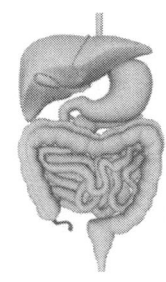

© 3drenderings | Dreamstime.com

The appendix is a tube approximately 10cm long with the distal end closed. It is connected to the caecum and is located near the junction of the small intestine and large intestine.

Appendicitis is inflammation of the appendix. It causes pain, nausea, vomiting, anorexia and a fever. Constipation is usual but diarrhoea may also occur. A fast pulse is an indication of any infection in the body.

It is estimated that 10% of the population will have Appendicitis at some point, the peak being in males between 10 and 20 years of age.

A life threatening problem will occur if the appendix ruptures and faeces enters the peritoneum this will cause peritonitis (an inflammation of the peritoneum). Untreated in 95% of people it will cause death.

Classically the pain starts as vague central abdominal pain, which may grumble on for 24-48 hrs. The pain then localises to a much sharper and discrete pain in the right iliac fossa. The pain from appendicitis is characterised by tenderness to palpation and rigidity (guarding) and pain when you press then let go (rebound tenderness) in the right iliac fossa. Laughing, coughing or movement may aggravate the pain. A good test is asking the patient to hop on their right leg being able to do this without making the pain worse, reduces the chance of it being appendicitis. Patient may alos experience tenderness in their left flank.

Unfortunately an abdominal exam may not always show the signs mentioned above particularly if the bowel nearby (caecum) is distended or the appendix lies within the pelvis. Old patients may also react to tests for appendicitis.

Gastroenteritis

An inflammation of the stomach, small intestine and colon. It can be categorised as bacterial or non-bacterial dependant on cause.

Signs

The smaller the child the more vulnerable they are to dehydration, remembers the elderly are also at risk.

Always perform an abdominal examination. Appendicitis can start with gastroenteritis and even if there is no sign of an acute abdomen at the time of the examination, be prepared to repeat the examination as signs can appear later.

Symptoms;

Symptoms can include; Sudden onset of diarrhoea, cramping abdominal pains, Temperature, Dehydration and vomiting.

Incubation periods can vary widely depending on cause, if a meal outside home is suspected, then contacting other dinners to check for symptoms is advisable and will help with diagnosis.

Diarrhoea with blood is more likely to be from a bacterial infection as does a patient with a temperature. Check if patient has travelled abroad recently. Children however often have a temperature and vomit for a variety of illnesses. Severely altered bowel habits in the elderly can also be a sign of cancer.

Possible causes

Rotavirus - incubation period 1 to 3 days, duration 3 to 8 days.

Norovirus, (Norwalk virus)

Salmonella species – incubation period 8 to 48 hours; lasts 2 to 5 days.

Campylobacter – incubation period 2 to 5 days, illness 2 to 5 days

Cholera produces profuse "rice-water" diarrhoea.

Urinary tract infection (UTI)

Urinary tract infections are very common in women, but very rare in men. The severity and treatment depends on where in the urinary tract they occur. Lower UTIs either affect the bladder (Cystitis), or the urethra (Urethritis). Upper UTIs either affect the kidneys (Pyelonephritis), prostate (*prostatitis*) or ureters and are the more serious of the two types.

Rare complications of untreated UTIs include Kidney failure and sepsis.

Symptoms of a Lower UTI include,

- Burning pain during urination
- Increased frequency of urination (>6 time a day)
- Urgency to pass urine
- Urge to pass during night
- Lower abdominal pain
- Cloudy, smelly urine
- Blood in Urine
- Back pain or tenderness in the pelvic area
- Incontinence
- Confusion

Symptoms of a upper UTI include,

- As above plus
- Rapid onset 1-2 days
- Temperature 38°C +
- Fever
- Nausea and/or vomiting
- Diarrhoea

- Fast Pulse (Tachycardia)
- Pain may be in your side, back or groin and usually one sided

Diverticulitis

Diverticulitis is a condition where small pouches form and protrude from the colon through weaknesses in the intestinal wall, if these diverticula become inflamed this is called diverticulitis.

It's a very common condition and generally affects people over 40, it is estimated that 50% of the population will have diverticula by the time they are 50 and 70% before the age of 80, although many people remain asymptomatic.

Symptoms can include;

- Severe Pain below navel, moving to the lower left quadrant of the abdomen.
- Pyrexia
- Frequent and/or painful urination
- Nausea and/or vomiting
- Constipation
- Rectal bleeding

Complications

In severe cases rectal bleeding may be severe and patient will need a blood transfusion.

Abscess may form. Colon can be narrowed causing blockages and fistulas can form between parts of digestive systems. Perforation of the colon often leads to peritonitis and sepsis.

Gallstones / Cholecystitis

Cholecystitis is inflammation of the gallbladder, which is a pouch that lies under the liver on the right side of the upper abdomen (RUQ) it stores bile which is produced in the liver and used in the gut to aid digestion. The cause of Cholecystitis is often attributed to gallstones but can be unknown. It can affect anyone but is more common in women.

Gastritis / GORD

Gastritis is caused when the lining of the stomach becomes inflamed and swells. It can happen briefly (acute) or be ongoing (chronic). Common causes are from long term use of NSAIDs, excessive drinking or bacterial infections. Some patients will have mild or no symptoms; others may have Epigastric pain, nausea and vomiting, loss of appetite. They may also vomit blood or pass it in stools

Gastro-oesophageal reflux disease (GORD/GERD) or acid reflux is caused by acid from the stomach into the oesophagus. It can be caused by a weakness in the sphincter leading into the stomach or by a hiatus hernia. The most common symptoms are heartburn (Epigastric pain), regurgitation, nausea and trouble swallowing. The pain may radiate into the chest and is often confused with cardiac pain.

Pregnancy

A diagnosis of pregnancy cannot be ruled out as a cause of abdominal pain in any sexually active women of child bearing age. If patient is young or potentially vulnerable a denial of sexual activity isn't conclusive.

Bowel Obstruction

The bowel is essentially a long tube extending from the mouth to the anus. A bowel obstruction occurs when it becomes mechanically obstructed. The clinical pattern and causes differ depending on if large or small bowel is affected.

Small bowel: This is usually caused by parts of the bowel sticking together (Adhesions) from previous surgery and presents with: vomiting, nausea and central abdominal pain and distension.

Large bowel: This is usually caused by cancer and can be more insidious in its onset. It presents with distension, pain and reduced or absent bowel sounds or wind. Untreated bowel becomes more distended; the blood supply is impaired by pressure and bowel wall loses its supply of oxygen (Infarcts) and dies. These areas of dead gut wall perforate and peritonitis develops.

Pancreatitis

Pancreatitis is the inflammation of the pancreas. It has many causes but the most common causes are gallstones (it shares a drainage system with the gallbladder) and alcohol.

The diagnosis is made in hospital by measuring the release of chemical called lipase from the pancreas. It should be considered in anyone with Epigastric pain, radiating to their back. The pain is normally more severe than for peptic disease, there may also be bruising of the flanks or around the umbilicus and sometimes a yellow tinge to skin and whites of eyes can occur (Jaundice).

Perianal Problems

Puritis: Puritis is itching around the rectum. The most common cause is poor hygiene / lack of hygiene but also skin conditions or irritation from stool or frequent loose stools (diarrhoea).

Haemorrhoids: These can be external (bulges in the external skin) or internal (hanging down from the inside of the anus). The medical distinction depends on if they originate above or below the dentate line, they are swellings and congestion of vascular cushions around the anal area and natural support deteriorates with age.
They present with swelling, itching and bleeding.

Peri-anal fissures: These are cracks in the skin around the anus. The skin splits and is slow to heal and results in very painful defecation. They can be caused by hard stools.

Peritonitis

Peritonitis is inflammation of the peritoneum which is a membrane sac covering the abdominal organs caused by an infection.

The peritoneum is usually germ-free so doesn't have capacity to fight off infection which can spread to the circulation system causing blood poisoning (sepsis) then to other organs causing organ failure and death.

Peritonitis can occur directly in the peritoneum or via damage to another organ allowing faeces to contact the peritoneum such as in a ruptured appendix or tears to the colon in diverticulitis.

Examine the abdomen it should move with breathing, ask the patient to 'suck' stomach in on inspiration then 'blow' it out on expiration. If the patient has peritonitis they will splint the abdomen and it will not move with breathing. In fact they will be trying to lie as still as possible as any movement will cause severe pain. On examination of the abdomen it will feel rigid like you are pressing on (Palpating) a piece of wood, known as Involuntary muscle rigidity (Guarding).

Rebound tenderness or Localised pain distant to site of pressure will me present. Bowel sounds may be absent and tickling or picking skin folds is very painful due to Cutaneous hyperesthesia.

Peritonitis is very serious and 10% of patients die even with full medical support in hospital.

Urology problems

Dehydration

Mild (5%):

- Thirst
- Decreased urinary output (in baby <4 wet nappies in 24hr)
- Dry mouth

Moderate (5-10%)

- Sunken fontanelle in infants
- Sunken eyes
- Fast Breathing (Tachypnoea) due to metabolic acidosis
- Fast Pulse > 100 (Tachycardia)

Severe (>10%)

- Decreased skin turgor on pinching the skin
- Drowsiness/irritability

Urinary retention

This is the inability to pass urine. It is most common in older men with prostate problems and is sometimes seen with urinary tract infections. It is a rare problem in women, but can occur when associated with a primary herpes attack.

Enlargement of Prostate

The prostate is a small gland located in the pelvis, between the penis and bladder, and surrounds the urethra. If it becomes enlarged it can place pressure on the bladder and urethra.

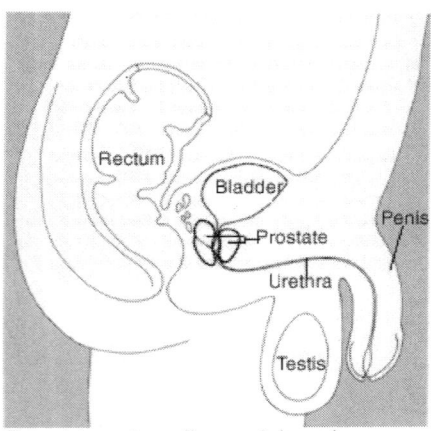

This picture shows the prostate and nearby organs.

Symptoms include;

- Difficulty urinating
- Increased frequent of urination
- Difficulty emptying the bladder

Abdominal Aneurysm

The differential diagnosis of a ruptured abdominal aneurysm needs to be considered. These are fairly common affecting more men than women at a ratio of 4:1 usually between the ages of 30 and 60.

Paraphimosis

This is the inability to replace a retracted foreskin. It usually occurs due to a chronically tight foreskin combined with extra congestion of the glans of the penis during sex or due to forgetting to retract it.

Testicular torsion

This is an abnormality in the position of the testis which leaves them prone to rotation. They tend to rotate towards the mid-line, twisting their blood supply and the testis dies. It is most common in young men 12-25 years. It usually presents a unilateral severe pain in the testicle.

Epididymo-orchitis

This is an Infection of testis and epididymis. It can be hard to differentiate between torsion and infection. Torsion is more likely in younger, not sexually active and is usually unilateral. Infection tends to be older men who are sexually active, can be bilateral. Often painful urination or increased frequency and may have urinary dip sticks consistent with a UTI. They may also be systemically unwell – fever, nausea, vomiting.

Chapter 12 Neurological Problems

Nervous System

The Nervous system consists of the Brain, Spinal Cord which make up the Central Nervous system and the Peripheral Nervous System which is made up of nerves which connect the Central Nervous system with limbs and organs.

Symptoms of Neurological problems.
Weakness in limbs or grasp on one or both sides
Loss of speech (Aphasia)
Inability to use appropriate words (Dysphasia)
Loss or reduction in senses
Numbness, pins & needles or altered sensation
Loss of balance (Ataxia)
Headache, Vertigo
Loss or decrease in level of consciousness (LOC)
Dizziness & blackouts
Seizures

Nervous system assessment

Questioning

Any headache? Where does it hurt?
Any fainting or dizziness?
Numbness, shaking, weakness or loss of sensation?
Any history of fitting (Seizures)?
Any problem with vision or hearing?
Are you unsteady on your feet?
Are you ok with heights? (Vertigo)

Examination

Eyes (PERLA)

After the primary assessment look for pupil symmetry and reactivity to light by shining a pen torch in the patient's eyes.

When shining a light into each eye, the pupil should become smaller (constriction). Move the torch up, down, left and right have the patient follow the movement with their eyes whilst keeping their head still.

A simple way of assessing a patient you think may have had a neurological problem is through the FAST acronym.

(F)ace

Look for facial droop of eye or mouth, dribbling etc

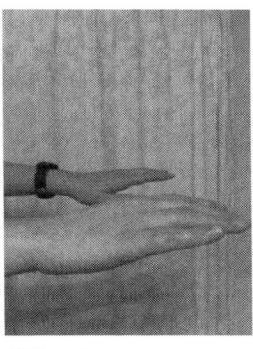

(A)rms
Ask them to raise both arms, close their eyes then keep them held in front of them, look for arm drift. Ask them to squeeze both your hands with theirs; feel for a difference in strength between body sides.

(S)peech
Listen for slurring, confusion and use of inappropriate words.

(T)est

Muscle

Tone: (Passive Movement)
Test tone in each limb by gently moving them for the patient the limb should neither be limp (flaccid) or be rigid with resistance.

Power:
Test power in Upper and Lower limbs by having patient raise and hold limb in air. Then the patient should push and pull against resistance. (Active & Resisted Movement)
The power of movement is graded using the scale below;

Power Classifications
0 – No muscle contraction is detected
1 – Some contraction is detected
2 – Able to move when gravity is eliminated.
3 – Moves against gravity but not resistance
4 – Able to move against some resistance from the examiner.
5 – Moves and overcomes the resistance of the examiner.

Tests for Coordination

Heel to Shin
Next have the patient perform the heel to shin test. With the patient lying supine, instruct them to place their right heel on their left shin just below the knee and then slide it down to their foot without dipping to either side.

Point-to-Point Movement
Ask the patient to extend their index finger and touch their nose, and then touch your finger with their finger. Go back and forth between their nose and your finger to perform correctly they must touch the tip of your finger. Once this is done correctly a few times at a

moderate speed, ask the patient to continue with their eyes closed. Normally this remains accurate when the eyes are closed. Repeat and then compare to the other hand.

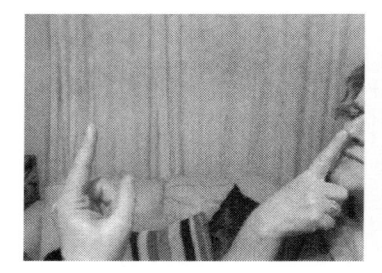

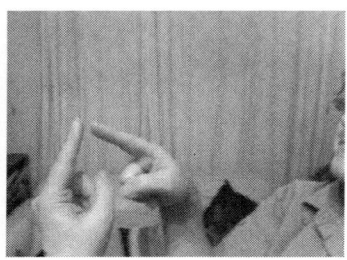

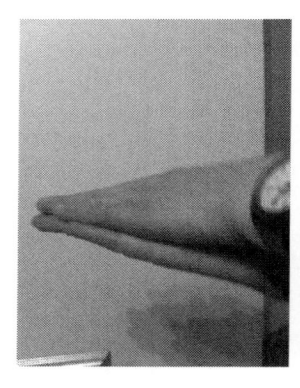

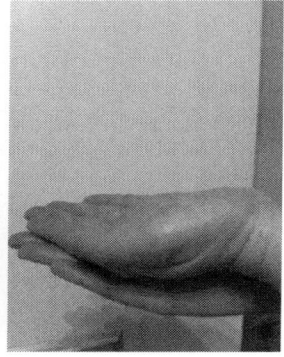

Flapping Hands
For the next task ask the patient to hold their non dominant hand palm upwards then place the dominant hand on top of it. Now ask them to turn the top hand rapidly from palm down to palm up, observe for coordination then repeat with hands the opposite way up.

Romberg test
Have the patient stand still with their heels together close their eyes. If the patient loses their balance they fail the test. An adaption of this is too give them a very gently push to the shoulder and observe if this puts them off balance.

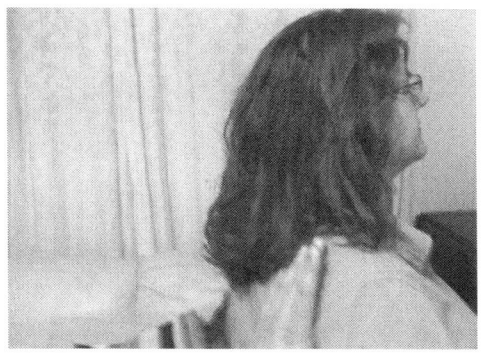

Gait
Gait is checked by having the patient walk across the room first normally then heel to toe, then on their toes only and finally on their heels only. Have them walk between 3 and 5 Meters turn around and return.

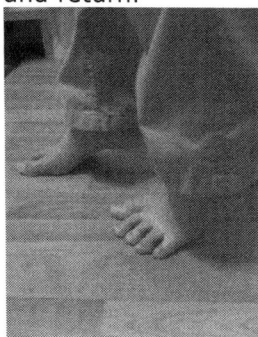

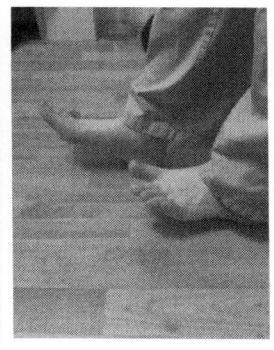

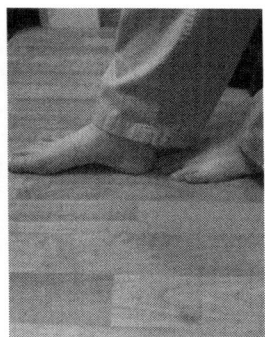

Heel to Shin
Next have the patient perform the heel to shin test. With the patient lying supine, instruct them to place their right heel on their left shin just below the knee and then slide it down to their foot without dipping to either side.

Reflexes

Reflexes are involuntary reactions to stimuli, if you place your hand on a hot surface the reflex arc will retract it, this is accomplished quickly as the signal from the sensory nerves enters the spinal cord and a signal is immediately sent from the spinal cord to a motor nerve which retracts the muscle. The brain isn't involved as this would slow the process.

To successfully test a reflex the patient must be completely relaxed and the joint flexed. Distract the patient by asking them to look at a point across the room. Compare each side as you move down the body.

Grade reflexes as;
0   Absent
+1   Diminished
+2   Normal
+3   Increased / Normal
+4   Hyperactive

A strong contraction indicates a 'brisk' or hyperactive reflex, and a weak or absent reflex is known as 'diminished', 'Dull' or Hypoactive reflex. Brisk reflexes can be found in lesions of upper motor neurones, and absent or reduced reflexes are found in lower motor neurone lesions.

The nine reflex levels with their nerve roots are listed below the first six are more commonly tested the anal and abdominal reflexes are generally only assessed by specialists. An unusually dull or brisk reflex indicates a problem along the nerve path, at the nerve root or above that point on the spinal cord. Some reflexes cause a noticeable jerk whilst others are more subtle and cause a slight muscle movement which is felt it not seen.

Biceps reflex arc C5 / C6 (musculocutaneous nerve)
The test is performed by using a tendon hammer to quickly depress the biceps brachii tendon below the biceps. This activates the stretch receptors inside the biceps brachii muscle to induce a reflex contraction of the biceps muscle and jerk of the forearm.

Triceps reflex arc C7 / C8
The test is performed by using a tendon hammer to quickly depress the triceps tendon above the elbow. This activates the stretch receptors inside the muscle to induce a reflex contraction of the triceps muscle.

Supinator / Brachioradialis reflex arc
The test is performed by using a tendon hammer to quickly depress the radial tendon above the hand. This activates the stretch receptors inside the muscle to induce a reflex contraction of the hand and flexion of the elbow.

Knee (Patellar) reflex arc L2, L3, L4
The patient sits with his leg swinging freely. The test is performed by using a tendon hammer to quickly depress the tendon below the Patellar. This activates the stretch receptors inside the muscle to induce a reflex contraction of the quadriceps muscle causing a leg jerk.

Ankle (Achilles reflex) arc S1
Bend the foot up (dorsiflexion), the test is performed by using a tendon hammer to quickly depress the tendon above the ankle. This activates the stretch receptors inside the muscle to induce a reflex contraction of the muscle causing the foot to move down (plantarflexion).

Plantar reflex arc S1 (Babinski's)
Rub the outside sole of the foot with a blunt instrument from the heel along a curve to the toes. In normal reflexes there is either no response or the toes curl inward and the foot everts. If there is damage to the nervous system then the big toe bends backwards and the rest of the toes fan out instead of curling.

Upper Abdominal reflex arc T8, T9, T10
Lower Abdominal reflex arc T10, T11, T12
Test the abdominal reflexes by stroking from the edge to the midline above and below the navel. The navel should move towards the stimuli.

Anal and bulbospongiosus Reflex S2, S3, S4
Anal reflex is a contraction of the anal sphincter triggered by a painful stimuli. The bulbospongiosus reflex is a similar contraction in response to firmly squeezing the penis head or clitoris.

Sensation
The sensation test involves the patient lying down with their eyes closed. It tests pain sensation (pin prick), light touch sensation (brush).
Alternatively touch the patient with the needle and the brush at intervals of roughly 5 seconds and ask which they feel. Work downwards towards the feet. Ask if they notice a difference in the strength of sensation on each side of their body.

Alternating between pinprick and light touch, touch the patient in the following 13 places. Touch one body part followed by the corresponding body part on the other with the same instrument. The corresponding nerve root for each area tested is indicated in parenthesis.

1. Back (posterior) of the shoulders (C4)
2. Outside (lateral) of the upper arms (C5)
3. Inside (medial) of the lower arms (T1)
4. Tip of the thumb (C6)
5. Tip of the middle finger (C7)
6. Tip of the pinky finger (C8)
7. Chest at nipple level (T5)
8. Chest at navel level (T10)
9. Upper part of the upper leg (L2)

10. Lower inside (medial) part of the upper leg (L3)
11. Inside (medial) lower leg (L4)
12. Outside (lateral) lower leg (L5)
13. Sole of foot (S1)

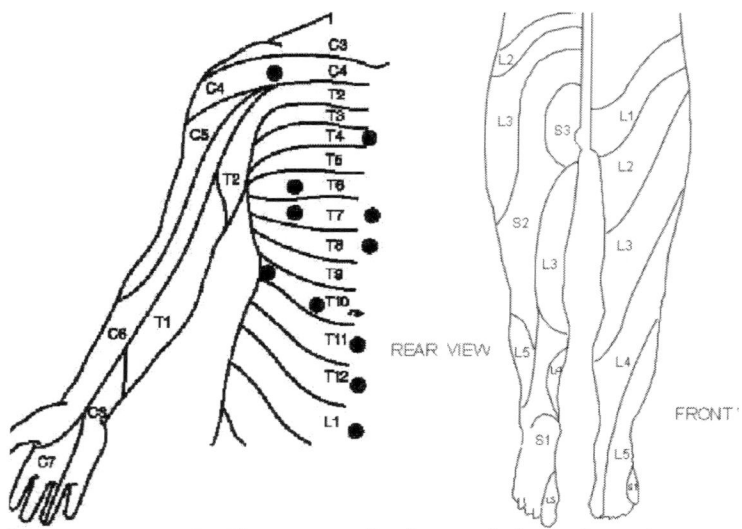

Major nerves in the upper limbs and their functions.

Nerve	Area of sensory loss	Motor function test
Axillary	Outer shoulder & top of upper arm	Abducting the arm against resistance
Musculo-cutaneous	Outer forearm	Flexing the forearm against resistance
Median	Lateral three and half digits	Abducting the thumb at right angles to the palm against resistance
Ulna	Medial one and half digits	Abducting the little finger against resistance
Radial	Back of the forearm to the first web space posteriorly	Maintaining extension of the metacarpophalangeal joints against resistance

Major nerves in the lower limbs and their functions

Femoral	Front of the knee	Extending the knee against resistance with the leg flexed at both hip and knee
Sciatic	Foot and inner calf	Flexing the knee against resistance
Posterior tibial	Sole of the foot	Pushing the foot downwards at the ankle against resistance
Deep peroneal	First web space on the top of the foot	Pulling the foot upwards at the ankle against resistance

Cranial nerves

There are 12 pairs of cranial nerves are nerves that emerge directly from the brain. The first two pairs come from the cerebrum; the other ten pairs come from the brainstem. They receive information from the bodies' senses and control movement of the Eyes, face, mouth, jaw, shoulders etc.

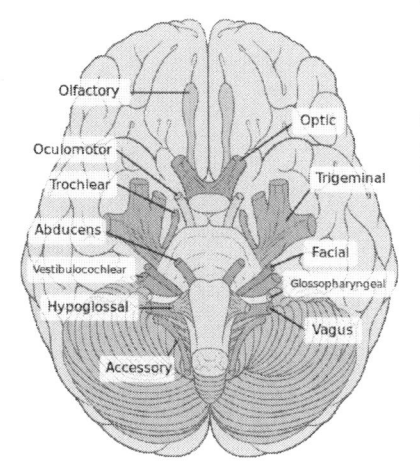

Original artwork by Patrick J. Lynch, medical illustrator; C. Carl Jaffe, MD, cardiologist, modifications by Dwstultz / Beao

There are a number of different tests for each nerve do what is reasonable and practical to your situation.

I- Olfactory Nerve (Sense of Smell)

Can the patient smell a strong scent?, test each nostril.

If optic nerve is damaged the patient may not be able to smell anything and may have decreased sense of taste. Ask the patient if they normally have a problem or if nose is blocked by congestion. Examine for any rashes, deformity or injury.

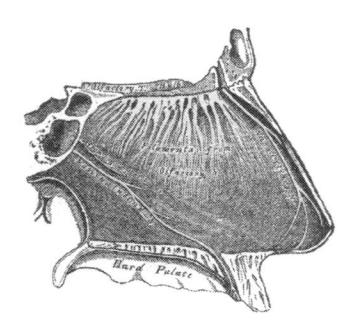

II- Optic Nerve (Sense of Sight)

Can the patient count the number of fingers that are being held up?

Examine back of eye (Optic Fundus) with Opthalmascope this is a specialist examination but is aiming to look for bleeding, foreign objects, abnormal or pulsating blood vessels.

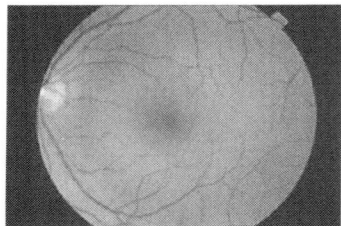

National Eye Institute

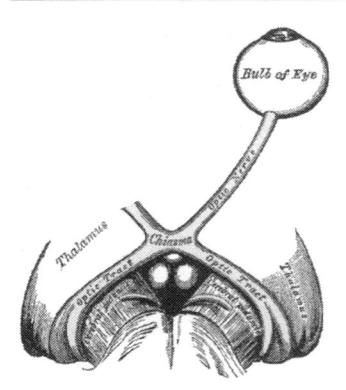

Test vision (visual acuity) have the patient read a script or number plate at a distance using glasses if they normally wear them..

Test peripheral vision (visual fields) by wiggling a finger to the left, right, above and below at 6 points in a 'H' pattern at about 30cm (1') from patient whilst they look ahead, note any differences in visual fields.

Test pupil's reaction to light by shinning a light in them, they should constrict to the light stimuli and dilate if in a dark environment.

Test pupil's ability to track movement (accommodation) place finger in front of patients, ask patient to look at your finger and move finger toward the patient, eyes should converge slightly and constrict).

If optic nerve is damaged the patient may lose sight in one or both eyes with no long standing disease or injury.

III- Occulomotor, IV- Trochlear, VI- Abducens (Nerve that controls muscles that move the eyes, eyelids and pupils)

Look at pupil shape and relative size.

Observe for drooping of the eyelid (ptosis).

Ask them to follow your finger with their eyes, check they can open their eyes; look up and down and to each side?

  (Lateral movement of eye=VI, Upper medial movement of eye= IV, All other eye movements III).

Do they complain of seeing double?, does covering one eye improve it. Check for involuntary eye movement (nystagmus) this can affect vision may be normal for patient

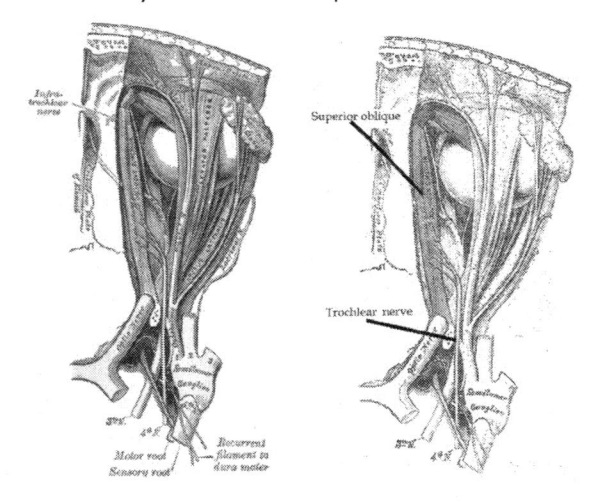

V- Trigeminal (Sensation to the face).

Test temporal and masseter muscle strength by moving jaw from open to clenched teeth.

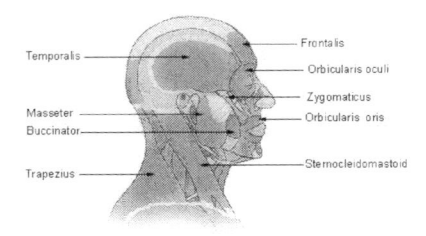

Test forehead, cheeks and jaw for sensations using dull and sharp object.

Test corneal reaction both sides (i.e. brush with cotton wool) the eye should move up and away from stimulus.

Touch the patient's face lightly with soft cloth on each side and assess soft touch on both sides?

Damage to the trigeminal nerve can cause numbness in an isolated area, across a one side or cause pain.

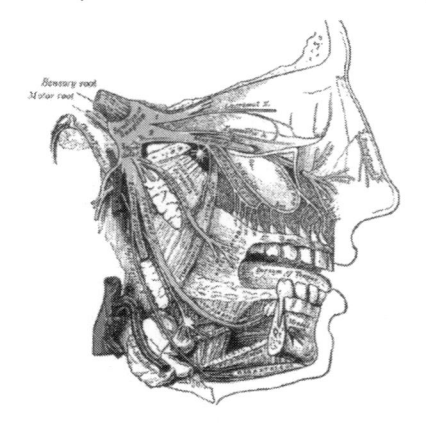

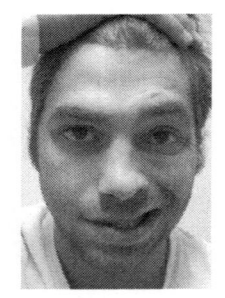

VII- Facial Nerve (That control Muscles that allow face to move.)

Check for any facial droop, weakness, slow response or asymmetry in facial movement.

Test the following movements; raise eyebrows, close both eyes to resistance, smile, frown, show teeth and puff out cheeks. The eyebrows on the same side as the weak face will also be weak if this is a cranial nerve problem.

A person attempting to show his teeth and raise his eyebrows with Bell's palsy (VII Injury) on his right side by James Heilman, MD

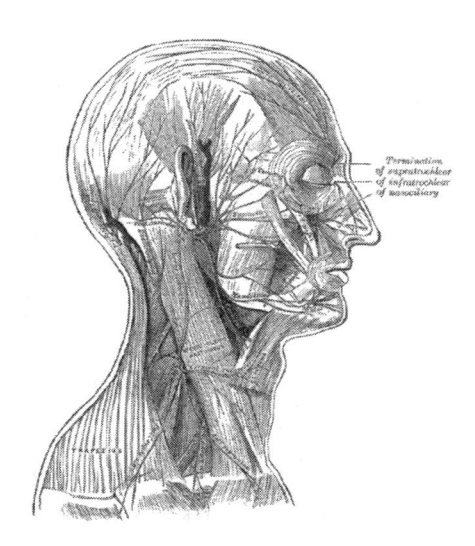

VIII- Auditory Nerve (Sense of Hearing and Balance)

Assess hearing, this is often only undertaken briefly to assess for major deficits.

Test the patient's hearing by holding hand at arms length either side the patients ears on one side rub fingers together and ask them which side they heard the noise. Ask them a question but do not let them watch your lips move. In children, have someone call their name softly from across the room.

Damage to cranial nerve VIII cause instabilities of balance, ringing in the ears and may appear to be drunk Examine ears look at external auditory canals and eardrums.

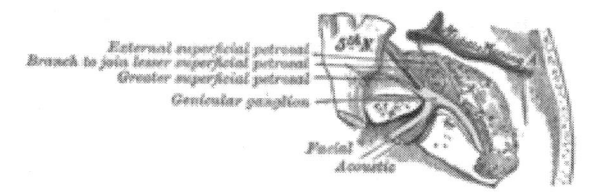

IX- Glossopharyngeal, X- Vagus Nerve (Controls muscles that move the palate and control swallowing)

Listen to the patient's voice. Is it hoarse or nasal?

(Hoarseness may indicate paralysis of vocal cords, nasal may indicate paralysis of the palate).

Is there any difficulty in swallowing?

Ask the patient to say "Ah". The palate and uvula should rise symmetrically, and the posterior pharynx should move medially.

You can stimulate the gag reflex by gently stimulating the back of the throat on each side they should have a gag reflex (Controlled by Nerves IX and X)

Watch the patient take a sip of water, can they swallow normally is there any dribbling?

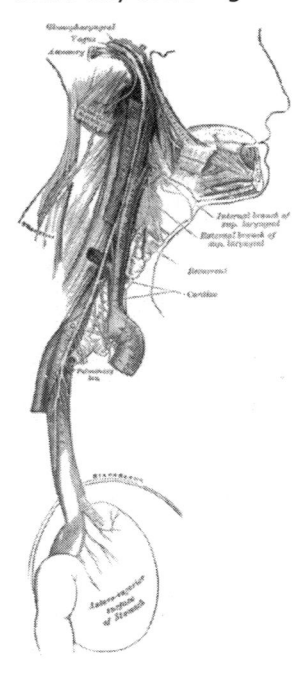

XI- Accessory Nerve (Controls Muscles that move the shoulders)

From behind the patient inspect the trapezius muscles for weakness, wasting or asymmetry.

Ask the patient to shrug their shoulders against resistance, noting any weakness or asymmetry.

Ask the patient to turn their head against resistance, watch and palpate the sternomastoid on the opposing side, noting inequality and weakness. Ask the patient to shrug their shoulders.

XII-Hypoglossal (Nerve that controls muscles that move the tongue and form speech)

Listen to the way the patients speaks (Articulation).

Look at the way the tongue as it lays in the mouth ask the patient to stick it out and move to either side. Look for asymmetry, weakness or deviation from mid-line.

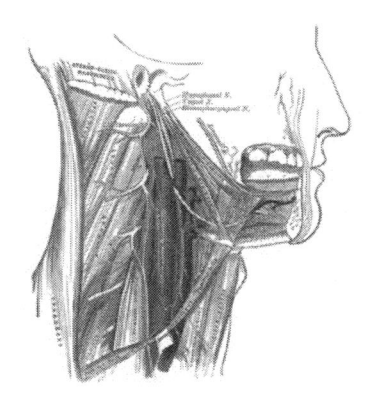

Abbreviated mini-mental test
To test cognitive function perform an abbreviated mini-mental test score (amts). A score of less than 7 indicates a problem.
Give random address to remember

1. Ask patients age?
2. Ask what time it is to nearest hour?
3. What year is it?
4. Ask who two people nearby are?
5. Ask date of birth?
6. Dates of Second World War?
7. Name of Reigning Monarch/President?
8. Ask them where they are now?
9. Ask them to count backwards from 20 to 1
10. Ask them to recall address given at the start?

Central Nervous System Red flag Indicators
Red flag indicators if found usually indicate the patient needs further possibly life saving medical assessment and treatment beyond what is normally provided in the pre-hospital environment. If available this should be sought as soon as possible.

- The 'worst headache ever'
- Sudden onset and or severe headache
- Not relieved by simple painkillers
- Headache associated after being knocked out
- Unwell, temperature, neck stiffness, rash? Meningitis
- Visual problem, dizziness, limb weakness
- New headache in patient over 60 years old.

Symptoms of Neurological Problems

CVA   Cardiovascular Accident
Hypo Hypoglycaemia
DKA   Diabetic Ketoacidosis

Symptoms of Neurological Illnesses

Information derived from Keith Hopcroft and Vincent forte (2008) Symptom Sorter 3rd Ed, Oxford: Radcliffe Publishing **(P=Possible)**

	Hypoxia	Infection	CVA	Hypo'	DVA
Cyanosis	Y	N	N	N	N
Fever	P	Y	N	N	P
Weakness	N	N	P	P	N
Fast Resps	Y	Y	N	N	Y
Sudden Dizziness		N		Y	
Irritable		N		P	
Relief on Lying down		N		N	
Episodic		N		Y	

Stroke (CVA)/TIA

A stroke (Cerebral Vascular Accident (CVA)) is an interference with normal brain function caused either by a clot (85%) or bleeding (15%) causing an interruption to blood flow to the brain. Depending on the severity and location of the damage the patient will exhibit different signs and symptoms. They may lose the use of their arms and legs on one side of the body, or there may be a decrease in strength and power on the affected side or just a heavy feeling in the limbs. Patients can become disorientated and confused, speech may be slurred, absent or they lose the ability to select appropriate words to form sentences (Dysphasia). They may have unequal pupils or develop a facial droop. A headache and high blood pressure often are present..

A Transient Ischemic attack is similar to a stroke, but the symptoms resolve without intervention normally within 24 hours and frequently within minutes or a few hours. Although separate parts of function may return at different times.

A simple way of assessing a patient you think may have had a stroke is through the FAST acronym. It stands for FACE, ARMS, SPEECH, TEST.

FACE

Look for facial droop, dribbling etc

ARMS

Ask them to squeeze both your hands with theirs, feel for a marked difference in strength between body sides. Ask if they can raise their legs and assess in the same way.

SPEECH

Listen for slurring, confusion, using inappropriate words.

Stroke (CVA)/TIA

A stroke (Cerebral Vascular Accident (CVA)) is an interference with normal brain function caused either by a clot (85%) or bleeding (15%) causing an interruption to blood flow to the brain. Depending on the severity and location of the damage the patient will exhibit different signs and symptoms. They may lose the use of their arms and legs on one side of the body, or there may be a decrease in strength and power on the affected side or just a heavy feeling in the limbs. Patients can become disorientated and confused, speech may be slurred, absent or they lose the ability to select appropriate words to form sentences (Dysphasia). They may have unequal pupils or develop a facial droop. A headache and high blood pressure often are present..

A Transient Ischemic attack is similar to a stroke, but the symptoms resolve without intervention normally within 24 hours and frequently within minutes or a few hours. Although separate parts of function may return at different times.

A simple way of assessing a patient you think may have had a stroke is through the FAST acronym. It stands for FACE, ARMS, SPEECH, TEST.

FACE

Look for facial droop, dribbling etc

ARMS

Ask them to squeeze both your hands with theirs, feel for a marked difference in strength between body sides. Ask if they can raise their legs and assess in the same way.

SPEECH

Listen for slurring, confusion, using inappropriate words.

Seizures

These can vary in intensity from brief periods of absence where the patient appears to be distracted to prolonged full body convulsions and repeated fits. Many things can cause seizures; epilepsy, CVAs, head and spinal injuries as well as other medical problems. It is believed that 30% of seizures as caused by heart problems when sufficient oxygen is not been delivered to the brain.

Three broad types of Seizures exist;
- Absences (Petit Mal)
- Tonic Clonic (Grand Mal)
- Focal (Jacksonian)

Focal seizures may only affect a single limb and do not necessarily require emergency treatment.

If the patient is known to have seizures and they are generally short in duration (<1 min), let the seizure run its course, protecting the patients head, don't try and restrain them and never put anything in their mouth.

A Tonic Clonic Seizure generally follows four stages;
- Indication of Seizure (Aura)
- Patient becomes Rigid (Tonic)
- Seizure activity (Clonic)
- Recovery Phase (Post Ictal)

Headaches
Headaches are very common and most are minor and go away.

Classically divided into:
Primary headache syndromes :
- Migraine
- Tension
- Cluster

Secondary causes:
- Infections
- Space occupying lesion
- Unknown cause

Information derived from Keith Hopcroft and Vincent forte (2008) Symptom Sorter 3rd Ed, Oxford: Radcliffe Publishing **(P=Possible)**

	Tension	Sinusitis	Migraine	Spondylosis	Eye Strain
Worse on Lying	N	Y	N	P	N
Congested	N	Y	P	N	N
Neck movement	N	N	P	Y	N
Tender	P	Y	N	N	N
One sided	N	P	P	N	P

One off mild-moderate severity headache
Causes include sleep deprivation, stress, dehydration or a viral illness.

More serious headaches
These include meningitis (infection around the brain), bleeding around the brain and space occupying lesions such as brain tumours. More concerning symptoms of a serious cause include;
- Increasing severity of the headache
- More than a mild fever
- Aversion to light (photophobia)
- Neck stiffness
- Repeated vomiting
- Altered conscious state such as confusion

Meningitis
This is an infection of the covering of the brain. Also possible are brain abscess or infection in the brain itself (encephalitis). Consider this diagnosis if severe headache and high temperature and has an aversion to light (Photophobia), a stiff neck, muscle aches and back ache.

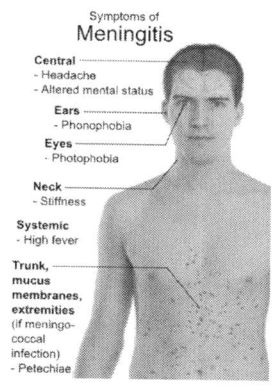

Symptoms of Meningitis
- Central
  - Headache
  - Altered mental status
- Ears
  - Phonophobia
- Eyes
  - Photophobia
- Neck
  - Stiffness
- Systemic
  - High fever
- Trunk, mucus membranes, extremities (if meningococcal infection)
  - Petechiae

© Mikael Häggström

Migraine
Not so much serious as severe. Migraines are common, affecting less men than women and as common as 1:6 people. Frequency of the attack can vary from weeks to every few years. The classical syndrome is of severe one sided (unilateral) headache, often associated with vomiting. Recurring warning signs prior to the onset of the headache called an aura (Prodrome) is common.

Subarachnoid haemorrhage
This is bleeding from blood vessels on the surface of the brain and is often fatal. It usually presents with a sudden onset and very severe headache, often with nausea and vomiting. Signs associated with a bad outcome are a reduced conscious state or the presence of neurological signs similar to a stroke.

Brain tumour / Space occupying lesions
This can be the cause of recurrent worsening headaches which may be worse in the morning or associated with nausea, as it progresses they develop neurological signs such as one sided (Unilateral) weakness or altered sensation.

Sciatica

Sciatica is an umbrella term used to describe a group of diseases causing specific symptoms. Commonly involves shooting pain travelling from the base of the spine down the legs. Pain can be intermittent or continuous, ranging from mild to severe.

Two useful tests for cause of sciatic pain are the straight leg raise with the patient lying flat if this produces pain the likely cause is from a herniated disk. If this can be achieved without discomfort then have them place the leg on the effected side over the opposite thigh with their foot placed down flat, if this causes pain the likelihood is that the sciatic nerve is trapped in the pelvis.

Fainting

This is a common problem and young women the most commonly affected group. A faint is characterised by brief loss of consciousness with a warning sign (Aura/Prodrome). This may be a feeling of light-headedness, feeling very hot or a feeling vision is closing in like looking through a black tunnel or a combination of all these. It can be triggered by emotional stress, sudden standing up, a hot environment or standing still for prolonged periods (soldiers' on parade). There is no specific treatment and recovery is usually rapid. Always consider the diagnoses of an ectopic pregnancy as a cause for fainting in a sexually active woman. There is a greater risk for a serious cause being present if the patient is over 60 years, has a history of heart disease and or is sudden with no warning signs.

Chapter 13 Common Infectious Diseases

Chickenpox

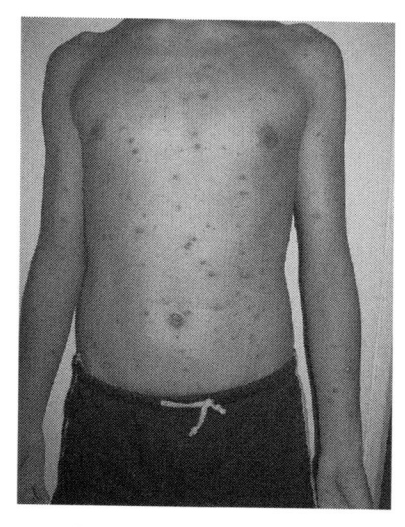

© Camiloaranzales

It starts with vesicular skin rash on the body and head which becomes itchy, raw pockmarks, which mostly heal without scarring unless scratched.

It takes from 10 to 21 days after initial infection for the disease to develop is infectious 1-2 days before the rash appears and remains contagious until all lesions have crusted over at 6 days.

Initial symptoms vary and can include; myalgia, itching, nausea, fever, headache, sore throat, pain in both ears, complaints of pressure in head or swollen face, severe lower pain back, loss of appetite and malaise in adolescents and adults. Temperatures 38 °C and 42 °C have been noted.

Rarely fatal, although more serious in adult males, pregnant women and immune-compromised patients.

In very rare cases chickenpox can cause strokes (CVA) in children. A more common complication is shingles appearing decades after the initial disease.

Clostridium botulinum – aka botulisim (W)

This is a very potent form of food poisoning usually through the ingestion of contaminated water or food such as raw fish, poorly canned vegetables or syrups causing botulism in humans. The bacteria itself is relatively harmless, the damage is caused by a toxin produced by the bug. It has many symptoms which include a sore dry mouth and throat causing difficulty in speaking and swallowing, Blurred vision, abdominal cramps and pain, nausea and/or vomiting, breathing problems, generalized weakness and can lead to paralysis. It is also used in biological warfare. It is not contagious unless exposed to the same contaminated food source or bioweapon.

Escherichia coli (E coli) (W)

E.coli is a common cause of gastroenteritis. It can also cause urinary tract infection or septicaemia.

Malaria

Malaria is spread via mosquito bites and on rare occasions by blood to blood contact and remains a large cause of death in the third world. There are different strains of Malaria the most virulent being Falciparum malaria. The disease has a variable incubation period usually from 7 days to one month but can appear much later, so patients often don't become ill until after they have returned from travelling. Patients experience some or all of the following;
Fever, shivering (Rigors), muscular pain, headache, diarrhoea, nausea, cough, lowered blood pressure, loss of appetite and general fatigue.

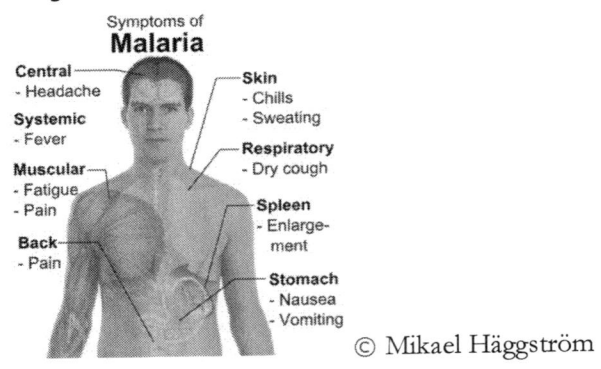

Symptoms of
Malaria

Central
- Headache

Systemic
- Fever

Muscular
- Fatigue
- Pain

Back
- Pain

Skin
- Chills
- Sweating

Respiratory
- Dry cough

Spleen
- Enlargement

Stomach
- Nausea
- Vomiting

© Mikael Häggström

In severe cases patient may become jaundiced, lose consciousness, experience seizures, have lowered blood sugar, become shocked and develop breathing problems.

It should always be considered in any patient with a history of exposure (ie travel) and a fever. The presence of confusion in addition to fever should be Falciparum malaria until proven otherwise.

Measles

In our modern world most childhood diseases that were common years ago have all but disappeared in the Western world. Worldwide 800,000 children die from measles each year, the majority of which live in developing countries. It is the leading cause of blindness in African children. Sadly due to poor vaccination levels in some communities we are see a recurrence.

In 2005 there were only 77 cases of measles reported in the UK. Unfortunately a year later this had risen to 449 cases. A boy's death from the disease in April 2006 was the first UK fatality in 14 years. The rise in cases was due to parents who were worried about side effects of vaccines not getting their children vaccinated with the triple MMR (Measles, mumps and Rubella). Measles is probably the most infectious disease in the UK and it is hanging around waiting for enough people without immunity to cause an epidemic.

Measles has been a notifiable disease in since 1940's, and notifications varied between 160,000 and 800,000 cases per year in the UK, the peaks occurring in two-year cycles. Before the introduction of measles vaccination in 1968, around 100 children a year in England and Wales died from the disease.

Early warning signs last 2 to 4 days and include irritability, a runny nose, conjunctivitis (pink eye), a hacking cough and an increasing fever that comes and goes. These symptoms may last up to 8 days.

Additionally, 'Koplik' spots which are highly characteristic of the early phase of measles may be spotted in the mouth on the inside of the cheek opposite the 1st and 2nd upper molars one or two days before the rash appears. The spots look like tiny grains of white sand, each surrounded by a red ring. However, these are difficult to see.

The typical measles rash appears from day four with the fever usually peaking at this time. The rash usually starts on the forehead and spreads down over the face, neck and body and consists of flat or raised red or brown blotches which flow into each other. The rash lasts for between four to seven days.

Symptoms develop 9 to 11 days after becoming infected and last up to 14 days from the first signs until the end of the rash. However, the illness can last longer if complications develop.

Measles is highly contagious and can be transmitted from four days prior to the onset of the rash to four days after the rash appears. It is most infectious just before the rash appears and so people tend to spread the virus before realising they are infected. It is estimated that 90% of susceptible close contacts of someone infected with measles will also become infected with the virus.

This would mean that a person could be contagious before any symptoms appear at all.

The virus resides in the mucus of the nose and throat of someone infected and is spread by coughing and sneezing which causes droplets of infected mucus to be sprayed into the air. These droplets are then breathed in by others or transferred to the mouth by fingers which have handled a surface contaminated by infected droplets. The virus remains active and contagious on surfaces for up to two hours.

After exposure to the virus it usually takes around 10 days (7-18 days range) for the first symptoms to appear.

In the UK, complications are quite common even in healthy people and approximately 20% of reported measles cases experience one or more complications. Complications are more common among children under 5 years of age, those with weakened immune systems, children with a poor diet and adults.

Common complications of measles include:
Diarrhoea and vomiting, conjunctivitis (eye infection), laryngitis (inflammation of the voicebox), inner ear (otitis media) infection, febrile convulsions, pneumonia.

Less common complications are:
Meningitis, hepatitis (inflammation of the liver), encephalitis (inflammation of the brain) which can lead to permanent deafness, mental retardation and can be fatal, bronchitis and croup, squint as the virus can affect the nerves and muscles of the eye.

On rare occasions measles can lead to:
Serious eye disorders, heart and nervous system problems, and very rarely (1 in 8000 cases in children under two and 1 in 25,000 cases in older persons), a progressive and fatal brain infection called subacute sclerosing panencephalitis (SSPE) sometimes many years after the first bout of measles. Death occurs in 1 in 5000 cases. Catching measles in pregnancy can also cause miscarriage, premature labour or a baby with a low birth weight.

Meningitis
Meningitis is inflammation of the meninges which covers the spinal cord and the brain. Signs and symptoms include a sudden onset of fever, severe headache, photophobia, neck stiffness and a rash which doesn't disappear when pressed on with a glass. Transmission is via droplet secretions, incubation period is between 2 and 10 days. Patients are no longer infectious 24hrs after start of therapy. Untreated it can progress to seizures, coma and death.

Mumps (Epidemic Parotis)

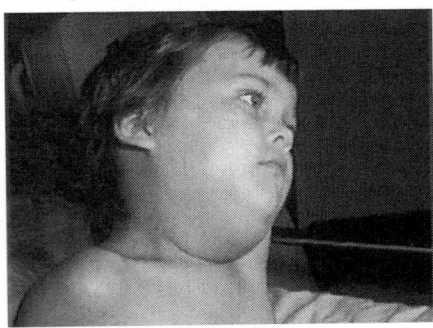

© Patho

Before the development of a vaccine mumps was a common childhood illness, even today with concerns over vaccine side effects have resulted in infection of unvaccinated children.

Infection risk starts 6 days before the onset of symptoms until about 9 days after symptoms start. The incubation is typically 16–18 days.

Fever, malaise, anorexia and headache can occur before swelling occurs.

It presents as painful swelling of the salivary particularly the parotid gland particularly when eating and can effect one or both sides. Other symptoms fever, dry mouth, headache, sore face and/or ears and occasionally in more serious cases, loss of voice. and. Painful testicular swelling (orchitis) and rash may also occur. The disease is generally self-limiting and no treatment other than pain killers are generally required.

Roseola

Caused by the herpes virus, causes a rose-colored transient rash. Other symptoms include fever lasting 3-5 days, runny nose, irritability and tiredness. As the fever subsides a maculopapular rash may appear on the face and body. It commonly occurs between 6 months and 3 yrs, but can occur up to the age of 18.

Rubella (German measles)

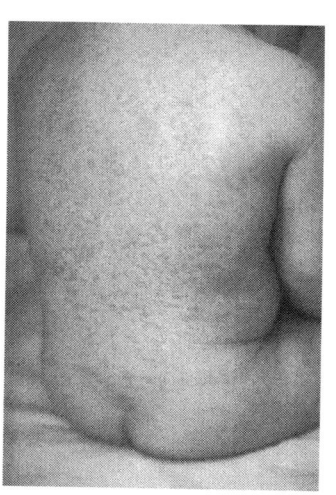

© Patho

A mild form of measles sometimes patients can be affected and are unaware. Lasting 1-3 days.

Children recover more quickly than adults. If the patient is in the first 20 weeks of pregnancy can cause serious problems with the baby known as congenital rubella syndrome (CRS) this causes 1 in 5 pregnancies to be aborted,

The disease has an incubation period of 2 to 3 weeks. Then causes flu like symptoms; low grade fever, swollen glands, joint pains, headache and conjunctivitis. Followed by a pink or light red itchy rash on the face which spreads to the trunk and limbs and usually fades after three days.

Forchheimer's sign occurs in 1 in 5 cases, as small, red papules on the area of the soft palate.

Shingles (Herpes zoster)

Adults have had chicken pox as children can get shingles as adults, often with difficulty in sleeping due to pain (postherpetic neuralgia)

Even after the shingles rash has disappeared, pain can continue in the area affected by the rash.

Tetanus (W)
Tetanus is caused by the bacteria Clostridium Tetani. It is transmitted through a puncture wound. Onset can take up to two months, but usually takes around 7 days. Early sign is jaw stiffness (hence the common name Lock Jaw), muscle stiffness, headache, fever and spasm. It is fatal in 40% of cases, death occurring due to failure of respiratory muscles.

Tuberculosis (TB) (W)
Tuberculosis (TB) is very infectious and transmitted by droplet infection. A primary pulmonary lesion usually leads to lymph node involvement. There may be no initial symptoms but the patient may be symptomatic from the lung lesion and have a cough, thick sputum, haemoptysis, pneumonia, pleura effusion, fever, rigors, lethargy and anorexia.

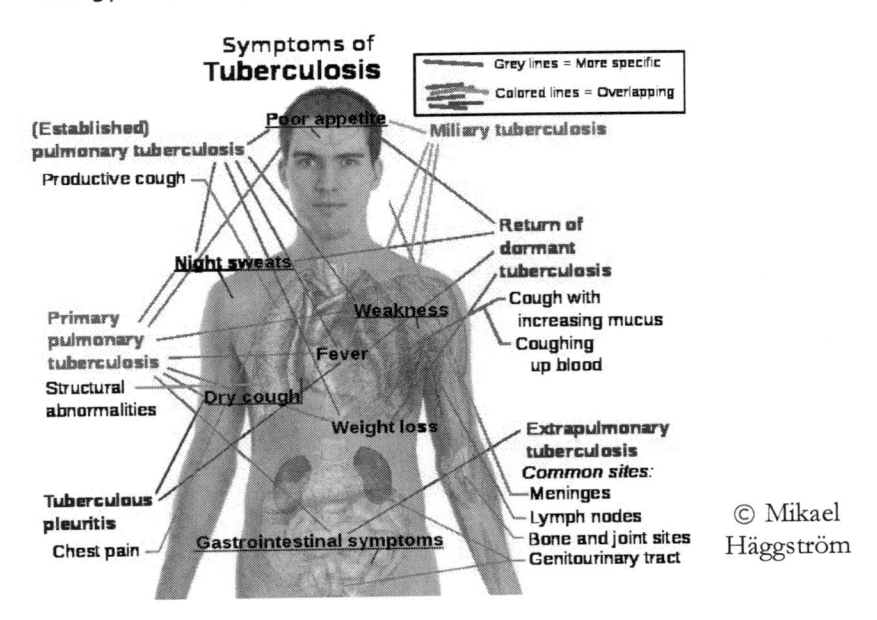

Symptoms of Tuberculosis

Grey lines = More specific
Colored lines = Overlapping

- (Established) pulmonary tuberculosis
  - Productive cough
- Poor appetite
- Miliary tuberculosis
- Night sweats
- Return of dormant tuberculosis
  - Cough with increasing mucus
  - Coughing up blood
- Primary pulmonary tuberculosis
- Weakness
- Fever
- Structural abnormalities
- Dry cough
- Weight loss
- Extrapulmonary tuberculosis
  Common sites:
  - Meninges
  - Lymph nodes
  - Bone and joint sites
  - Genitourinary tract
- Tuberculous pleuritis
  - Chest pain
- Gastrointestinal symptoms

© Mikael Häggström

The disease may reactivate as post-primary TB, exhibiting the initial symptoms or spreading to other organs and producing relative symptoms.

Chapter 14 Diabetes

There are currently over 2.8 million people with diabetes in the UK and there may be up to another 750,000 people who have the condition and do not know it. It has now become a standard test if you have contact with medical professionals. Undiagnosed or poorly treated diabetes is a cause of much disability and contributes to early death.

There are two different kinds of diabetes mellitus these are commonly known as type 1 or type 2 diabetes. The type you have determines the body's ability to produce and metabolise the hormone insulin. Insulin is required for the body to make use of sugar in our diet. Most bodily functions rely on fuel in the form of fat and sugar to work. The brain however relies on sugar only.

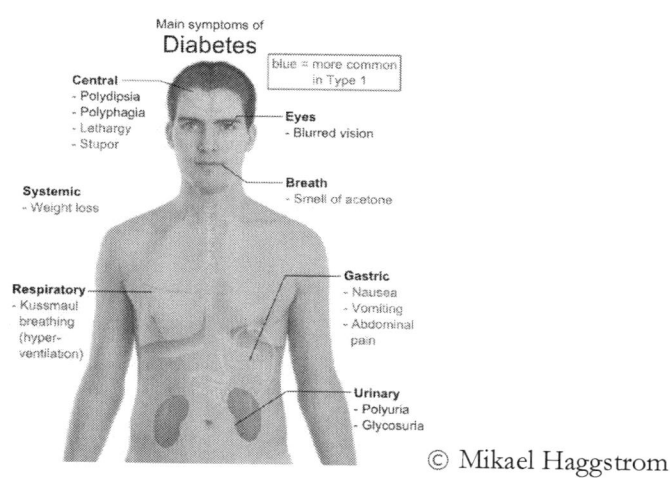

Main symptoms of Diabetes (blue = more common in Type 1)

- Central: Polydipsia, Polyphagia, Lethargy, Stupor
- Eyes: Blurred vision
- Breath: Smell of acetone
- Systemic: Weight loss
- Respiratory: Kussmaul breathing (hyperventilation)
- Gastric: Nausea, Vomiting, Abdominal pain
- Urinary: Polyuria, Glycosuria

© Mikael Haggstrom

Type 1

Type 1 diabetes affects between 5 – 15% of people that have the disease. Type 1 diabetes was formerly called early onset diabetes as it was developed in childhood or before the age of 40. These patents are unable to produce their own insulin. This type of diabetes is therefore controlled with daily subcutaneous insulin injections and regular blood glucose monitoring. These patients learns to vary the amount of insulin they need based on what they eat, their level of activity and blood glucose measurement.

Type 2

Type 2 diabetes usually occurs later in life, when the body can still make some insulin, but not enough, or when the insulin that is produced does not work properly (known as insulin resistance). Triggering factors include obesity, lack of exercise, poor diet, high blood pressure, high cholesterol and genetic disposition. It can develop earlier in life if these risk factors are prevalent. The onset of Type 2 diabetes can be delayed with lifestyle choices, but is incurable once developed and the condition is on the rise. Type 2 diabetes is controlled by diet, exercise, tablets and sometimes insulin.

Insulin

Insulin is a hormone which enables cells to absorb glucose from the blood stream which can then be distributed around the body via the circulatory system. Predominantly used to treat type 1, insulin may be prescribed to type 2 patients who are deteriorating or not responding to anti-diabetic meds. The problem with insulin is it cannot be taken orally as a pill (it is broken down in the stomach) and its storage requires a refrigerator.

If the body is unable to metabolise the sugar it stays in the blood stream, this can damage the vessels and organs it comes in contact with.

Glucose monitoring

Only a drop of blood is needed to gain a blood sugar reading. This is usually taken from the end or side of a finger. The normal blood glucose level is between 4 -7 mmol/l before meals, and less than 10 mmol/l two hours after meals, mmol/l means millimoles per litre and is a way of defining the concentration of glucose in the blood.

Symptoms

The blood sugar begins to rise (hyperglycaemia) and results in Lethargy, with aching legs being the first indicator.

The next symptom will be increased urine output coupled with extreme thirst. This is because the glucose left sitting in the blood has to be discharged via the kidneys.

After that the patient will rapidly begin to lose weight as the body will have burnt up all of its fat reserves, and become much more lethargic due to the decrease in reserves.

The next stage comes about because the body begins trying to burn protein in the form of muscle-mass as a last-ditch attempt at fuelling itself and the patient will literally waste away, stones lost in days. The by-products of this process are called ketones. If ketones are in the blood they turn acidic and rapidly bring about a condition called ketoacidosis.

The patient's breath may start smelling of ketones which is a 'fruity' or 'pear drops' smell similar to Acetone, however this is a well documented but an unusual symptom.

Hypoglycaemia 'Hypo'

This is when the blood glucose level falls too low. The actual level at which the patient become symptomatic varies between cases but a reading below 3.5 mmol/l is concerning. A hypo occurs when blood glucose drops to such a point that there is not enough to fuel the brain. This has various causes:

- Too much medication
- Not enough food eaten
- Over exertion
- Illness

or a combination of any or all of these.

A patient suffering from a 'Hypo' will gradually become more confused, irritable, aggressive, disorientated and uncooperative. A diabetic 'Hypo' is often confused for intoxication. This can rapidly lead to unconsciousness and seizure, followed by coma and then death.

Chapter 15 Poisoning

Fatal mushroom & plant poisoning is rare but some species can cause unpleasant diarrhoea and vomiting (D&V), which in itself can lead to dehydration and shock through loss of fluids (Hypovolemic).

As a general rule the time between ingestion and onset of symptoms gives a clue to the seriousness. Interestingly those that cause symptoms early (within 6 hours) are less likely to be serious than those with a delayed onset. Although anyone who is seriously ill with lasting D&V should be considered a serious case.

Two particular poisonous mushrooms, *Amanita phalloides* (Death Cap) *and Amanita virosa* (destroying Angel) both contain a poison called amatoxin. These are pictured below;

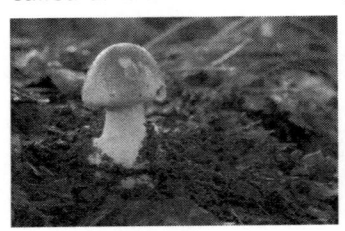

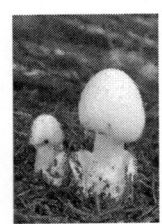

Other common species can cause hallucinations, D&V and abdominal pain.

Poisonous plants such as belladonna, yew and elder all have different effects in addition to possibly causing D&V.

Other rarer symptoms particularly from fungi can include;

Convulsions

Decrease Respiratory Effort

Chapter 16 Shock

Shock

If you've ever injured yourself significantly (or given blood) in addition to the pain you may have experienced being weak, dizzy, and nauseous, in which case you may have experienced a mild form of shock. In this case, the symptoms appeared immediately after the injury, but they may not show up for several hours dependant on the speed of the blood or fluid loss. Shock is a condition in which blood circulation is seriously disturbed. Crushed or fractured bones, burns, prolonged bleeding, asphyxia and dehydration can all cause Shock.

Shock may be slight or it may be severe enough to be fatal. Because all traumatic injuries result in some form of shock, you should learn its symptoms and know how to treat the casualty.

The best approach to Shock Prevention is to treat all casualties suffering from moderate and severe injuries for shock even if they are no showing immediate signs or symptoms.

Shock is defined as widespread poor blood supply (hypo-perfusion) of the tissues and cells resulting in not enough oxygen and nutrients arriving at the various parts of the body and not enough waste products produced in the cells is being removed. The organ that needs the best perfusion is the brain.

Shock is frequently the most serious consequence of an injury

Types of Shock

Shock can be caused by several different processes and a useful analogy is to consider the human vascular system as a houses heating system consisting of a pump (Heart) and pipes /heating circuit (Vessels) and radiators (Organs):

- Hypovolemic shock - (losing the fluid from the pipes)

There are several causes:

- Haemorrhagic – loss of blood due to either internal or external bleeding.
- Intestinal obstruction - results in the movement of large amount of plasma from the blood into the intestine.
- Severe burns - loss of large amounts of plasma from the burned surface.
- Dehydration - results from severe and prolonged shortage of water intake.
- Severe diarrhoea or vomiting - loss of plasma through the intestinal wall.

- Distributive shock: (dilation of the pipes) through either nerves (neurogenic shock) or local chemicals (anaphylactic or septic shock) causes the blood vessels to dilate or become leaky.

    - Neurogenic shock through a spinal cord injury causes rapid loss of contractibility of blood vessels (Vasomotor Tone) that leads to them expanding (Vasodilatation) to the extent that a severe decrease in blood pressure results. Anaesthesia also decreases the activity of the area of the brain that controls constriction and dilation of blood vessels (*medullary vasomotor*).

    - Anaphylactic shock - results from an allergic response that causes the release of inflammatory substances that increase vasodilatation and amount of leakage (Capillary Permeability).

    - Septic shock or "blood poisoning" - results from peritoneal, systemic, and gangrenous infections that cause the release of toxic substances into the circulatory system, depressing the activity of the heart, leading to vasodilatation, and increasing the amount of leakage (Capillary Permeability).

- Cardiogenic shock - (the pump itself is broken): Occurs when the heart stops pumping or performance is decreased in response to conditions such as a heart attack or a very rapid heart rate.

How to recognise Shock

A person who is going into shock may show quite a few different signs or symptoms, some of which are indicated below and are discussed in the following paragraphs. They reflect the effect of the poor blood supply (perfusion) or the various ways the body has to compensate for this poor blood flow. Remember that some signs of shock do not always appear at the time of the injury; and, in some very serious cases the symptoms may not appear until hours later. Shock is caused directly or indirectly, by the disturbance of the circulation of the blood. Symptoms of shock include the following:

- The pulse is weak and rapid.

- Breathing is likely to be shallow, rapid, and irregular, because the poor circulation of the blood affects the breathing centre in the brain.

- The temperature near the surface of the body is lowered because of the poor blood flow; so the face, arms, and legs feel cold to the touch.

- Sweating is likely to be very noticeable.

- A person in shock is usually very pale, but, in some cases, the skin may have a bluish or reddish colour. In the case of victims with dark skin, you may have to rely primarily on the colour of the mucous membranes on the inside of the mouth or under the eyelid or under the nail bed. A person in or going into shock has a bluish colour to these membranes instead of a healthy pink.
- The pupils of the eyes are usually dilated (enlarged).
- If the casualty is conscious, they may complain of thirst. They may have a feeling of weakness, faintness, or dizziness, or they may feel nauseous.
- The casualty may be very restless and feel frightened and anxious. As shock deepens, these signs gradually disappear and the victim becomes increasingly unresponsive to what is going on around them. Even pain may not arouse them. Finally, the victim may become deeply unconscious.

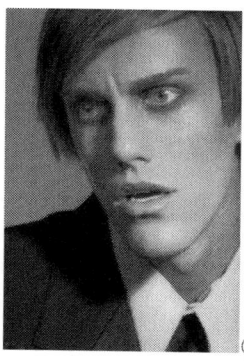

© Lev Olkha | Dreamstime.com

You are unlikely to see all the symptoms of shock in any one case. Some symptoms may appear only in later stages of shock when the disturbance of the blood flow has become so great that the person's life is in serious danger. Sometimes other signs of the injury may disguise the signs of shock. You must recognise which symptoms indicate the presence of shock, but don't ever wait for symptoms to develop before beginning the treatment for shock.

Remember, every seriously injured person is likely to develop serious shock!

Emotional Shock

Emotional shock (Faint) – is not shock in the true sense of the work. Sometimes strong emotions can cause strong parasympathetic stimulation of the heart and results in vasodilatation in skeletal muscles and in the viscera.

The impact of this type of shock will vary widely – sometimes there will be a powerful sympathetic nervous system response or times it may just present and anxiety. Comfort and reassurance coupled with rest and relaxation after you are clear of immediate dangers is very effective in management of the casualty suffering from emotional shock.

Clinical Signs of Shock

	Class 1	Class 2	Class 3	Class 4
Blood Loss Volume (mills) in adult	750mls	800 - 1500mls	1500 - 2000mls	>2000mls
Blood Loss % Circ. blood volume	<15%	15 - 30%	30 - 40%	>40%
Systolic Blood Pressure	No change	Normal	Reduced	Very low
Diastolic Blood Pressure	No change	Raised	Reduced	Very low / Unrecordable
Pulse (beats /min)	Slight tachycardia	100 - 120	120 (thready)	>120 (very thready)
Capillary Refill	Normal	Slow (>2s)	Slow (>2s)	Undetectable
Respiratory Rate	Normal	Normal	Raised (>20/min)	Raised (>20/min)
Urine Flow (mills/hr)	>30	20 - 30	10 - 20	0 - 10
Extremities	Normal	Pale	Pale	Pale & cold
Complexion	Normal	Pale	Pale	Ashen
Mental state	Alert, thirsty	Anxious or aggressive, thirsty	Anxious or aggressive or drowsy	Drowsy, confused or unconscious

Giving fluids

The mainstay of treatment in severe shock is the replacement of fluid. In order to safely do this, first there needs to be some understanding of how fluids behave in the body.

Basic homeostasis (how fluid work and move in the body)

Healthy kidneys are very good (better than any doctor) at maintaining a proper balance of salt, water and total volume of your fluids.

With a drop in blood pressure, the kidneys actively absorb more salt and water to correct the balance. Likewise, if the electrolytes such as potassium are too high or low, the kidneys have mechanisms to correct this.

Osmolarity: the amount of electrolyte (sodium, potassium, chloride etc) in the blood is not just a matter of how much of that electrolyte is there. It also has the effect of how much "saltiness" each electrolytes provides. The "saltiness" is osmolarity. Normal plasma is about 300 milliosmols per litre (equivalent to 0.9% saline). By comparison, seawater is about 1300 mOsmol/L (3.5% saline), and the kidneys can concentrate urine up to about 1200 mOsmol/L. Thus, drinking seawater is not an option for most humans, especially as we age and our kidneys become less efficient. "Hypertonic" means extra salty. "Hypotonic" means less salty than normal.

A good example of osmolarity: take a vegetable such as a carrot. Place it in slightly brackish or fresh water and it absorbs water. Even wilting plants can be brought back to a vigorous appearance this way. Placing a healthy plant in very salty water, on the other hand, causes it to wilt. This is because the water is drawn to the more salty solution. "Salt sucks" is the simple way to remember this.

This becomes of extreme importance when giving IV fluids: red blood cells will burst if **plain water** is given IV. This can be fatal. "Normal" saline (0.9% sodium chloride – 9gms of salt in 1000mls of water) is so called because it has a "normal" osmolarity, that is, it's saltiness matches plasma. An IV fluid which is too salty will draw water out of the body's cells, and potentially cause death.

A good experiment is to place a drop of blood into each of 3 test tubes: one tube is filled with water, another with normal saline, and a 3rd with hypertonic saline. The water-filled tube will lose the turbid cloudy appearance as the red blood cells burst in a few minutes. The 3 samples can be viewed under microscope: the burst cells will be obvious. The hypertonic (extra-salted) cells will appear shrunken and shrivelled.

The concentration of urine takes energy to produce, and the more concentrated, the harder it is for the kidneys to work. The saltier the water you drink, the more the kidneys have to work "uphill". Drinking seawater would be the same as trying to go up too steep a hill: it's just not going to work.

For an adult, the requirement to rid the body of wastes means a minimum of 500ml of urine per day. This is assuming the kidneys are working as hard as they can. By drinking extra water, the kidneys can create more dilute urine, but still rid the waste products without working too hard (and at less risk of kidney stones).

The kidneys are essentially like a huge recycling plant: good things are kept and returned to the bloodstream, bad things are tossed out in the urine. This can be simply due to the concentration of the substance, or by active excretion (e.g. ammonium) or reabsorption (e.g. glucose) of certain substances.

Ant diuretic hormone (ADH) causes water to be reabsorbed in the kidneys. ADH is released in response to low blood pressure of high osmolarity of the plasma. Alcohol inhibits this ADH from being released, hence the diuresis (lots of urine) as a result of alcohol.

Oedema:

It is possible to drown a patient if too much fluid is given too quickly. The heart gets overloaded with fluid, and a backlog of pressure can cause oedema (fluid build-up) in the lungs. This is more likely in patients with some heart problems, the elderly, or very small (e.g. Children). It is also more likely in the types of fluids easily obtained (e.g. Saline, Hartmann's) than in the more specialised fluids such as plasma or plasma substitutes.

An similar example of this situation is peripheral oedema, seen where heart failure patients have "puffy" legs, which can be dimpled with finger pressure, like pressing on an orange. A long bus trip can cause this in some people, as the fluid accumulates in the lower limbs.

If this happens to a patient, they may experience shortness of breath, and they may have pink frothy sputum when they cough. Listening to their chest with a stethoscope leads to a crackling sound (like wringing out a wet sponge), worse over the lower part of the lungs than the top.

Chapter 17 Ear, Nose and Throat (ENT)

Ear Problems

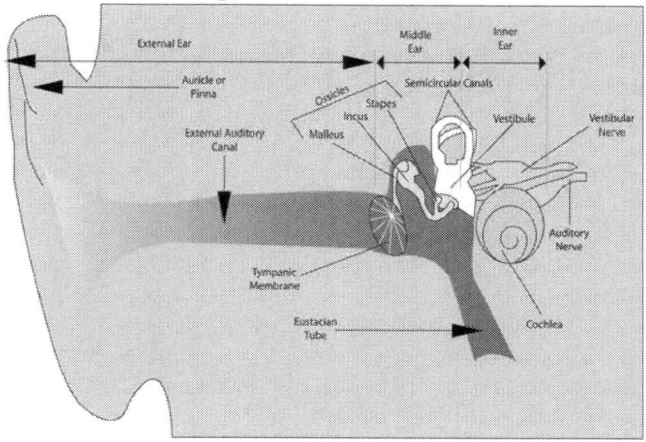

Diagram of a Human Ear

© Anita Potter – Dreamtime.com

When taking a history not any of the following as they constitute the main symptoms of ear disease and/or ear problems

Otalgia (Earache).

Record onset of pain, severity, aggravating & relieving factors and associated symptoms.

Otorrhoea (discharge)

The external ear will only produce minimal discharge, the middle ear will produce copious offensive discharge. The presence of blood indicate trauma, severe infection or the possibility of tumour.

Deafness.

To assess deafness cover one ear and whisper in the other one. Note onset and if any deafness is either unilateral or bilateral.

Tinnitus.

Note type of noise, duration, intensity, if it is worse at night (cmmon) and presence of background noise.

Vertigo

A sense of movement or "Spinning" sensation of the patients surroundings, patient may vomit or be nauseous. Can be benign in origin, caused by Labyrinthitis, Menieres disease or in rare cases an acoustic neuroma.

Examination

Check hearing by whispering in each ear. Feel the tragus, pinna and mastoid for tenderness. Inspect for wounds, scarring, ulceration, reddening, swelling, discharge or skin conditions and ask about any pain.

I was once told the smallest thing that should be put into a ear is an elbow. So in other words don't stick anything blindly in as it can cause damage.

An instrument called an Otoscope or auroscope is used to examine the ears and sometimes the nose. It consists of a cone with a magnifying lens and a light source. With it you can look for infection, reddening, traumatic damage, pus and wax build up in the canal and to examine the ear drum for reddening or fluid levels.

Examination best performed when patient and examiner are seated on same level. Hold otoscope like a pen near eyepiece end. Hold pinna between fore finger & thumb & gently pull back and away from head in adults. In children pull pinna back only. Move the ear with care as inflammatory conditions cause pain on movement of external ear. To protect the patients ear from sudden jolts steady the hand that holds the otoscope on their cheek.

Tympanic Membranes

Whilst examining the condition of the ear canal, look for flaking or redeemed skin, presence of wax, Foreign Object or discharge.

It is not always possible to see whole tympanic membrane in one single view so move otoscope about to view the whole of the membrane.

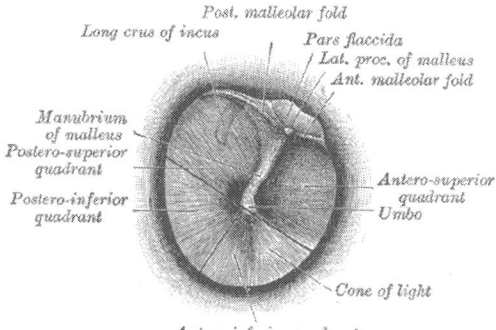

The normal tympanic membrane is approximately 1 cm diameter, a translucent pearly grey and bowed outwards. In normal anatomy you should be able to identify the following.

    Handle/lateral process of malleus

    Light reflex/cone of light.

    Pars tensa & pars flaccida(attic).

    It is sometimes possible to see:-

    Long process of incus,

    Chorda tympani

    Eustachian tube opening

Foreign objects

Insects are the most common foreign objects found in the ear, if they crawl in, then bite, sting or die in the ear they can trigger an infection. The safest way of removal is to irrigate with oil or water and allow the object to float out. If this is not possible use grasping or magil`s forceps to get it out, care must be taken not to rupture the tympanic membrane 'ear drum'.

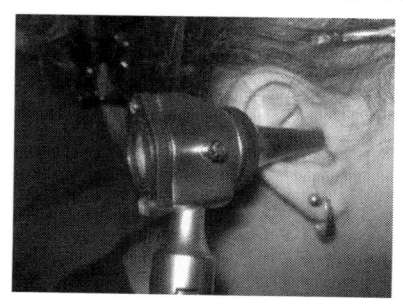

Symptoms of Ear Problems

1. Wax
2. Infection of middle ear 'ottis media'
3. Infection of outer ear 'ottis externa'
4. Glue Ear
5. Boils
6. Throat Problem

Information derived from Keith Hopcroft and Vincent forte (2008) Symptom Sorter 3rd Ed, Oxford: Radcliffe Publishing **(P=Possible)**

	1	2	3	4	5	6
Pain	P	Y	Y	N	Y	
Painful pinna traction	N	N	Y	N	Y	N
Discharge	P	P	Y	N	P	N
Deafness	Y	Y	Y	Y	N	N
Fluid on drum	N	N	N	Y		
Bulging Eardrum		Y	N		N	N
Pain swallowing		N	N		N	Y
Skin disease		N	p		P	
Tender Tragus		N	Y		Y	
Drum perforated		Y	N		N	
Vertigo		P	P			
Tinnitus		Y	Y			

Infection of outer ear 'ottis externa'

An inflammatory condition of the outer ear, ear canal or outer surface of the eardrum. Acute conditions can be localised or diffuse

Outer ear infections often occur in moist environments, such as with diving or in tropical regions. The auditory canal becomes red, itchy and there may be a discharge as well as hearing loss. Pulling on the ear lobe will be painful.

Furunculosis

An outer ear infection causes by bacterial penetrating hair follicles and producing a boil in the ear canal. These are very painful which is increased if the ear is touched or moved, lymphadenopathy may be present, pain is relieved if boil bursts.

Infection of middle ear 'ottis media'

Can be mild or severe, in mild cases the patient has mild ear pain, no severe systemic features, a temperature <39°C and no discharge.

In severe cases moderate or severe ear pain is felt, fever 39°C or above, bilateral, systemic symptoms (eg vomiting), severe local signs such as perforation or purulent discharge

Often associated with an upper respiratory infection with the inside of the ear being painful and usually decreased hearing. If you examine the ear with an auroscope the inside may be reddened or yellow and pus may be seen behind the tympanic membrane. The membrane can be swollen, opaque with loss of landmarks and absent light reflex. This condition is uncommon in adults , more often seen in children under 10 years.

A crying or feverish child will have a pink or red eardrum. Therefore changes in colour alone are unreliable.

Ear Wax

The presence of Ear wax can cause pain, but more so loss of hearing and a feeling of being underwater.

Glue ear/Middle ear effusion.

A non-purulent collection of fluid in the middle ear. Eustacian tube dysfunction results in failure to clear fluid after an acute episode of inflammation and the development of a persistant middle ear effusion.

Half of cases follow acute Infection of middle ear 'ottis media' other causes can include; Low grade viral or bacterial infections, Gastric reflux, Nasal allergies and overgrowth of lymphoid tissue.

Tuning fork tests

These test hearing in both ears & can help distinguish between a sensorinueral or conductive hearing loss. Ideally use a 512Hz tuning fork. Strike tuning fork against your elbow or knee to make it vibrate, striking against a metal object can introduce unwanted harmonic vibrations in the sound signal.

Tell patient what you are doing and what you want them to do before you put the fork against their head as talking to them while you are doing the test may confuse the result.

Weber test

Place the fork in the middle of the forehead.

Ask patient if they hear the sound equally in both ears or if it is louder on one side.

A patient with normal hearing should hear the sound equally in both ears.

If a patient has a unilateral conductive loss the sound will localise to affected ear.

If patient has a unilateral sensorineural loss the sound will localise to unaffected ear.

Rinne Test

Place the fork approx 2cm in front of the external auditory canal, then hold fork behind ear pressing on mastoid process (firmly).

In a normal ear the patient should hear tuning fork louder at front (rinne +ve).

If the patient has a conductive hearing loss it will be louder at back of ear (rinne −ve).

In a patient with a dead ear they will hear bone conduction louder as sound will be transmitted around skull and heard by the other cochlea (false-negative rinne).

Nasal Problem

Congestion

Congestion is usually caused by allergies, but is sometimes bacterial particularly if the patient has a fever.

Throat problems
Sore throat

A simple sore throat or upper respiratory tract infection doesn't usually require any treatment apart from symptomatic relief for congestion. Look for swelling of the uvula and tonsils or exudate on their surfaces be more suspicious if patient has a fever is drowsy or immune-compromised. Check for enlarged lymph nodes or a flat red patchy rash (mascular)

A lighted probe can be used with a mirror to examine the inside of mouth and back of throat be careful if Epiglotitis is suspected. Whilst examining the throat for inflammation look at the tongue it should be pink and moist.

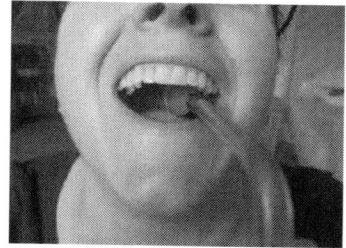

The 'Centor criteria' is often used to determine if a sore throat has a viral or bacterial cause. Presence of 3-4 signs suggests 40-60% likely to be bacterial an absence of 3 or 4 signs suggests 80% likely to be viral.

- Tonsillar exudate
- Absence of cough
- History of fever
- Tender anterior cervical lymph nodes

Tonsillitis

© Guniita| Dreamstime.com

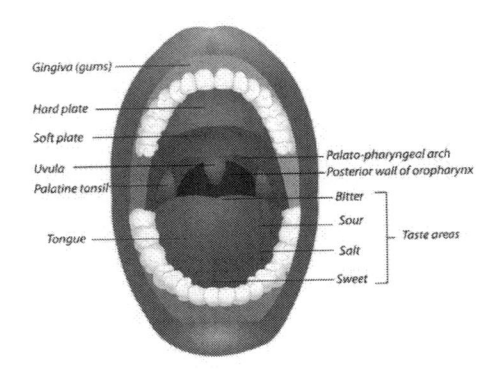

The tonsils are two small glands found at the back of the throat on each side. Tonsillitis is inflammation of the tonsils caused mostly by a viral or sometimes a bacterial infection.

The main symptom of tonsillitis is a sore throat and pain when swallowing, there may also be coughing, headaches and a fever. White pus-filled spots will be visible on the tonsils and swollen glands (lymph nodes) in the neck.

The incubation is between 2 and 4 days. It is spread through droplets in the air, hands or on surfaces etc, anybody can get tonsillitis but it is most prevalent in 5-15 year olds.

Glandular fever

In teenage patients consider glandular fever as a differential diagnosis. Symptoms include a high temperature, sore throat, swollen glands and malaise. The symptoms can last several weeks and are unpleasant but rarely dangerous.

Complications are uncommon, but can be serious and include:

- secondary infection of the brain or nervous system
- breathing difficulties caused by inflammation of the tonsils
- ruptured spleen

Quinsy

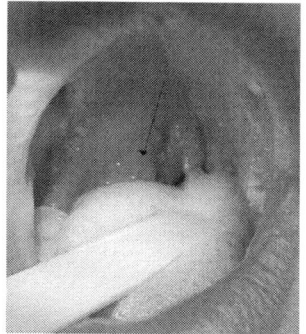

© James Heilman, MD

Quinsy is a collection of pus in the peritonsillar space, the patient starts experiencing the symptoms of one sided pain and difficult painful swallowing, two to eight days before the abscess forms. After abscess formation fever, malaise, headache, speech problems, problems opening mouth (trismus) and bad breath (halitosis) can occur.

On examination the neck will reveal enlarged lymph nodes and the patient may report ear pain. The back of the throat will show reddening and swelling of the area surrounding the tonsils. The uvula may be pushed towards the unaffected side.

Scarlet Fever (Scarlatina)

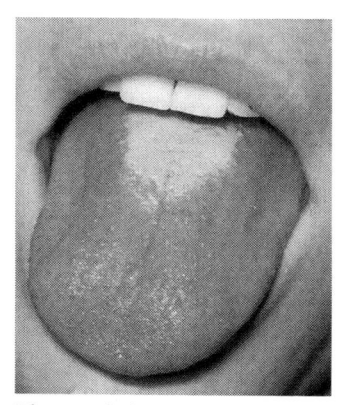

© Kronawitter

Presents with a Bright 'strawberry' red tongue, reddened sore throat, a temperature above 38°C, and swollen glands in the neck. and a rash starting on the chest, armpits, and behind the ears which is fine, red, rough and blanches upon pressure. Rash usually not present on face but appears 12-72 hours after the fever starts. In body creases, underarms and elbows it forms as red streaks. Areas of rash usually turn white when pressed on.

The rash begins to fade three to four days after onset and the skin starts to peel this is progressive and can last several weeks.

The tonsils and back of the throat may be covered with a whitish coating, or appear red, swollen, and dotted with whitish or yellowish specks of pus. Early in the infection, the tongue may have a whitish or yellowish coating. Also, an infected person may have rigors, body aches, nausea, vomiting, and loss of appetite.

When scarlet fever occurs because of a throat infection, the fever typically stops within 3 to 5 days, and the sore throat passes soon afterward. The scarlet fever rash usually fades on the sixth day after sore throat symptoms started, and skin begins to peel.

Although rarely fatal it can cause rheumatic fever, sepsis or pneumonia due to spread of streptococcus in blood but more often milder ear, throat and sinus infections are seen.

In rare cases, scarlet fever may develop from a streptococcal skin infection like impetigo. In these cases, the person may not get a sore throat.

Sinusitis

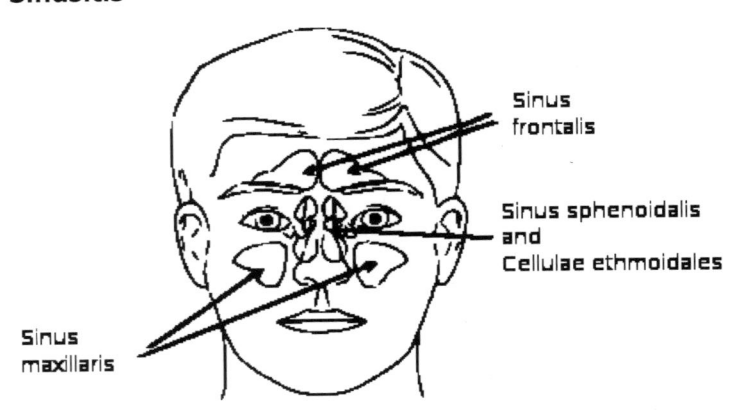

Sinus frontalis

Sinus sphenoidalis and Cellulae ethmoidales

Sinus maxillaris

Sinusitis is inflammation (swelling) of the lining of the sinuses, caused by infection. Other symptoms are headache, earache, tooth discomfort, high temperature, pain and tenderness in the face, and a blocked or runny nose. If the patient "looks down" or "stamp your foot" it can increase pain.

The sinuses are small, air-filled cavities behind your cheekbones and forehead; two sinuses behind the forehead, two at either side of the bridge of your nose, two behind your eyes and two behind your cheekbones. Your sinuses open up into the cavity of your nose and help control the temperature and water content of the air reaching your lungs.

Usually, the mucus in the sinuses drains into the nose the channels that carry it can become blocked when the sinuses are infected and inflamed. It is the sinuses behind the cheekbones that are most commonly affected.

Rhinitis

A condition where the inside of the nose become inflamed and irritation occurs and excessive mucous is produced this cause both dripping and congestion. Rhinitis is primarily caused by infection or allergic irritants (hay fever) such as pollen, mold and animal hair it also affects fluid production in the throat and eyes. A third type of non-inflammatory Rhinitis called vasomotor rhinitis exists triggered by smells, fumes, smoke, dusts or temperature changes. Lastly Rhinitis can also be triggered as a rebound effect to prolonged use of decongestants.

Epiglotitis

This is a medical emergency. Patients are generally unwell, high temperature, sore throat, hoarseness, noisy breathing, trouble swallowing (Dysphagia), difficulty breathing (dyspnoea), increased respiratory rate . They will often lean forward and hyperextend their necks to enhance air entry. Drooling is usually present and tongue hanging out. Don't examine back of throat as this cause spasm. Looking at the epiglottis is diagnostic and it will appear as beefy red, stiff and oedematous.

Chapter 18 Eye Problems

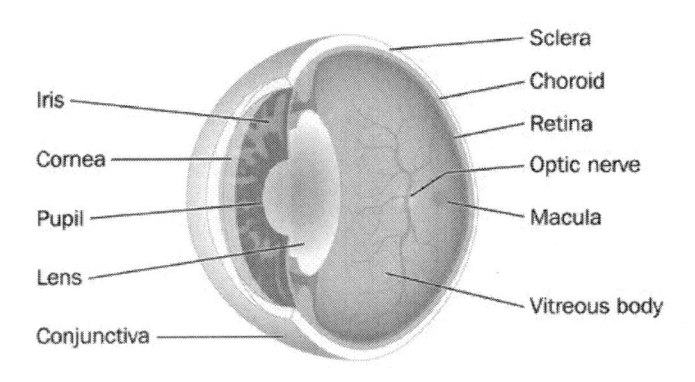

© Legger/ Dreamstime.com

Examination

Most eye problems are either visible or give clear symptoms for a closer and more detailed eye exam an ophthalmoscope can be used.

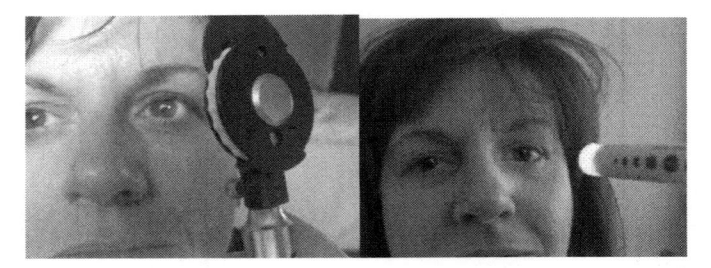

A pen torch with or without a magnifying glass could also be used.

- Do the pupils react to light?
- Check Vision is it normal for patient, compare both sides?
- What do the pupils look like, size and shape?
- What does the conjunctiva look like?
- What does the front part of the eye look like?

Eye Infections

Patients with Eye Infections don't necessarily need them covered unless blinking irritates the eye. If secretions or pus is present these need to be wiped away. If both eyes are affected use separate cloths for each eye. There are a number of infections that effect the eye and surrounding tissues.

Conjunctivitis

Conjunctivitis is an infection of the surface of the eye, it feels like having grit in your eye. See below for different presentation.

Signs of Bacterial Infection;

- Widespread Reddening of the eye
- Pus
- Fever, Enlarged Lymph Nodes in neck

Signs of Viral Infection;

- Watery excretions
- Blotchy Reddening of the eye
- Fever, Enlarged Lymph Nodes in neck
- Signs of Allergic Conjunctivitis;
- Reddening of the eye - Light pink in Colour
- Clear discharge
- Other allergy signs

Iritis

A more serious condition is Iritis, inflammation of the iris. A red circle is seen around the edge of the iris. If you shine a pen torch in to the eye it doesn't constrict and will be painful. If untreated the pupil will become misshaped and the eye becomes cloudy.

Always examine to eliminate a foreign object in eye.

Snow' Blindness

Snow blindness is caused by reflection of ultra-violet light off the ground, most often snow, but also water and desert conditions. Excessive ultra-violet exposure can also cause headache and cold sores. Any vision loss will heal itself usually within 72hrs but is very painful. Always examine to eliminate a foreign object in eye. Prevent Snow Blindness by wearing proper sunglasses which block ultra-violet light.

Eye Examination for foreign objects

If the eye is painful or feels gritty it should be checked for foreign objects. Perform a visual inspection of the visible surface, a magnifying glass may help. If any objects are visible they can usually be removed by using a damp cotton bud. If nothing is immediately obvious use a clean bud to roll up the top eyelid, this allows examination of both the top of the eye and inside of lid.

If an object is not removed it will form an ulcer on the surface and affect the patient's vision.

An ophthalmoscope can be used to examine the eye which allows for a greater magnified view of the surface, but is often not required.

If the eye is very painful Amethocaine 0.5% drops can be used to dull sensation. Either pull down lower lid and administer one drop, if the eye is too painful too open, one or two drops can be placed in the corner of the eye when the patient is lying on their back. Then have the patient blink this distributes the drug over the surface of the eye. The drops initially hurt but the pain quickly subsides. Shine a pen torch in to the eye and often the foreign object will glint or cast a shadow, some may be very small.

Fluorescein 1% strips can be used after Amethocaine to dye the eye, which gives foreign objects a greater contrast and makes them easier to remove.

Corneal Abrasion

Corneal abrasion are small scratch on the surface of the eye, can be caused by grit, contact lens removal or other trauma. Always examine to eliminate foreign object in eye.

Chapter 19 Dermatology

The skin is the largest organ of the body

- It Protects the body from infections
- Provides an interface by means of touch, sensation and temperature.
- Regulates your body temperature.

Assessment and Documentation

Use PQRST Adapting questions to dermatology

- Palliation/provocation
- Quality/quantity
- Region/radiation
- Severity
- Timing

Consider and document;

- Previous occurrences or Family history
- Occupation/hobbies/recent travel
- Recent medications or topical applications
- Sun exposure
- Systemic symptoms
- Distribution of rash
- Patients normal skin

General tips

Dermatology is the study of the skin and its structures. On one hand it is very simple and on the other it can be mind numbingly (unless you are a dermatologist) complicated. We will focus on the simple ! The first thing you will need is a good rash atlas – there are many. You also need to understand some broad dermatology terms which will make things more easy to understand the atlas will be.

Bulla
Raised, circumscribed lesion (>0.5cm) containing serious fluid.

Comedome
Plug of keratin and sebum in a pore. (Black Head)

Crusting
Varying colours of liquid debris (serum or pus) that has dried on the surface of the skin.

Eccymosis
Larger extravasion of blood into the skin

Erosion
Loss of the superficial layers of the epidermis.

Erythema
Blanching redness of the skin that can be either localised or generalised and is caused by dilation (but not leakage) of superficial blood vessels.

Induration
Dermal thickening that presents as the skin feeling thicker

Macule
A circumscribed change in skin colour without elevation or depression. Not palpable. (< 1cm, if greater than 1cm = **Patch)**

Nodule
Palpable solid lesion (>1cm round). Usually found in the dermis or SC tissue. Extends deeper than papule.

Papule
Superficial solid lesion. Palpable. <0.5cm. Confluence of papules is a Plaque

Plaque
Elevated area of skin, >2cm diameter, without substantial depth

Petechiae
Small non-blanching, erythematous macules (<<0.5cm), due to rupture of small blood vessels. If greater than > 0.5cm is a Purpura

Purpura
Larger (> 0.5cm) macule or papule of blood in the skin.

Pustule
Small (< 1cm) circumscribed superficial lesion, filled with purulent material.

Scaling
Visible fragments of stratum corneum as it is sheds.

Telangiectasia
Visible dilatation of small cutaneous blood vessels

Tumour
Solid, firm lesion > 1cm. Extend deeper than plaques.

Ulcer
A lesion with < 50% of its surface area broken down.

Urticaria
Elevated papules and plaques, often with erythematous, sharply defined borders and pale centres (wheals).

Vesicle
A small, superficial, circumscribed elevated lesion, < 0.5 cm, which contains serous fluid.

An approach to dermatology
Once you have the language to read the dermatology atlas book, you can start to think about the diagnoses. Rashes are common and often hard to diagnose. Below are some general tips:

Localised rash + fever - think cellulitis

Generalised rash + fever - think septicaemia if patient looks sick or a simple viral illness if less so.

Rashes in groin or between toes or arm pits - think fungal. Fungal infections very common and they like warm damp environments. The treatment is with topical anti-fungal such as clotrimoxazole

Localised rash + itchy - allergic dermatitis / eczema. Anti-histamines are useful for itch and steroid cream (such as hydrocortisone) for rash itself. - Moisturise skin → keep skin slightly oily

Small pustules / crusting - Staph or Strep bacteria and needs to treated like Cellulitis.
If it looks like it follows a dermatome (see assessment chapter) - think Shingles

Itchy erythematous rash in the web spaces of the fingers or sides of palms → think Scabies

Erythematous rash – sunburn, viral exanthema, allergic reaction, drug reaction, Antabuse reaction with alcohol or a chronic skin problem – eczema, psoriasis

Vesicular / blistering rash - Herpes Simplex, Herpes Zoster, Hand Foot Mouth Disease, Kawasaki Disease, Staph Scalded Skin Syndrome or Bullous Impetigo

Generalised red rash with a fever – measles, rubella, viral rash

Extensive purpura and skin infarction – Meningococcemia, Gonococcemia, Disseminated Intravascular Coagulation (severe infection with clotting system failing)

Sun damage
Very common in Australia and parts of the US. There is a long list of lesions caused as a consequence of sun damage. Most present as small lumps or small areas of dry peeling skin and are referred to as solar kurtosis.

There are however three you need to be aware of:
    Melanoma – malignant cancer
    Squamous cell carcinoma / Basal cell carcinoma → less malignant but slow growing and locally destructive. Any wound on sun damaged skin which will not heal are likely a melanoma or SCC or BCC. They need to be excised..

Melanoma
Melanoma is a true aggressive skin cancer. Sometimes the diagnosis is straight forward and sometimes tricky
    Consider if:
        Mole changes colour
        Becomes itchy
        Starts bleeding
        Becomes hard and nodular
If you think there is a high chance it is a melanoma its needs to be cut out.

Melanoma checklist *(SIGN guideline 72, 2003)*

7 point checklist

Major features

- Change in size
- Irregular pigment
- Irregular border

Minor features

- Inflammation
- Altered sensation
- Oozing or crusting
- Diameter >7mm

ABCDE system

- Asymmetry in two axes
- Border irregularity
- Colour variation
- Diameter >6mm
- Elevation

Cellulitis

This is an inflammation of the layers of the skin and is caused by a bacteria often introduced through open wounds, often affecting the face and lower legs

It is classically defined by swelling, redness, being hot to touch and pain. The patient may have fevers and feel generally unwell.

Impetigo

Impetigo is a superficial skin condition causing blisters that when they erupt form yellow crusted lesions, that spread rapidly and are highly contagious. It is also known as school sores.

Erysipelas

is a bacterial infection which is near the skin surface (more superficial) than cellulitis, causing reddening. In severe cases it can spread causing septicemia. Sudden onset, patient may feel unwell with fevers, chills and shivering, affected skin red, swollen, finely dimpled and may blister

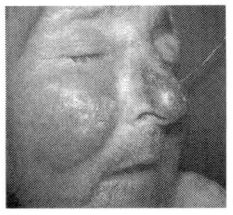

© Martin H.

Exanthems

A widespread rash with systemic symptoms. May be viral (chicken pox, measles, german measles, roseola, fifth disease) or bacterial (meningococcal, staphylococcal). The rash is a reaction to the toxin produced by the organism, skin damage by the organism, or an immune response. (See Infectious diseases)

Slapped cheek disease (parvovirus)

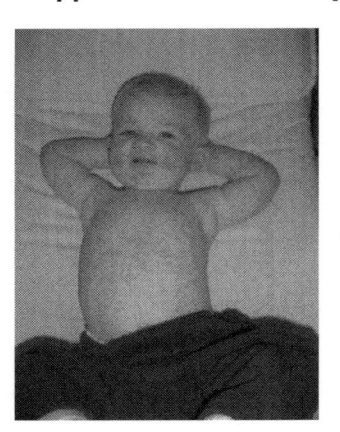

Causes bright red cheeks as a defining symptom of the infection in children the rash may extend over the nose or around the mouth. Patients often develop a red, lacy rash on the rest of the body and. an itchy rash that lasts a couple of days; some cases have been known to last for several weeks. Patients are not infectious once the rash has appeared. Other symptoms include painful joint swelling

© Andrew Kerr

Eczema

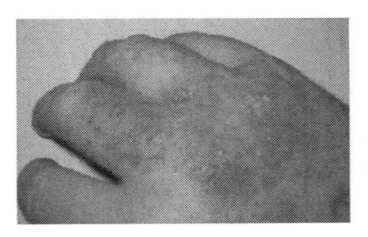

©Topbanana

Is a form of dermatitis, In the UK an estimated 5.7 million (1 in 9) will experience it at some time. The term applies to a range of skin conditions. These include dryness and recurring skin rashes that share are characterized by one or more of the following; redness, swelling, itching, dryness, crusting, flaking, blistering, cracking, oozing, or bleeding.

Chapter 20 Minor Medical Problems

Diarrhoea

Diarrhoea like constipation is usually brought on by a change of habits, different types of food or drinking contaminated water.. If in a relevant area and other symptoms (such as fever or blood in the stool) are present consider cholera or typhus.

Headache

Headache's have many causes; common ones include dehydration, heat exhaustion, tension, sinusitis, viral illnesses, migraine, lack of sleep and eye strain. Most headaches are fortunately benign. Rarer causes include very high blood pressure bleeding within the skull, strokes, TIAs, concussion, hypoglycaemia, meningitis, pre-eclampsia and menstruation.

Indigestion

Indigestion is often characterised by pain, nausea, belching, bringing up food or acid and a full feeling. Often self limiting goes away within the hour.

To reduce the effect of indigestion avoiding eating large meals particularly of fatty or greasy meals. Other things to avoid include smoking, alcohol, spicy foods, fizzy drinks and coffee. Drink plenty of water before and after meals. Antacids van also be used Those based on magnesium and aluminium are longer lasting than those based on calcium or bicarbonate. Drugs such as aspirin and steroids can cause ulcers or worsen there effects. if these steps fail to stop the pain it could indicate the patient has an ulcer rather than simple indigestion.

Nausea and/or Vomiting

There are many causes of nausea and vomiting – gastroenteritis, migraine, space occupying lesions of the brain, early pregnancy, drugs, poisoning, radiation sickness – the list is very long.

Chapter 21 Medication

Introduction

Within this section is information on common useful medication. Most are available only with a prescription, those freely available over the counter are marked (OTC), Those that can be dispensed by a Pharmacist are marked (P) and any Controlled Drugs are marked (CD).

It is beyond the scope of this book to go into detail on each drug, so information leaflets must be studied carefully and it is recommended you also purchase a reliable up to date Pharmacy Book, In the UK the British National Formulary (BNF) is published twice a year and is an excellent resource. If you ask you local chemists they may have some old ones they will give away.

Medicines are described here in generic context – specific applications of specific drugs are described in relation to specific conditions.

How medicines work

Pharmaceutical science is a huge subject, before any drug is taken or administered both parties need to have knowledge of its use, side effects, interactions and contra-indications. Patients with other existing conditions or who are taking other medication must be particularly careful when starting new ones. Both parties need also be vigilant in case serious side effects occur and know how to counter them.

A basic understanding of how medications is important to their safe use in a remote or remote situation.

Pharmacology is the study of how drugs work. It can be broadly divided into:

Pharmaceutics ("what is it?" i.e. preparation, packaging, storage, reconstitution, etc).

Pharmacokinetics (what the body does to the drug)

Pharmacodynamics (what the drug does to the body)

Indications and contraindications (when you do/<u>do not</u> use it)

1. Pharmaceutics:

Drugs come in various forms. These can be natural, unprocessed raw materials (e.g. willow bark for aspirin, tobacco leaves for nicotine), powders, liquids, tablets, capsules or gasses. These can be further divided into those ready for use (e.g. tablets to be swallowed "as is") or powders for reconstitution before use (some children's medicines to be mixed with clean water to form a liquid suspension).

Some powders will dissolve well in the right solvent, whilst others will form a chalky mixture which needs to be shaken well immediately before use. For this reason, certain drugs will also need specific solvents (e.g. Alcohol vs. water. Iodine will not dissolve well in water, so it is made as a "tincture", which is an alcoholic solution).

Some liquids will dilute well with solvents, while others are made as an emulsion (fatty globules of drug suspended in water, making a milky appearance, such as the anaesthetic drug propofol).

Most of the decisions of a drug's form will depend on considerations such as shelf life, cost, ease of use, and physicochemical properties such as whether it is an acid/base, an oil-soluble or water-soluble compound and likely size of dose to be used.

It is important that drugs not be mixed without knowing what will happen. For example, Lignocaine (a local anaesthetic drug) is dissolved in a weak acid solution, owing to the drug's own pKa (its' tendency to act like an acid)*. Thiopentone (a general anaesthetic drug) is a highly alkaline solution. If the 2 are mixed, it will cause sediment to form in the container, rendering the mixture potentially useless.

If in doubt, give one drug at a time, and wait for it to work. Using too many at once will cloud the clinical picture, resulting in a confusing array of effects and side-effects to be dealt with.

(Footnote (for those with an interest) *pKa is best thought of as "the pH the drug wants to achieve if left to its own devices". To do this, it will act as an acid or as a base (alkali). Whether it does so by donating an ion (e.g. Hydrogen) or accepting one, it will gain/lose electrical charge. This will affect how well it enters/leaves tissues. See "distribution" below.)

2. Pharmacokinetics (what the body does to the drug)

-Absorption

-Distribution

-Metabolism

-Excretion

Absorption:

Drugs can be given via oral/rectal route (enthral), intravenous/intramuscular (parenteral), absorbed via skin (cutaneous), inhaled, or topically. Some are also given vaginally or under the tongue (sublingual).

Drugs which are highly broken down if ingested are usually not given orally, as the liver will breakdown much of the dose. The amount which reaches the circulation is referred to as "bioavailability". An intravenous injection has 100%, while many oral drugs have about 30% bioavailability (e.g. morphine). For this reason, oral doses are often very different from intravenous/intramuscular doses, depending on the drug in question.

E.g. Tramadol has a high oral bioavailability (70-100%). Glyceryl trinitrate (GTN) is used under the tongue for angina, as it is almost entirely eliminated by the liver when ingested, with very little reaching the circulation (very low oral bioavailability).

There is further discussion on routes of administration in chapter xx (pg)

Distribution:

Drugs will spread into various areas of the body, depending on a number of factors.

A water-soluble drug with no charge (not positively or negatively charged), will spread everywhere, (e.g. glucose, ethyl alcohol).

A lipid (fat) soluble drug will cross cell membranes relatively easily.

Drugs with an electrical charge will not easily cross the membranes of cells, or even be absorbed via the gastrointestinal tract.

Aspirin is a WEAK acid, so in the stomach (full of strong acid), it does not have the opportunity to act like an acid and become charged. As a result, when swallowed it is lipid-soluble, and will enter the bloodstream easily.

Some drugs need to reach certain areas, e.g. Entering the brain means crossing the "blood-brain barrier" (BBB). Ethanol, as mentioned above, does this quickly, but many drugs do not. If treating meningitis, for example, a suitable antibiotic drug must be given, in high enough doses, and early enough, that a sufficient amount crosses the BBB.

Passive transport involves drugs flowing down their concentration gradient, from an area of high concentration to low concentration. Putting salt into one end of a swimming pool, without stirring it will see some salt slowly reach the far end of the pool, for example. Drinking plain water will see some water absorbed from a less salty area (stomach full of water) to a more salty area (bloodstream when dehydrated).

Active transport: some chemicals are absorbed via channels in cell membranes. This can be done even against concentration gradients, at a cost of using some energy. E.g. rehydration solutions: The Gastrointestinal Tract (GIT) actively absorbs sugar and some salts, which then cause water to be absorbed into the bloodstream. For this reason, properly made rehydration solutions can be better to rehydrate someone than plain water.

Metabolism

The liver is responsible for much of the body's metabolism, and will have a large part to play in breaking down drugs, into either inactive or active forms. The subsequent products may be passed out of the body in urine or faeces.

"First pass metabolism": the blood returns from the GIT into the rest of the bloodstream, after passing through the liver. This enables the liver to process raw materials as well as breaking down any potentially harmful substances prior to them reaching the main circulation. This is known as "first pass metabolism". For this reason, some drugs, as mentioned above, will almost entirely be removed by the liver if ingested orally (or rectally, to a varying degree).

Some drugs are ingested in the inactive form, and only activated after passing via the liver (e.g. Oral contraceptive pill). These drugs should NOT be given parenterally, as they will have limited effect.

People with severe liver failure may not be able to process certain drugs, or the duration of the drug may be extended. These people often have smaller or less frequent doses, if no alternative drug is available.

Newborn infants under one month of age do not have the capacity to break down certain drugs, which can remain active for dangerously long periods in their bodies.

The liver has a vast array of enzymes which break down different drugs. For this reason, certain combinations can be either beneficial or dangerous. If the liver is overloaded with breaking down one drug, other drugs may pass through with little effect. Overdoses committed with combinations can be lethal for this reason alone (as well as the combined effects of the drug at the target organs).

Excretion

Renal (kidneys) excretion is an important factor in many drugs, especially doses and frequency of dosage.

Drugs made water-soluble by the liver are excreted renally, and this can vary according to the acidity of the urine, as well as the volume (and normally functioning kidneys). An acidic chemical can be excreted more readily by making the urine alkaline. A good example is that of uric acid (causes gout and kidney stones) being cleared more easily in patients taking urinary alkalisers ("ural" or "citravescent").

People who are badly dehydrated or shocked (e.g. Blood loss) will often not be able to excrete drugs via urine. In addition, they may be very susceptible to doses of any drug which causes sedation.

3. Pharmacodynamics (what the drug does to the body)

-Effects of drug

-Dose-response relationships

-Side effects

Effects of drug

Drugs act via several different ways:

4 main targets:

Enzymes, e.g. Aspirin and similar drugs

Carrier proteins, e.g. Proton Pump Inhibitors (powerful anti stomach-acid drugs)

Receptors (a type of "switch" see below)

Ion channels, (block flow of electrolytes) e.g. Local anaesthetics have direct action in blocking these.

Also: unknown, e.g. Inhaled anaesthetics, placebo effects.

Other mechanisms:

- absorption/chelating other chemicals, e.g. Charcoal for poisoning.

- neutralising, e.g. Antacids

- structural analogues, false substrates, which subvert normal metabolic pathway. e.g. folate or folic acid is mimicked by the antibiotic trimethoprim. Other drugs will increase/decrease absorption or metabolism of some drugs, interfering with each other.

- colligative properties, (raises osmotic pressure and boiling point. Lowers vapour press and freezing point) Due to *number* of particles of solute.

Receptors exist on cell surfaces. These act like an ignition switch, where the drug (or natural chemical in the body) is the "key". Some drugs will be a perfect fit and mimic the body's normal actions (and increase the activity of the receptor), e.g. Adrenaline and salbutamol (Ventolin) have varying activities on adrenoreceptors, causing the heart to increase rate, the blood pressure to rise, and bronchioles in the lungs to dilate.

The degree of effect of each drug (and exact effect) will depend on how close a fit the drug is to the receptor. In higher doses, this becomes less important, e.g. Salbutamol dilates bronchioles to treat asthma, but in bigger doses, it then affects the heart.

Adrenaline and noradrenaline are naturally occurring neurotransmitters, which are responsible for the sympathetic ("fight or flight") response, leading to dry mouth, fast pulse, high blood pressure, and blood vessels in skin constrict.

Other drugs will block the receptor (like jamming sand in the ignition slot), and decrease the body's normal chain of events. Acetylcholine is a chemical which generally does the opposite of adrenaline (e.g. Slows the heart, causes salivation).

Acetylcholine is the chemical responsible for the parasympathetic ("rest and digest") response. It encourages the GIT to move normally, for example.

Blocking the acetylcholine receptor causes the heart to race and the mouth to go dry. Atropine is the classical drug for doing this, thus it is "anticholinergic". Buscopan (hysocine butylbromide) is a mild anticholinergic, which help relieve crampy-type gut pains, as it decreases the activity of the gut.

Dose-response relationships

Effect of a drug depends on how much is able to reach the effect site in the active form.

Beyond a certain point, no further effect is noted. This is one reason for maximum doses (besides side effects).

The ratio between effective dose and dose required to do harm is known as the 'therapeutic window", i.e. the range in which a drug can be usefully given without serious side effects.

Synergy: some combinations of drugs will achieve a better effect (or similar effect at lower dose) than a single drug used alone. For example, when using Flucloxacillin to treat an infection, a small dose of gentamicin is sometimes given (well below the dose of gentamicin alone). This combination is more effective at killing some bacteria. Another example is to add a small dose of sedative when using pain killers, as the sedative effect relaxes the patient, so the analgesia is more effective. This can be more effective than even large doses of analgesia alone (but must be used with caution!)

Side effects

These can be uncomfortable, or even dangerous. They can also be useful e.g. promethazine, an antihistamine, has sedative effects. The sedation is unwanted if operating machinery, but useful if a patient needs help with anxiety.

Drugs can also interfere with each other's metabolism (see above). This can mean increasing or decreasing the breakdown of the other drug, with resulting increase/decrease in drug effect. Many herbal/alternative remedies can interfere with some drugs, which is why mainstream medicine is often wary of combinations (especially when the person giving one drug is unaware of the other drugs/herbs being used).

Drugs can also affect their own metabolism, by "upregulation" of liver enzymes. Heavy alcohol users, for example, will process alcohol and some other drugs more quickly than someone who never drinks (although will frequently still be legally over the limit for driving when they think otherwise!)

4. Indications and contraindications

Indications:

A broad list, varying from drug to drug but some examples:

-analgesics for pain relief

-antibiotics for infections susceptible to that antibiotic

-antiviral for viral infections

-sedatives for anxiety

Contraindications:

Allergy to the drug OR any ingredients in its formulation.

Sedation

Age (infants or very old may be quite susceptible to sedative or heart-related side effects).

Combination with other drugs (e.g. Tramadol and antidepressants can cause 'serotonin syndrome' where the patient can become hot, twitchy and confused.

Patient refusal (may not wish to take the drug).

Any unwanted interference with body systems (e.g. Drugs which are excreted via kidneys vs. patients with kidney failure. Patients who are already sedated vs. drugs which reduce breathing).

Antibiotics

Microbiology is the study of bugs causing human disease. It is a complicated subject area and not appropriate for this book, but some broad information about bugs and how antibiotics work will help with choosing the right one.

There are multiple different antibiotics and they work best depending on the bacteria causing the infection and the location of the infection. What follows is an overview designed to give you a better understanding of what works for what.

Antibiotics only work in bacterial infections and some parasitic infections. They do not work in treating viral infections which accounts for the vast majority of coughs, colds, flu's, earache, sinus, and chest infections which people suffer from every winter. While there are some specific antiviral medications most viruses do not have a specific drug to treat infections caused by them.

There is no one antibiotic that works in every situation and giving the wrong antibiotic can be worse (long-term) than not giving one at all. Each organism has one or two antibiotics that are specific for that organism and that is the antibiotic which should be used.

The Bacteria:

A basic understanding of how bugs (read bacteria) cause infections is required to appropriately use antibiotics. There are hundreds of millions of different species of bacteria; most do not cause illness in man.

There are four main classes of bacteria

- Gram-positive (+ ve)
- Gram-negative (- ve)
- Anaerobes
- Others

Gram-positive bacteria stain blue and gram-negative bacteria stain pink when subjected to a gram staining test. They are further subdivided by their shape (cocci = round, bacilli = oval) and if they form aggregates or not. This is relatively low tech and learn – all basic microbiology textbooks cover this. Anaerobic bacteria are ones which require no oxygen to grow. The 'other' group is a group of very diverse bacteria who do not clearly fit in another group.

Gram-Positive Bacteria (Gram +ve)

* Staphylococcus: Commonest pathogen is S. aureus; Gram-positive cocci in clumps. Causes boils, abscesses, impetigo, wound infections, bone infections, pneumonia (uncommonly), food poisoning, and septicaemia. Generally very sensitive to Flucloxacillin as first choice drug, and Augmentin, and the cephalosporin's. A

strain which is resistant to the above known as MRSA (Methacillin resistant staph aureus) – fortunately it is sensitive to agents like co-trimoxaxole.

* Streptococcus: Gram-positive cocci in pairs or chains. Most are not pathogenic in man except Strep pneumonia and the Strep pyogenes. Strep pneumonia causes pneumonia, ear infections, sinusitis, meningitis, septic arthritis (infected joints), and bone infections. Strep pyogenes causes sore throats, impetigo, scarlet fever, Cellulitis, septicaemia (blood poisoning)and necrotising fasciitis (severe rapidly spreading infection below the skin). Streps are usually very sensitive to penicillin's, cephalosporin's, and the quinolones.

Gram-Negative Bacteria (Gram -ve)

* Neisseria meningitidis: Gram-negative cocci in pairs. Common cause of bacterial meningitis, may also cause pneumonia and septicaemia. Can be rapidly fatal. Sensitive to penicillin's, cephalosporin's, quinolones, Co-trimoxazole, and tetracycline's.

* Neisseria gonorrhoea: Gram-negative cocci in pairs. Causes gonorrhoea. Sensitive to high dose amoxicillin (single dose), Augmentin, and also cephalosporin's, and quinolones.

* Moxella catarrhalis: Gram-negative cocci in pairs. Common cause of ear and sinus infections, also chronic bronchitis exacerbations. Sensitive to Augmentin, cephalosporin's, quinolones, Co-trimoxazole, and tetracycline's.

* Haemophilus influenzae: Gram-negative cocci-bacilli. Can cause meningitis (esp. in children under 5), Epiglotitis, Cellulitis, and a sub group causes chest infections. Sensitive as M.catarrhalis

* Escherichia coli: Gram-negative bacilli. Normally found in the bowel. Causes urinary infections, severe gastroenteritis, peritonitis (from bowel injury), and septicaemia. The antibiotic of choice has traditionally been a quinolones or cephalosporin. However E.Coli is becoming increasingly resistant to both (although in many areas they work fine – that is why it is important to understand local resistant patterns which can be obtained from the microbiology labs at your local hospital).We recommend Co-trimoxazole as a first choice – especially for urinary tract infections.

* Proteus species (sp).: Gram-negative bacilli. Lives in the bowel. Causes Urinary tract infections (UTI's), peritonitis (from bowel injuries), and wound infections. Drug of choice is the quinolones.

Anaerobes

* Bacteroides sp.: Gram-negative bacilli. Normal bowel flora. Commonly causes infections following injury to the bowel, or wound contamination, causes abscess formation. Treated first choice with metronidazole or second with Chloramphenicol or Augmentin. Chloramphenicol is moderately high risk with high doses (>4gm/day) causing bone marrow suppression which rarely can be fatal – but it is cheap, readily available, and complications are rare. Metronidazole and cefotaxime IV combination is good for Bacteroides fragilis. Zosyn or imipenem is a good single agent therapy.

* Clostridium sp.: Gram-positive species produce spores and toxins:

I. C. perfringens/C. septicum - common cause of gangrene; treat with penicillins or metronidazole

II. C. tetani - tetanus damage is from toxins, not the bacteria themselves.

III. C. botulinum – botulism

V. C. difficille - causes diarrhoea following antibiotic dosages; treat with metronidazole

Others:

* Chlamydia sp: Includes C. pneumonia; responsible for a type of atypical pneumonia and C. trachomatis; responsible for the sexually transmitted disease Chlamydia. It is best treated with tetracycline's or as second choice a macrolide.

* Mycoplasma pneumonia: A cause of atypical pneumonia. Treated best with a macrolide, second choice of tetracycline.

Commonly Prescribed medication

It is beyond the scope of this book to go into detail on each drug, so information leaflets must be studied carefully and it is recommended you also purchase a reliable up to date Pharmacy Book, In the UK the British National Formulary (BNF) is published twice a year and is an excellent resource.

I'm constantly amazed at the number of patients I visit that when asked what past medical history or problems they have, claim to have none or very few, but when looking at their prescriptions they are taking a considerable amount of medication.

So why is this, I believe it is due to a number of factors;

- Patients don't consider a condition to be a problem if it is well controlled, such as Hypertension or Diabetes.

- Patients are unaware of exactly why a doctor may have prescribed a particular medication as they 'trust' them to do the right thing.

- They may be embarrassed by a particular problem such as urinary incontinence or fungal infections and not mention them.

Practically all drugs have one or more potential side effects in some cases they may be unpleasant such as causing diarrhoea or dizziness. But contrary to popular belief not all medication is harmful if taken in excess.

Medication which has a sedation effect, lowers blood pressure or alters pulse rate or rhythm may itself be the cause or contributing factor to why the patient has called for assistance.

In the table below you will find a selection of the 300+ most prescribed medications and their common use. In some cases both generic and common brand names are listed to aid identification. Always check with the patient the listed use is what is intended for that patient, as some have multiple uses that are less common.

Drug Name	Uses
Aciclovir	Antiviral, Herpes
Adalat	(See Nifedipine)
Adcal-D3	Calcium supplement
Adipine	(See Nifedipine)
Adizem-XL	(See diltiazem)
Alendronic Acid	Osteoporosis
Alfacalcidol	Vitamin D deficiency, Kidney
Alfuzosin	retention, incontinence, Prostate
Allopurinol	Gout, Kidney stones
Alverine Citrate	IBS, diverticula or painful periods
Aminophylline	Bronchodilator
Amiloride	Hypertension, CHF
Amisulpride	Antipsychotic, Depression
Amitriptyline	Anxiety, depression, pain
Amiodarone	Abnormal heart rhythms
Amlodipine	Angina
Amoxicillin	Antibiotic
Anastrozole	Breast Cancer
Aricept	Alzheimer's disease.
Arimidex	Breast Cancer
Arthrotec	Diclofenac/Misoprostol (NSAID)
Asacol	Ulcerative colitis, Crohn's disease
Asasantin Ret	Anti-thrombolytic
Aspirin	Antiplatelet, Anti-Pyretic, Analgesia
Atenolol	Hypertension
Azathioprine	Immunosuppressive
Atorvastatin	Lowering blood cholesterol
Baclofen	MS, Alcoholism
Bendroflumethiazide	Diuretic, Hypertension
Betahistine	Anti-vertigo, Balance Problems
Bezafibrate	Hyperlipidaemia
Bisacodyl	Constipation, Bowel Dysfunction
Bisoprolol Fumar	Hypertension
Bumetanide	Diuretic, Heart failure
Buprenorphine	Addiction, Pain
Buccastem	Nausea, Vertigo, Antipsychotic
Buscopan	abdominal cramps
Calc & Ergocalciferol	Calcium & Vitamin D
Calc & Colecal	Calcium
Calc Carb_Tab Chble	Calcium
Calceos	Calcium
Calcichew	Calcium
Candesartan Cilexetil	Hypertension
Carbamazepine	Epilepsy, bipolar disorder, Pain
Carbimazole	Hyperthyroidism.
Carbocisteine	Reduces the viscosity of sputum
Carvedilol	Congestive heart failure.
Cefaclor	Antibiotic

Cefalexin	Antibiotic
Cefradine	Antibiotic
Celecoxib	(NSAID)
Cerazette	Contraceptive
Cetirizine	Antihistamine
Chlordiazepoxide	Sedative
Chlorphenamine	Antihistamine
Chlorpromazine	Antipsychotic
Cilest	Contraceptive
Cinnarizine	Antihistamine, Nausea & Vomiting
Ciprofloxacin	Antibiotic
Citalopram	Depression
Clarithromycin	Antibiotic
Clobazam	Seizures
Clomipramine	Tricyclic antidepressant
Clonazepam	anticonvulsant, muscle relaxant
Clonidine	Hypertension, Pain, Insomnia
Clopidogrel	Antiplatelet
Co-Amilofruse	Diuretic
Co-Amilozide	Hypertension, CHF
Co-Amoxiclav	Antibiotic
Co-Codamol	Codeine/Paracetamol Analgesia
Co-Cyprindiol	Prostate problems
Co-Careldopa	Parkinsons
Co-Dydramol	Dihydrocodeine & paracetamol
Co-Fluampicil	Antibiotic
Co-Proxamol	Paracetamol & Aspirin, Analgesia
Co-Tenidone	Hypertension
Codeine Phosphate	Analgesia
Coracten XL	(see Nifedipine)
Creon 10000	Assists digestion
Cyanocobalamin	pernicious anemia; vit B_{12} deficiency
Cyclizine	Nausea & Vomiting
Desloratadine	Antihistamine
Desogestrel	Contraceptive
Detrusitol	Urinary incontinence.
Dexamethasone	Anti-Inflammatory
Dianette	Prostate disorders
Diazepam	Anxiety, insomnia, seizures
Diclofenac	Analgesia
Digoxin	Atrial fibrillation, Atrial flutter
Dihydrocodeine	Analgesia
iltiazem	Hypertension, Angina, Arrhythmia
Dipyridamole	Anti-thrombolytic
Docusate Sod	Laxatives, Stool softener
Domperidone	Nausea and Vomiting

Drug	Use
Donepezil	Alzheimer's disease.
Dosulepin	tricyclic antidepressant
Doxazosin	Hypertension, Urinary retention
Doxycycline	Antibiotic
Duloxetine	Depression
Dutasteride	Prostatic problems
Enalapril	Hypertension
Epanutin	Antiepileptic.
Epilim Chrono 500	Anticonvulsant
Eprosartan	Hypertension
Erythromycin	Antibiotic
Escitalopram	Anti-depressant
Esomeprazole	Peptic Ulcer / GORD
Ethinylestradiol	Contraceptive
Etodolac	NSAID
Etoricoxib	Anti-Inflammatory
Exemestane	Breast cancer
Ezetimibe	High cholesterol
Felodipine	Hypertension
Femodene	Contraceptive
Femulen	Contraceptive
Fenofibrate	High cholesterol
Ferrous Fumar	Iron deficiency anemia
Ferrous Gluconate	Iron deficiency anemia
Ferrous Sulphate	Iron deficiency anemia
Fexofenadine	Antihistamine
Finasteride	Prostate Problems
Flecainide Acet	Anti Arrhythmic
Flucloxacillin	Antibiotic
Fluoxetine	Ant Depressant
Folic Acid	Vitamin B
Forceval	Multi-vitamins
Fosamax	Osteoporosis
Fluconazol	Fungal Infections
Fludrocort Acet	Addison's Disease
Furosemide	Diuretic
Gabapentin	neuropathic pain, fibromyalgia
Gaviscon Advance	GERD
Glibenclamide	Diabetes
Gliclazide	Diabetes
Glimepiride	Diabetes
Glipizide	Diabetes
Glucophage SR	Diabetes
Glucosamine	Osteoarthritis
Glyceryl Trinitrate	Angina
Half-Indera	Anxiety

Drug Name	Uses
Haloperidol	Aantipsychotic
Hydrocortisone	Steroid
Hydroxocobalamin	Vitamin B12
Hydroxychloroquinine	Rheumatic
Hydroxyzine	Antihistamine
Hyoscine Butylbrom	Biliary Colic
Ibandronic Acid	Osteoporosis
Ibuprofen	Anti-Inflammatory
ICaps	Multi Vitamins
Imdur Durule	Angina
Imipramine	Anti depressant
Indapamide	Hypertension, Cardiac Failure
Indometacin	NSAID
Indoramin	Hypertension
Irbesartan	Hypertension
Isosorbide Mononitrate	Angina
Isotard 60 XL	Angina
Itraconazole	Fungal Infection
Kapake	(see co-codamol)
Lacidipine	Hypertension
Lamotrigine	anticonvulsant
Lansoprazole	Ulcers, GERD
Lercanidipine	Hypertension
Letrozole	Breast Cancer
Levetiracetam	Epilepsy
Levocetirizine	Antihistamine
Levonorgestrel	Contraceptive
Levothyroxine	Hypothyroid
Lisinopril	Hypertension, CHF
Lithium Carbonate	Depression
Loestrin 20	Contraceptive
Lofepramine	Anti depressant
Logynon	Contraceptive
Loperamide	Anti diarrheal
Loratadine	Antihistamine
Lorazepam	Anxiety, Sedation
Losartan Potassium	Hypertension
Lymecycline	Antibiotic
Marvelon	Contraceptive
Mebeverine	Irritable bowel syndrome
Mefenamic Acid	NSAID
Mepradec	Indigestion
Mercilon	Contraceptive
Mesalazine	ulcerative colitis
Metformin	Diabetes
Meloxicam	NSAID
Methadone	Opioids Substitute

Drug Name	Uses
Methotrexate	Ectopic Pregnancy, Abortion
Metoclopramide	Nausea and vomiting
Metoprolol Tart	Hypertension, CHF
Metronidazole	Antibiotic
Microgynon 30	Contraceptive
Micronor	Contraceptive
Minocycline	Antibiotic
Mirtazapine	Antidepressant
Montelukast	Hay Fever, Asthma
Monomax XL	Angina
Morphine Sulphate	Analgesia
Moxonidine	Hypertension
Mst Continus	Analgesia
Naftidrofuryl Oxal	Circulatory Problems
Naproxen	NSAID
Naratriptan	Migraine
Nebivolol	Hypertension
Nefopam	Analgesia
Nicorandil	Analgesia
Nifedipine	Hypertension, Angina
Nitrazepam	Sedative
Nitrofurantoin	Antibiotic, UTI
Norethisterone	Contraceptive. Breast Cancer
Noriday	Contraceptive
Nortriptyline	Antidepressant
Olanzapine	Antipsychotic
Olmesartan	Hypertension
Omacor	Fish Oil
Omeprazole	Indigestion, peptic Ulcer
Orlistat	Obesity
Ovranette	Contraceptive
Oxazepam	Sedative, Anxiety, depression
Oxybutynin	Urinary and bladder difficulties
Oxytetracycline	Antibiotic
Pantoprazole	GORD
Paracetamol	Analgesia
Paracetamol/Tramadol	Analgesia
Paroxetine	Antidepressant
Pentasa	Ulcerative colitis, Crohn's
Perindopril Erbumine	Hypertension, Heart Failure
Peppermint Oil	IBS
Phenobarbital	Sedative
Phenoxymethylpenicillin	Antibiotic
Phenytoin	antiepileptic
Phyllocontin Continus	bronchodilator
Pioglitazone	Diabetes
Piriton	Antihistamine

Drug Name	Uses
Pizotifen Malate	Migraine
Pravastatin	High Cholesterol
Prednisolone	Steroid
Pregabalin	Anticonvulsant
Premarin	HRT
Priadel	Bipolar disorder, depression
Prochlpzine Mal	Nausea, anti psychotic
Procyclidine	Parkinson's disease
Promethazine	Antihistamine
Propranolol	Hypertension
Pseudoephed	Decongestant
Quetiapine	antipsychotic
Quinine Bisulph	Cramps
Quinine Sulphate	Cramps, Malaria
Rabeprazole Sodium	Ulcers, GERD
Raloxifene	Osteoporosis
Ramipril	Hypertension, Heart Failure
Ranitidine	Peptic Ulcer
Risedronate	Osteoporosis
Risperidone	Antipsychotic
Rizatriptan	Migraine
Rosiglitazone	Diabetes
Rosuvastatin	High Cholesterol
Salazopyrin	Lower Bowel Inflammatory Diseas
Senna	Laxative
Sertraline	antidepressant
Sibutramine	appetite suppressant
Sildenafil	erectile dysfunction
Simvador	High Cholesterol
Simvastatin	High Cholesterol
Sinemet-Plus	Parkinson's disease
Sitagliptin	Diabetes
Sodium Bicarbonate	Antacid
Sodium Valproate	Anticonvulsant
Solifenacin	Overactive Bladder
Solpadol	(see Co-codamol)
Sotalol	Hypertension, arrhythmias
Spironol	Diuretic
Spasmonal	GI Muscle Relaxant
Sulfasalazine	Arthritis
Sumatriptan	Migraine
Sulpiride	Antipsychotic
Tabphyn	Prostate, Urinary Retention
Tadalafil	Erectile dysfunction
Tamoxifen Cit	Breast Cancer
Tamsulosin	Prostate, Urinary Retention
Tegretol Ret	seizures, nerve pain, bipolar disorder
Tibolone	osteoporosis

Tildiem	Hypertension, Arrhythmia, Angina
Telmisartan	Hypertension
Temazepam	Sedative
Terbinafine	Fungal nail infections
Thiamine	Vitamin B
Tolterodine	Urinary incontinence
Tramadol	Analgesia
Tranexamic Acid	Prevents Blood Clots
Trazodone	Antidepressant
Trifluoperazine	Antidepressant
Trimethoprim	Antibiotics
Trospium Chlor	Urinary retention and incontinence
Tylex	See Co-codamol
Uniphyllin Continus	Bronchodilator
Valsartan	Hypertension, CHF
Varenicline Tart	smoking cessation
Venlafaxine	Antidepressant
Verapamil	Hypertension, Anginaa
Warfarin	anticoagulant.
Xismox	Angina
Yasmin	Contraceptive
Zapain	(See Co-Codamol)
Zolmitriptan	Migraine
Zolpidem Tart	Sedative
Zopiclone	Sedative

Chapter 22 Vaccines (Immunisation)

The following information is taken from the UK NHS website and shows recommended vaccines based on age and exposure risk. As part of a patient assessment it is important to know what immunisations they have received. If your differentials include diseases that may have been vaccinated against.

Children (Routine)

DTaP/IPV/Hib or 5-in-1 vaccine
Protects against: diphtheria, tetanus, pertussis (whooping cough), polio and Hib (Haemophilus influenza type B). Given at: 2, 3 and 4 months of age.

Pneumococcal (PCV)
Protects against some types of pneumococcal infection. Given at: 2, 4 and 12-13 months of age.

Meningitis C (MenC)
Protects against meningitis C (meningococcal type C). Given at: 3 and 4 months of age.

Hib/MenC (booster)
Protects against Haemophilus influenza type b (Hib) and meningitis C. Given at: 12-13 months of age.

MMR
Protects against: measles, mumps and rubella.
Given at: 12-13 months and at 3 years and 4 months of age, or sometime thereafter.

DTaP/IPV (or dTaP/IPV) 'pre-school' booster
Protects against: diphtheria, tetanus, whooping cough and polio.
Given at: 3 years and 4 months of age or shortly thereafter.

Children (Optional)

Varicella
Protects against: chickenpox.
Given: from one year of age upwards (one dose for children from one year to 12 years. Two doses given 4-8 weeks apart for children aged 13 years or older).

BCG (Bacillus Calmette-Guerrin)
Protects against: tuberculosis (TB). Given: from birth to 12 months of age.

Flu
Protects against: seasonal flu. Given: from six months and over in a single jab every year in Oct / Nov.

Swine flu
Protects against: swine flu. Who needs it: children with long-term health conditions or weakened immune system. Given: as part of the swine flu programme in 2009/10.

Hepatitis B
Protects against: hepatitis B.
Who needs it: children at high risk of exposure to hepatitis B, and babies born to infected mothers.
Given: at any age, as four doses given over 12 months. A baby born to a mother infected with hepatitis B will be offered a dose at birth, one month of age, 2 months of age and one year of age.

Teenage (Routine)
Teenagers are advised to get the following if complete courses were not received as a child.

Teenage booster (Td/IPV)
Protects against: tetanus, diphtheria and polio.
Given at: between ages 13 and 18.

Cervical cancer vaccination (HPV, or human papillomavirus vaccination)
Protects against: human papillomavirus, which has been shown to cause cervical cancer in women.
Given at: 12-13 (girls only) and also, for the time being, to girls aged between 13 and 18 as part of a catch-up programme.

Teenagers (At Risk or missed in Childhood)

Meningitis (MenC) vaccine
MMR vaccine
Flu/Swine Flu vaccine
Hepatitis B vaccine

Adult (For at Risk groups)

Seasonal / Swine flu vaccine
Pneumococcal vaccine (PPV)
Varicella (chickenpox) vaccine
Hepatitis B (hep B) vaccine
BCG - Tuberculosis (TB)

Other Vaccines available for foreign travel

Typhoid, Cholera, Hepatitis A, Yellow Fever, Rabies, Japanese / tick-borne encephalitis, Meningitis, Plague

Chapter 23 Environmental Problems

Sunburn

Prevention of sunburn is better than cure, wear loose fitting cool long sleeved tops, wide brimmed hat, sun glasses and sunscreen. Too much sun can damage the skin, usually it's only superficial but severe sunburn may cause partial thickness burns with blistering

Severe sunburn is commonly underestimated – once blistering has occurred sun burns by definition become a partial thickness burn and need to be managed accordingly.

Heat Exhaustion

Heat exhaustion is caused by loss of water and essential salts from the body. The patient develops a headache and may become dizzy and confused. Show signs of shock including sweating, pale clammy skin, nausea, rapid weak pulse and fast breathing. They also may have cramps in limbs and abdomen.

Extreme Heat exhaustion can be life-threatening

Heatstroke

Heatstroke is caused by a long period of heat and can follow on from heat exhaustion and really are part of the same spectrum. Unconsciousness can develop quickly. The patient develops a headache and may become dizzy and confused. Show signs of hot, flushed and dry skin, full bounding pulse and a fever of 40 degrees plus.

Dehydration

Dehydration like Heat exhaustion is caused by loss of water and essential salts from the body. A person should drink at least 2.5 litres of fluid a day, more in hot climates to replace fluids due to heat and exercise.

The patient develops a headache and may become dizzy, confused, feel nauseous and they may also have cramps in limbs.

Hypothermia

Hypothermia starts when the body's temperature falls below 35 Degrees Celsius and can be caused by cold weather or immersion in cold water. A person will begin shivering as the body attempts to generate heat. Their skin becomes cold, pale, dry and they become lethargic. As Hypothermia progresses both breathing and heart rate slow and weaken. Once core temperature falls below 30 Degrees Celsius the patient rarely recovers and may eventually go into respiratory and cardiac arrest.

Frostbite

Frostbite occurs when tissues freeze, in severe cases can lead to tissue death and the loss of digits or limbs. Most common in toes, fingers, nose and cheeks. First signs are altered sensation 'pin-and-needles' followed by numbness then stiffening of skin. Frostbite can also cause blood poisoning (Septicaemia).

In severe frostbite the toes or fingers may die and dry gangrene can develop. It can take several months to know if frost damaged tissues will survive or not.

Frostnip

Frostnip is a more of a temporary discomfort but if left untreated, can eventually turn into frostbite.

High Altitude Problems

Several problems affect people at high altitude;
- Decreased Atmospheric Pressure
- Decreased Oxygen Levels
- High Winds and Cold

Oxygen Levels in Blood start reducing after 2500m, above 5500m the atmospheric pressure is half what it is at sea level. To acclimatise to high altitude may take several weeks and it's recommended that once you reach 2500m you do not ascend more than 300m a day and drop down 100m before sleeping, as this will make breathing easier.

There are three conditions that affect people who do not acclimatise slowly;
- Acute Mountain Sickness (AMS)
- High Altitude Pulmonary Oedema (HAPE)
- High Altitude Cerebral Oedema (HACE)

Acute Mountain Sickness (AMS)

This can affect anybody who arrives at high altitude without acclimatisation. Effects usually take 6-12 hours to manifest. Initially AMS shows as a headache and feeling generally unwell, without an obvious cause. Other symptoms include anorexia, nausea and vomiting, fatigue, dizziness, and sleep disturbances. Signs may include Peripheral Swelling (Oedema), fast heart rate, diffuse crackles whilst listening to chest, and a slightly raised temperature.

High Altitude Pulmonary Oedema (HAPE)

This occurs 2-4 days after arrival at altitudes above >2500m, fast ascents make it worse and dropping down before sleeping lessens it.

HAPE causes alveoli to swell and fill with fluid, and this reduces exchange of gases.

Symptoms include; becoming short of breath on exertion, productive cough, blood in sputum, pleuritic chest pain, breathlessness when lying down, confusion, and other symptoms of AMS.

Signs are; Mild fever, fast breathing and pulse, crackles in base of lungs when listening to chest. Blueness(Cyanosis) in severe cases.

High Altitude Cerebral Oedema (HACE)

HACE is rare but potentially fatal, it follows on from AMS and takes 3-4 days to manifest. It is caused by a lack of oxygen which causes the brain to swell.

Symptoms include; Headache, Nausea, Confusion, Disorientation and Hallucinations

Signs; Unsteady on feet (ataxia), Low oxygen levels (Hypoxia), unusual behaviour, Pulmonary Oedema (HAPE) and in extreme cases Coma may occur.

In some cases at high altitude over 4300m, Retinal Haemorrhages may occur, no treatment is usually required but if vision is affected descending to a lower altitude will alleviate the symptoms . High altitude cachexia (HAC) is extreme weight loss affecting people above 5000m. At these altitudes between 5000-6000 Kcal is required per day with 55% coming from carbohydrates, 35% Fats and 10% protein. Vitamin input is three times normal and high fluid intake is required.

Blisters

As with all things prevention of blisters is better than cure. For feet, wearing correctly fitting, supportive, comfortable footwear and either thick socks or two pairs of thinner ones is a must. If a raw spot starts to develop, place a piece of adhesive or surgical tape over the area, this will stop friction and a blister developing.

Trench Foot

When feet become wet for an extended period of time such as in swamps or jungles or they become very cold without it turning into frostbite, they can be affected by reduced circulation and become numb.

Chapter 24 Bites, Stings and Parasites

Bites

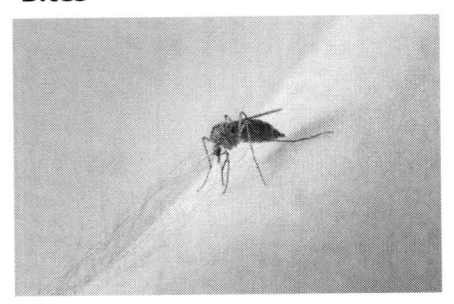

Mosquito: © Stocksnapper | Dreamstime.com

Prevention is better than cure, if in an area where biting insects are prevalent use a strong repellent that contains 30% DEET. Cover skin with suitable clothes treated with Permethrin. Natural remedies such as citronella can be used but are less effective.

A number of insects bite, including mosquitoes, midges and some other flies and bugs.

Effects vary but the following are common dependant on type;

- Local Irritation and Itching
- Raised reddened lumps
- Swelling
- Possible wound Infections
- Secondary infections transmitted via touch to eyes etc
- Transmission of disease
- Allergic or Anaphylactic reaction

Stings

There are several stinging insects such as Wasps, Bees and Ants, complications are rare unless the patient develops anaphylaxis.

Ticks

Ticks transmit diseases whilst sucking blood, but if removed within 24 hours this can usually be avoided. © Melinda Fawver | Dreamstime.com

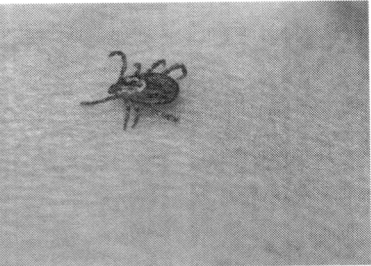

Poisonous Bites

In the UK there are only a few poisonous animals, but in hotter climates many poisonous species do exist and in Australia many of the worlds deadliest snakes are endemic. However the risk from snake bites has often been over exaggerated. Often a bite is from a non poisonous snake, or the snake will either inject insufficient venom to harm the patient or not inject at all. Frequently the bite is a consequence of annoying the snake.

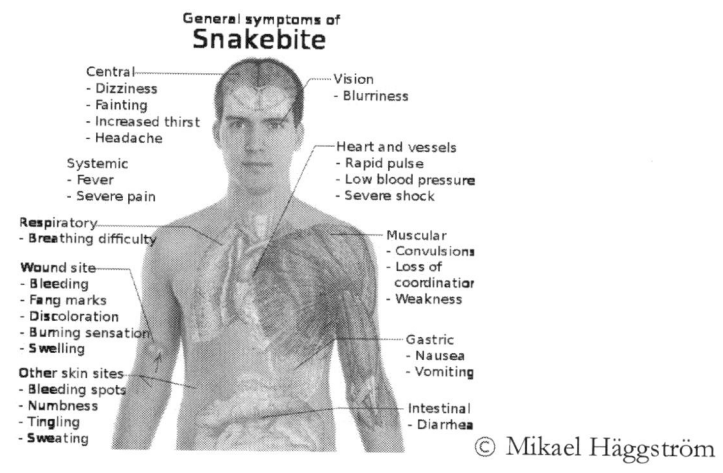

General symptoms of **Snakebite**

Central
- Dizziness
- Fainting
- Increased thirst
- Headache

Systemic
- Fever
- Severe pain

Respiratory
- Breathing difficulty

Wound site
- Bleeding
- Fang marks
- Discoloration
- Burning sensation
- Swelling

Other skin sites
- Bleeding spots
- Numbness
- Tingling
- Sweating

Vision
- Blurriness

Heart and vessels
- Rapid pulse
- Low blood pressure
- Severe shock

Muscular
- Convulsions
- Loss of coordination
- Weakness

Gastric
- Nausea
- Vomiting

Intestinal
- Diarrhea

© Mikael Häggström

Scorpion Stings

© Nico Smit | Dreamstime.com

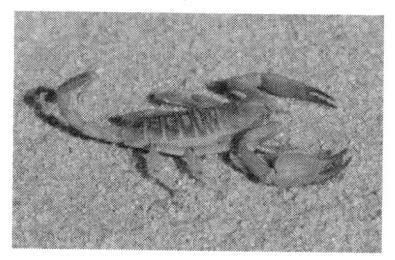

Scorpions are found in deserts and hot, dry locations around the world.

Stings are very painful and can be fatal. Effects vary and should be treated symptomatically, with anti-venom being administered where appropriate.

Black Widow Spider Bites

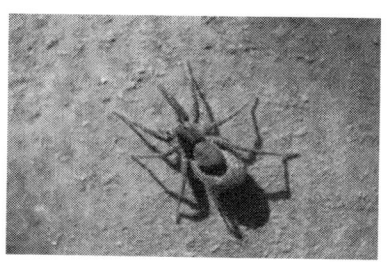

© Dmitriy Gool | Dreamstime.com

Black Widow spider bite, starts affecting the patient within 15 minutes, starting with a dull cramping pain which then spreads to affect the whole body. Other symptoms include muscle spasms, rigid abdomen, nausea, vomiting swelling of eyelids, weakness, anxiety, and pleuritic chest pain. Symptoms are debilitating but rarely fatal in a healthy adult.

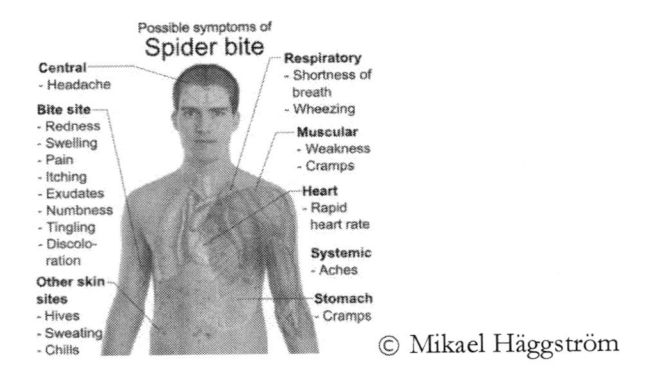

Possible symptoms of Spider bite

Central
- Headache

Bite site
- Redness
- Swelling
- Pain
- Itching
- Exudates
- Numbness
- Tingling
- Discoloration

Other skin sites
- Hives
- Sweating
- Chills

Respiratory
- Shortness of breath
- Wheezing

Muscular
- Weakness
- Cramps

Heart
- Rapid heart rate

Systemic
- Aches

Stomach
- Cramps

© Mikael Häggström

Lizards

Some lizards can deliver a poisonous bite, but there are no anti-venoms for these.

Fish

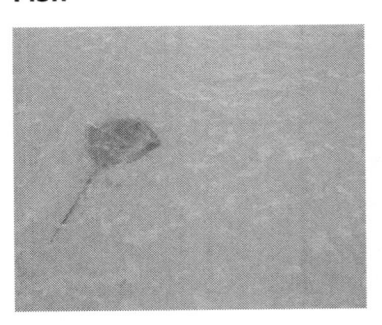

© Yobro10| Dreamstime.com

Many species of tropical fish have poisonous spines which can affect people who try to handle them, or inadvertently step on them. Commonly known species include scorpion fish, stingrays, mantas, catfish and dogfish.

Stings can be very painful and deep penetration can cause serious injuries to lungs and other organs although this is very rare. Other effects, though rare may include such things as, vomiting diarrhoea, irregular heartbeat, sweating, low blood pressure, seizures and paralysis.

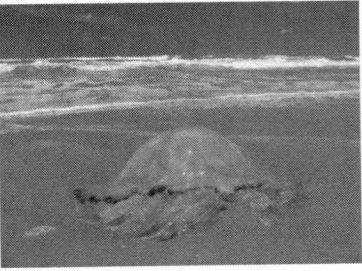

Untreated or grossly contaminated wounds can become infected from pathogens in the water.

© Vaclav Janousek| Dreamstime.com

Other marine stings

Jellyfish, Portuguese man of war, sea coral and sea anemones cause painful blisters through contact with stinging hairs on their surfaces. Effects can continue for an extended period in some people. The sting of the box jellyfish and can cause cardiac arrest within minutes - an anti-venom is available which can be given via IM injection. Other species cause severe pain, anxiety, trembling, headache, sweating, painful erections (priapism), fast heart rate, high blood pressure and fluid on the lungs (Pulmonary oedema).

Scabies

Scabies is a contagious skin infection that effects humans and other animals and is caused by a mite that burrows under the skin, causing itching and a rash.

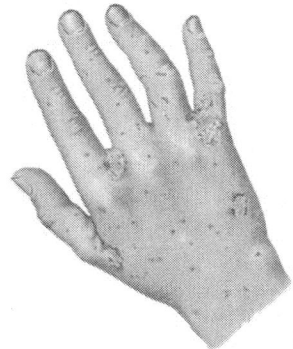

© Walker, Norman Purvis (1905)

Infection can be transferred via fabric or directly from another host and has an incubation period of 4-6 weeks. Although if cured and re-infected itching can start again within a 2-3 days. However, throughout this time, you can infect other people. Unfortunately symptoms continue for a period after mites have been killed. Infected areas often include areas between fingers, toes and in skin folds, around the genital area, buttocks and under the breasts of women. The pattern of mites burrows show as straight or s-shaped tracks in the skin, often with rows of small bites.

In order to prevent re-infection, the patient's family and any others who have had skin to skin contact must also be treated at the same time.

Lice

Lice that effect humans come in three types;

Head Lice

Head Lice are transmitted by close contact, Patient will be itchy and both eggs and lice will be visible.

Body lice

Spread by poor hygiene. Patient will be itchy, both eggs and lice will be visible on clothes and/or skin.

Pubic Lice (Crab Lice) spread by sexual contact.

Infects all body hair, causes bluish staining and itching.

Lice eggs (nits) are oval, yellowish-white in colour, are hard to see and may be confused with dandruff. They take about a week to hatch. The empty egg cases remain after hatching.

Nymphs hatch from the nits. The baby lice look like the adults, but are smaller. They take about 7 days to mature to adults and feed on blood to survive.

Adults can live up to 30 days and feed on blood. Head lice cannot jump, hop or swim.

The itch takes from one week to 2-3 months to develop. Itching may also occur due to an allergic reaction to the bites. Sores can develop due to scratching the bites which can then become infected.

Fleas

Patients can be infected by both human and animal fleas. Rat fleas in tropical countries can transmit plague and Typhus. Their bites show in small groups and are very itchy.

Threadworms (pinworms)

Threadworms are white cotton like worms found on the skin around anus or in stools. They cause anal irritation and discomfort. When the person scratches the area the eggs are transferred via the fingernails to the mouth and swallowed. They can also be picked up from infected clothes and linen.

- Seeing worms, (which appear like threads) on the anus, or in the faeces
- Itching, redness and soreness around the anus
- Irritability
- Disturbed sleep

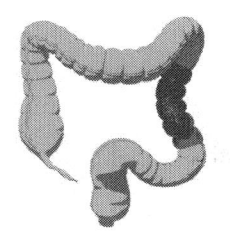

© Sebastian Kaulitzki | Dreamstime.com

Worms only live for around 6 weeks and good hygiene should prevent re-infection or cross infection. Washing, vacuuming and discouraging scratching is the best way to stop spread. In very rare cases they may cause Appendicitis

Bed Bugs

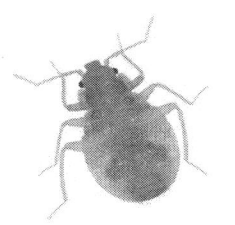

© MorganOliver | Dreamstime.com

Bed bugs do not fly, but can move very quickly. They are nocturnal, and feed at night. They can be found in crevices and cracks in wallpaper, furniture, bed frames and mattresses, even in clothes.

They are difficult to kill, bedding should be washed at the highest temperature for the fabric, and tumble dried on a high setting. Thoroughly vacuum mattresses and steam clean carpets. Powerful chemicals will be required.

Red weal's appear, which are very itchy, and are often in an orderly row. Occasionally, blisters may form with swelling around the bite.

Although unpleasant, they do not carry disease. But if you are bitten and then scratch the area, this could introduce bacteria from under your nails into the wound.

Chapter 25 Clinical Observations &Tests

Recording a Blood Pressure

The first higher figure (Systolic) is the pressure of blood leaving the heart; the second lower figure (Diastolic) is the pressure of blood in your arteries between heart beats. Blood Pressure is measured as millimetres of mercury, expressed as mmHg

An average normal adult has a blood pressure of 120/70 mmHg. As we get older our blood pressure tends to rise. The treatment threshold at which patients are Hypertensive (have High Blood Pressure) and are usually medicated is 140/85 mmHg. Pressures between 120/70 mmHg and 140/85 mmHg are referred to as pre-hypertensive blood pressures, and above 140/85 mmHg as Hypertensive pressures. People who have had a stroke, heart attack, have coronary Artery disease (CHD) or diabetes should maintain their blood pressure below 130/80 mmHg.

Blood Pressure for Children varies as follows:

New Born	Systolic 70-90	Diastolic 45
6 Months	Systolic 70-90	Diastolic 55
1 Years	Systolic 70-90	Diastolic 60
2-4 Years	Systolic 80-100	Diastolic 60
6-8 Years	Systolic 90-110	Diastolic 60
10-12 Years	Systolic 90-110	Diastolic 65
14 Years	Systolic 100-120	Diastolic 65

Ultimately people die due to decreased cerebral perfusion, which is a decrease in the amount of oxygen going to their brain. This is generally caused by clinical shock which itself has a number of causes and is discussed in more detail in the chapter on shock.

- Hypovalemia - Loss of Blood, plasma or severe dehydration
- Cardiogenic – Damage to the heart
- Obstructive - Damage to the heart or Lungs
- Septic – Bacterial, viral, fungal infections
- Neurogenic – Due to head or spinal injury
- Anaphylactic – Due to vasodilatation , blood vessels getting bigger

To measure blood pressure you either need a manual or automatic sphygmomanometer. Automatic ones can be affected by a number of things, so best practice is to use a manual one.

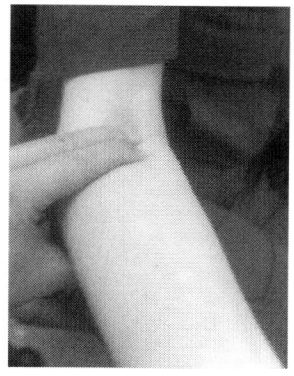

Apply the cuff of the sphygmomanometer to the upper arm

Straighten arm with palm up

Feel for the brachial pulse on the inside of the elbow

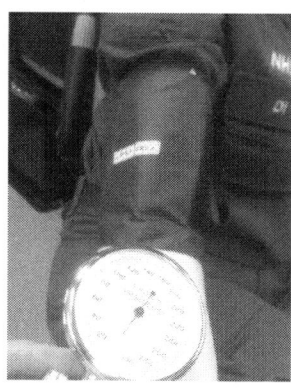

Close the valve, Inflate until you can no longer feel the pulse then increase by 30mmHg

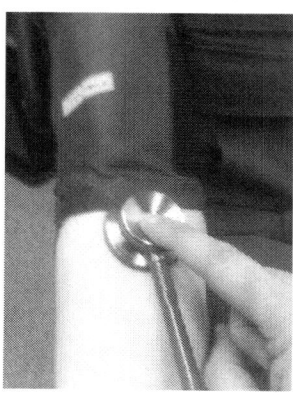

Place the stethoscope over the pulse

Open the valve then slowly release the air.

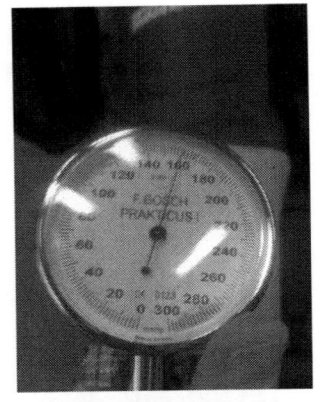

Listen for the sound of blood passing through the vessel (systolic)(thump-thump-thump)

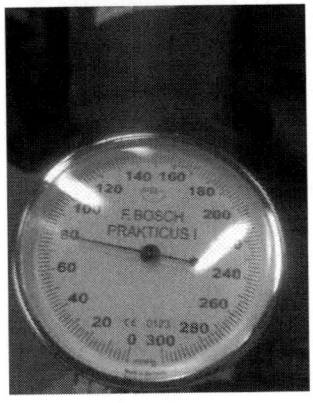

Listen for when it stops. (Diastolic)

Pulse Oximetry and Oxygen Therapy

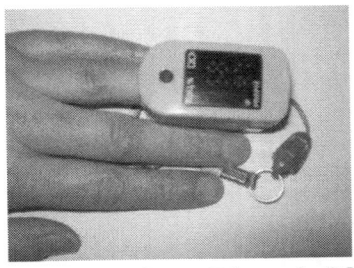

Pulse Oximetry is a way of monitoring the oxygenation of the patient's haemoglobin in their blood. A sensor is placed on a thin part of the patient's body, usually a fingertip, toe or earlobe. These devices are cheap and reliable and very useful.

Measuring Blood Glucose levels

See diabetes in Medical Conditions. Low blood glucose levels are also present in casualties that are starving, intoxicated or exhausted. Low blood glucose known as Hypoglycaemia is potentially a life threatening condition.

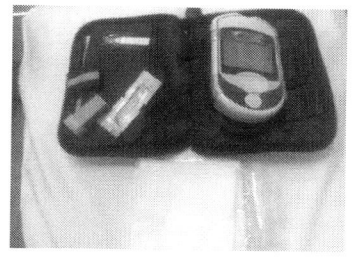

To measure a blood sugar level you will need a Blood Glucose Meter these cost around £30, a test strip and a finger pricker

You need something to prick the finger to obtain a drop of blood. Special safety devices are available but in an emergency a clean, sterile pin or needle will suffice.

Place test strip in meter the display will say "apply blood" or something similar.

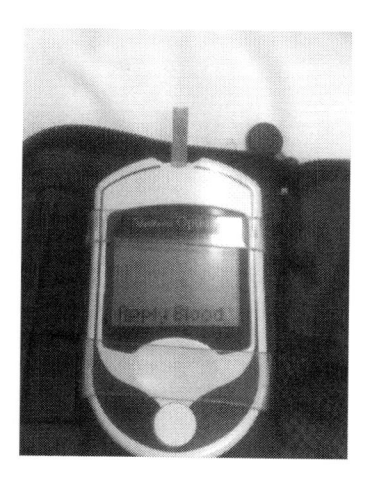

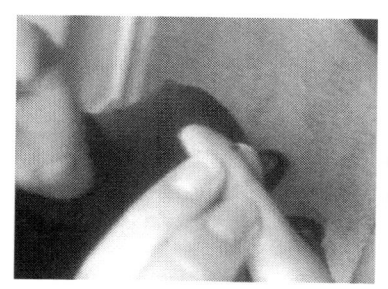

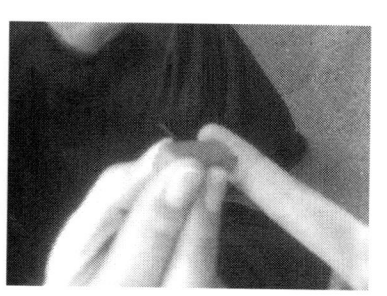

Prick finger, hold finger downwards and apply slight pressure to produce a drop of blood. Stroking the finger with firm pressure will help if blood isn't immediately forthcoming.

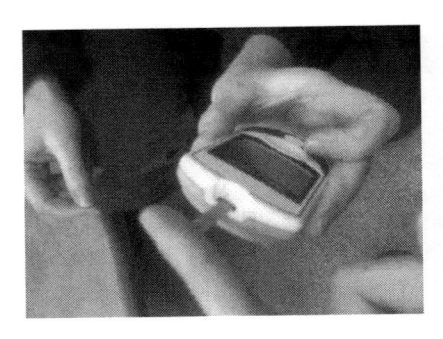

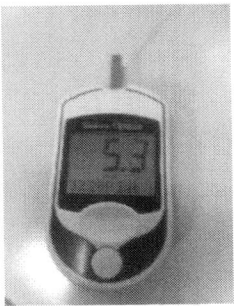

Apply a drop of blood to the top of the strip and wait for the meter to count down, Different models take different amount of time. The model shown takes 20 seconds to analyse the sample.

Read and record the blood glucose measurement. If actively treating a patient the level will change quite quickly and can be rechecked ever few minutes.

The basics of a diagnosis can generally be reached by a careful history and physical examination. Modern medicine relies heavily on laboratory investigations.

Urine Dip Sticks

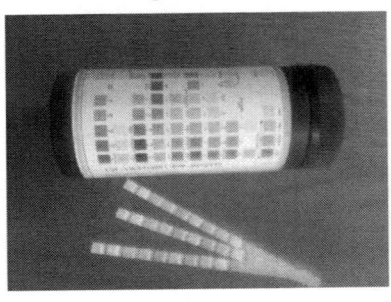

The strips are designed to analyse a number of different values either 1,2,5,8,10 or 12 tests can be performed from a single strip making them a very useful aid. Each stick has a row of reagent pads which change colour according to the amount of the substance present.

Prices vary according to suppliers but you can easily get 100 x 10 tests Test Strips for under £10 a set.

Urinalysis

For urinalysis its best to obtain a mid stream sample first thing in the morning if possible before the patient eats or drinks.

Collect urine in suitable container, before testing check the colour and odour. Normal urine in straw coloured and clear. Cloudy urine or with debris indicates a disease process.

Normal urine has very little odour, if left standing will smell like ammonia. Infected urine has a strong 'fishy' smell and from a diabetic with high ketones will have a sweet pear drop smell. However smell isn't particular sensitive for disease.

An abnormally coloured specimen may be due to food consumed such as beetroot turning urine pink. If no food source can be traced see table below;

Red, Pink or orange	Blood
Green or blue-green	Liver or gall Bladder disease
Bright yellow or yellow-orange	Kidney problems
Cloudy urine	Phosphates, carbonates, stones

Next dip the urine with a reagent strip, wipe off excess urine and then leave on a dry surface. Check manufactures guideline but most tests make 1 to 2 minutes to complete. Sections on the strip change colour according to the amount of substances present in the urine. The relevance of positive findings need to be considered with all the available clinical information (history and exam) and shouldn't be considered in isolation

Bilirubin

Raised levels may indicate a problem with the biliary system. If Urobilinogen is also raised may indicate liver disease.

Blood

Blood in urine may be due to infection, injury to the kidney or urinary tract, renal stones or cancer.

Glucose

Present in urine if problem with kidneys or in patients such as diabetics who have high blood sugar level.

Ketones

Caused by breakdown of fatty acids, can indicate diabetes

Nitrite

Indicates infection although a negative test does not rule out UTI

Protein

Can indicate High Blood Pressure, infection, pre-eclampsia or diabetes.

Urobilinogen

Raised levels indicate problems with liver or breakdown of red blood cells.

pH 4.6 to 8.0, with an average of 6.0

Specific Gravity 1.006 and 1.030

Leucocytes esterase (LE)

These are not conclusive tests but aid in the diagnosis of Urinary Infections, Kidney Disease, Liver Function, Diabetes and traumatic injuries.

Urinary Tract Infections (UTI)

If either nitrite or leucocyte esterase (LE) dipstick tests are positive, diagnose UTI otherwise If both nitrite and LE dipstick tests are negative, exclude UTI.

Blood and protein are sometimes found in the urine when there is a UTI, but their presence or absence does not help in making the diagnosis. Also haematuria is common in uncomplicated cystitis, and resolves with treatment.

Samples for testing should be obtained by the 'clean-catch, mid-stream urine' method.

Dipstick tests cannot be relied on to definitely exclude or confirm a diagnosis of UTI. Urine culture provides the definitive diagnosis and guides choices for antibiotic therapy.

Pregnancy Tests:

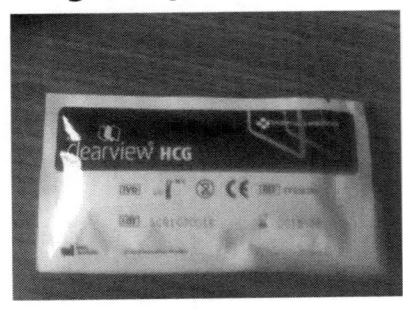

The ability to accurately diagnose pregnancy may be important both for psychological reasons and for practical reasons. Currently available pregnancy test kits will test urine for the presence of the hormone Human chorionic gonadotrophin (HCG). They require only a small amount of urine and are accurate from 10-14 days from conception. The tests available in stores are nearly as sensitive as a laboratory test, in fact many Emergency Departments rely on this type for their rapid tests. These tests are inexpensive and widely available. Follow directions included with packaging.

Chapter 26 Dental Problems

Dental Pain:

Pulpitis

Inflammation of the dental pulpcommonly called toothache. This pain is often referred to surrounding area or radiates to other teeth. It can be difficult for patient to ID the exact tooth which is originating the pain. The tooth is usually not sensitive to percussion or palpation but maybe sensitive to heat, cold, sweets. Frequently there is obvious cause, e.g. a large cavity.

Periapical Inflammation

Inflammation, but not infection, at the apex (root base). The involved tooth is usually is easily located. The tooth may protrude a bit and/or cause pain with chewing. Usually there is no obvious external swelling as is the usual case with infection.

Aphthous Ulcers

Painful small lesion on oral mucus membranes, cause unclear. There are often multiple ulcers lasting 7 – 15 days. May be triggered by trauma, stress. Management is with standard dental first aid. Topical steroids may shorten course of healing

Muscle Pain & Spasm

Chewing muscle dysfunction due to teeth grinding, jaw clenching, heavy chewing, etc.

Other Causes

Infections (discussed below), facial nerve pain, herpes zoster, vascular pain-migraine, sinus pain, referred pain can all cause pain localized to the face.

Infections:

Herpes Labialis (viral)

These are the classic "cold sores" on lips, tongue, gingiva, palate. Often triggered by sunburn, stress, and trauma. The patient often has a "prodrome" or tingle/pain before lesion presents.

Oral Candidiasis (fungal)

Thrush; caused by overgrowth of yeast normally found in the mouth. Often seen in the very ill, immunocompromised, or those on/recently taking antibiotics. It looks like white spots or patches throughout mouth, may have a "cottage cheese" appearance, can be rubbed off, the patient's mouth and throat often very sore & red.

Bacterial Infections

Many different organisms can cause infections often mixed aerobic and anaerobic bugs that are normally in the oral cavity. Infections can be life threatening if the infection spreads to deep tissues or into the brain. Fever, local swelling, and lymph node swelling is common.

Apical Abscess/Cellulitis – Infection of the pulp extending down to the bone & gum. The gum and tooth base appear normal. This is an infection at the very apex of the roots that has eaten through the thin bone of the jaw. Notable for fever, pain, often an abscess/pus pocket, or swelling will form where the gum tissue joins the lip, no sensitivity to heat or cold.

Gingival/Periodontal Abscess – Infection between the gum and the tooth. The abscess is usually on the cheek side. The tooth is usually sensitive to percussion but not heat or cold.

Pericoronitis – Infection of the gum overlying a partially erupted tooth such as a wisdom tooth. It often occurs in the back reaches of the mouth. It can mimic a peritonsillar abscess or pharyngitis although there usually is no drainage or purulence with this. Muscle spasm in the chewing muscles is common also.

Deep Tissue/Fascia Infections – Any intraoral infection can spread quickly through the relatively loose tissue planes to other areas in the neck causing tissue breakdown, bleeding, and obstruction of the posterior pharynx and airway.

Dental Trauma

Related Head & Neck Injury

Any blow or force strong enough to cause dental injury is potentially severe enough to produce injury to the head, other facial structures, and/or neck

Crown Chip

Small lines or "crazing" in the enamel. These are harmless.

Simple Crown +/- Root Fracture

The tooth is fractured but no pulp is exposed. This is usually not a problem although sometimes it can be cold sensitive.

Complicated Crown +/- Root Fracture

The pulp is exposed but the root is intact.

Root Fracture

A fracture below the gum line involving one or more roots. May be difficult to distinguish between this and luxation of the entire tooth (see below).

Subluxation & Concussion

The tooth remains in normal position. In subluxation the tooth is abnormally loose due to damage of the periodontal ligament and gingiva; in concussion the tooth is only tender not loose.

Lateral Luxation

The tooth is intact but the root has been displaced breaking the surrounding bone. Often there is a bulge of the gum tissue indicating where the root has been pushed out of the socket. There may be a high metallic ring on percussion.

Intrusion

The tooth is driven deeper into the socket.

Extrusion

The tooth is partially pulled down out of the socket.

Tooth Loss

The tooth is knocked completely from the socket.

Segment/Jaw Fracture

Fracture of the bony structure of the jaw with 2 or more teeth involved. The teeth move independently of each other.

Injuries To Primary "Baby" Teeth

Normally these are not repaired unless needed for comfort care of the patient.

Soft Tissue Injuries

The tongue, gums, and oral mucus membranes are often injured at the same time as the teeth. The excellent blood supply promotes rapid healing, and infection is rare.

Chapter 27 Sexually Transmitted Diseases (STD)

Many sexual diseases are symptomatic in males but not in females. For some general rules of thumb:

- Painful crops of small vesicles (fluid filled pimples) on the genitals = herpes
- Non-painful single ulcer = syphilis
- Greeny grey urethral or vaginal discharge = gonorrhoea

Gonorrhoea

Incubation time 2 to 8 days. Symptoms in men: greenish-yellow discharge from penis, lowered urine output.

Syphilis

This disease is a great mimic and may present (especially in the 3rd stage) looking like a whole host of other diseases. Always think of it and ask about painless genital ulcers which have healed or a widespread rash which affected hands and feet which also went away by itself.

Stage 1: Incubation time 2 to 6 weeks.

Painless ulcerated sore, non-tender enlarged lymph nodes. Lasts several weeks and heals spontaneously.

Stage 2: Incubation time after 6 weeks.

General skin rash especially on soles of feet and palms of hands, not itchy. It is important to think of it in any spread papular rash – often the recent presence of a penile or vulval ulcer will on be disclosed on direct questioning.

Stage 3: Incubation time after several years.

Multiple Organ Failure or progressive dementia or neurological problems.

Chlamydia

Incubation time 7 to 28 days.

Symptoms in men; clear discharge from penis.

Herpes simplex

Symptoms: painful genital ulcers.

Vaginal Discharge/Itching (Monilia)

Symptoms: white discharge with lumps like cottage cheese, itching, burning, increase in amount or foul odour.

Vaginal Discharge/Itching (Trichomonas)

Symptoms: frothy greenish-yellow, itchy discharge, itching, burning, increase in amount or foul odour.

Chapter 28 Obstetrics and Gynaecology

It is really important to have a good understand of obstetrics and gynaecology.

The Pregnant Patient

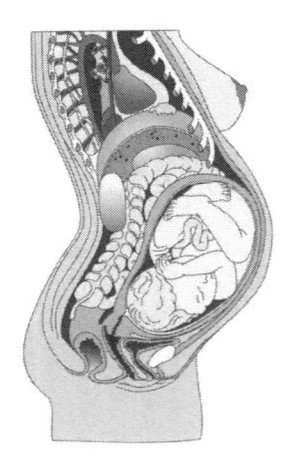

© Maryna Melnyk | Dreamstime.com

The female body goes through many changes when pregnant. Anatomical changes make managing the airway more challenging. They are more prone to gastric reflux of acid and other stomach contents. Changes in shape of the ribs and physiological changes make them mildly breathless and increase respiration rate. The heart enlarges which can make their ECG appear abnormal and they are often mildly anaemic. Systolic BP is slightly reduced with a larger decrease in diastolic BP.

Due to the size and position of the uterus when the patient lies flat the blood returning to the heart is reduced due to compression of the vena cava. Therefore the patient should be laid leaning to the left (Left Lateral Position) with support under the right buttock.

As they have a larger blood volume for them and the baby, signs of haemorrhage and shock won't start until they have lost a third of their blood volume by which time both will be in serious trouble.

The diagnosis of pregnancy

Urine pregnancy test
> Test's for the presence of a hormone produced in the early placental tissue – HCG. These test kits are small, lightweight and cheap; and worth stocking up on.

Clinical
> The clinical diagnosis of pregnancy is usually a combination of things:- a missed period (or 2), trying to get pregnant or "feels pregnant" (sore breasts, unexplained nausea)

When is the baby due?
> The baby is due approximately 288 days from the patients last period (LMP) - (LMP + 15 days) – 3 months. E.g. (1st April + 15 days) – 3 months = 16th January

Early pregnancy problems
Miscarriage

Around 4 in 10 women experience bleeding or cramping within the first 20 weeks of pregnancy, this is best treated with limited rest. 2 in 10 women will abort the foetus within this period and there is nothing that can be done to prevent it.

If the foetus and afterbirth are all passed the pain and bleeding will stop. In some women the bleeding will be torrential – this is likely due to the afterbirth becoming stuck in the cervix – it can be removed with your fingers. This will usually stop heavy bleeding. Low level bleeding for several weeks in inconvenient but will usually stop by itself.

Watch for signs of fever and abdominal pain, which may indicate endometritis (and infection in the uterus) or septicaemia - a life threatening condition.

Ectopic Pregnancy

An ectopic pregnancy is one which implants and starts to grow anywhere but in the uterus (where it is supposed to be) – most commonly in a fallopian tube and erodes blood vessels and causes the tube to rupture.

The pain is classically unilateral pain +/- vaginal bleeding in someone who is 8-14 weeks pregnant. They may present with shoulder pain and abdominal pain – which is classical "referred" pain and is due to blood running in the abdominal cavity upwards to the diaphragm and causing irritation (which is felt as shoulder pain)

The diagnosis in hospital is by blood test (measuring the HCG hormone) and ultrasound.

Ante-partum problems (problems after 20 weeks)
Placenta Praevia

When the placenta implants near or across the cervical opening. There are several degrees and in the milder forms the mother may be able to push the baby past and out – provided blood loss can be managed in labour. However in the severest form with the placenta fully over the cervix, the only option to perform a caesarean section.

Symptoms: painless. Heavy bleeding after 24 weeks.

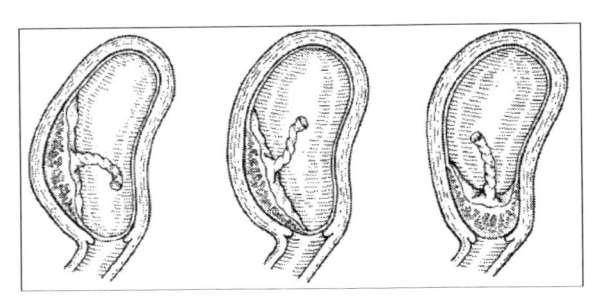

WHO(2003)P.236

Placenta Abruption

This occurs when placenta partially separates from the wall of the uterus causing heavy bleeding. There are milder forms where just a tiny fraction separates and bleed is light and self-limiting. For the remainder if delivery isn't imminent then caesarean is the only option to save mother and baby.

Symptoms: lower abdominal pain, vaginal haemorrhage, uterus tender and rigid, sign of shock, reduced/absent foetal movement or heartbeat.

Pre-Eclampsia

This is a unique disease of pregnancy. It is a disease of abnormal placental implantation. The disease itself is complex, but the outcome is high blood pressure, leaky kidneys (protein in the urine) and oedema (extra fluid in the tissues leading to swollen ankles and hands).

Symptoms: Over 20 weeks gestation and diastolic BP>95mmHg or BP>140/90. You also can see swelling (due to oedema) and in severe cases; upper abdominal pain, headache and visual disturbance. If untreated it can lead to inter-uterine death and/or eclampsia.

Eclampsia

This is fitting in Pregnancy, occurring as a consequence of pre-eclampsia and due to High Blood Pressure.

Pre-term labour

This is labour before 38 weeks. Survival after 34 is likely.

Child Birth

Normal Labour

There are three stages of labour

> First stage – from the establishment of regular contractions with dilation of the cervix to full dilation
>
> Second stage – from full dilation to delivery of the baby

Third Stage – from delivery of the baby to delivery of the placenta.

With each stages comes possible problems and complications and we have addressed these at each stage.

First Stage of labour

This is from the establishment of regular contractions (2-3 minutes) that cause changes to the cervix (you need both to be in labour). It can be associated with a 'show' of blood stained mucus, rupture of the membranes and descent of the head into the pelvis.

The initial flattening (effacement) of the cervix and the first 3cm dilation can take several hours to a day, but after that it should progresses at roughly 1cm/hr for a single baby and 2cm/hr for multiple births if the women's first pregnancy. Many midwifes become concerned at allocating times to these processes and think that they should be allowed to "take as long as it takes". This approach is fine but you need to have a continuous awareness of how tired the mother is, any evidence of fetal distress and signs they aren't progressing (not dilating). In second and subsequent pregnancies it is hugely variable, but is usually much faster.

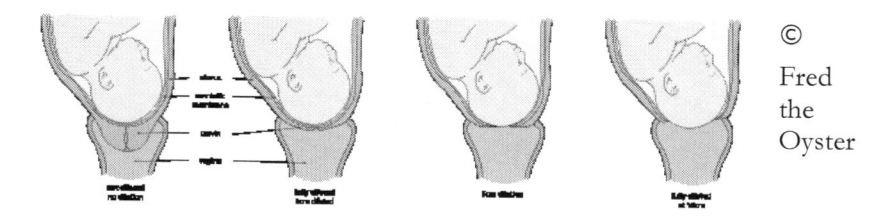

© Fred the Oyster

The first stage ends when the cervix is fully dilated about 10cm.

Problems in the first stage

Failure to progress is the biggest problem with the first stage and is discussed below together with failure to process in the second stage.

Second Stage of labour

The second stage of labour lasts from full dilation until the baby is delivered. Usually lasts between 1-2 hours, usually begins with an urge to push. It is worth checking internally when the women has a dire to push, that the cervix is fully dilated. Pushing against a cervix not fully dilated can cause it to become swollen and slow the process.

The usual position the baby is at the start of labour – occiput anterior (or OA). As the baby's head appears at the vulva. Its head rotates to face towards the mothers back. The back of the head delivers first followed by the face. The head then turns sideward to allow the shoulders to pass.

The shoulder nearest the front is delivered first followed by the other. The rest of the baby is then delivered.

Problems in the second stage

Prolonged second stage

Usually once the cervix is fully dilated and the pushing starts the head (or presenting part) begins to descend through the pelvis and out of the birth canal. This process normally takes less than an hour, but 1-2 hrs at most. Slow descent often means the head is presenting abnormally. Instead of the occiput being at the front (OA), it may be at the rear (OP) or off to one side. This may also slow the first stage of labour and some women do not get to the second stage before requiring a caesarean section due to abnormal presentation.

The most important element here is time. With time the women will usually rotate the baby's head with contractions so it can be delivered.

Prolapsed cord

If the cord is visible through the vulva this is a life-threatening emergency for the baby, as the foetal circulation may be effected.

Breech Presentations

If the babies bottom instead of the head presents this is known as a breech presentation. The problem is that the head is biggest part of the baby, and usually stretches the birth canal before delivery. If the bottom comes first then that dilation doesn't occur and there is risk of the head getting stuck.

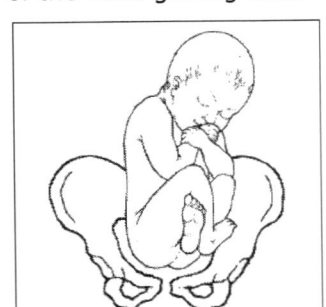

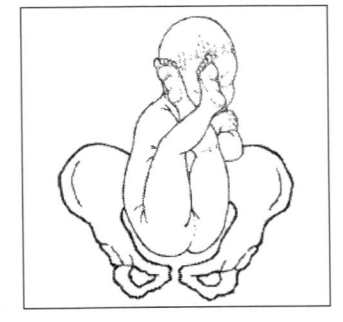

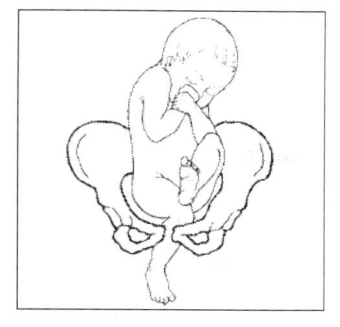

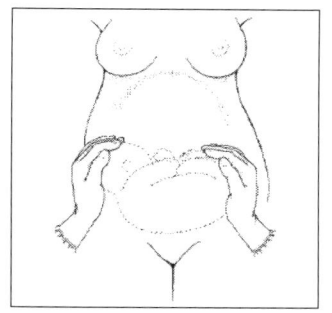

WHO(2003)P.210

You may see baby's buttocks, genitalia, soles of feet or any limb. There are three types of breech:

    Complete / Full – fully flexed foetus

    Frank – extended legs

    Footling / Incomplete – 1 or both thighs extended

A complete breech is the best sort and a footling breech the worst.

The diagnosis of breech can be tricky and even experienced midwives and obstetricians. Some signs of a breech include a longitudinal lie (not lying up or down, lying across), a hard head at fundus, the heart heard above the umbilicus. Ask mum where she feels the most kicks – up is good, down is bad. On a vaginal examination you don't feel the head in the pelvis and may feel a soft buttock or even an anus.

Shoulder Dystocia

This is when the shoulder facing forward becomes stuck under the pelvic bone.

Third Stage of Labour

The placenta 'after birth' will deliver within 20 minutes. Placenta delivery is stimulated by putting baby on mothers breast, which stimulates the release of oxytocin.

Problems with the third stage

Post-Partum Haemorrhage (PPH)

At the time of delivery the uterus has a blood flow of 250-300mls/min. Postpartum haemorrhage is defined as blood loss of greater than 500(+) mills, of blood, a major PPH is greater than 1000ml. If it occurs within 24 hours of the delivery it is known as a primary PPH, after 24 hours it is known as a secondary PPH.

Primary PPH:

There are four Main Causes:- a floppy uterus that is tired and wont contract, retained tissue, damage to the vagina or vulval region or a clotting problems

The risk factors for a primary PPH are a prolonged labour, a large uterus (big baby, twins, too much fluid), several previous labours, previous PPH, pre-eclampsia or a uterine abnormality.

The area should be examined with a good light source and an assistant to help you.

Retained Tissue

The placenta should be allowed to pass naturally.

To record the level of the baby's response and to monitor its responsiveness the APGAR score is used.

Sign	0 Points	1 Point	2 Points
(A)ctivity	Absent	Arms and Legs Flexed	Active Movement
(P)ulse	Absent	< 100 bpm	> 100 bpm
(G)rimace	No Response	Grimace	Sneeze, cough, pulls away
(A)ppearance	Blue-gray, pale all over	Normal, except for extremities	Normal
(R)espiration	Absent	Slow, irregular	Good, crying

A score is taken at 1, 5 and 10 minute if required/

A score of:

7-10 is normal,

4-7 may require some resuscitation.

3 or below requires immediate resuscitation.

Gynaecology

Gynecology is the study of women's health problems. The main broad areas are:

> Pelvic pain
>
> Pelvic infection
>
> Abnormal bleeding
>
> Contraception

Pelvic pain

This is a very common presentation. You need to determine if the pain is acute (new and sudden) or chronic (old and recurrent). The acute causes include ovarian pain, an appendix (RLQ) or infection.

Toxic Shock Syndrome

Is a special type of infection. It is introduced by tampon into the vagina (usually forgotten or lost), and usually occurs 2-4 days after period. The symptoms: fever, circulatory collapse, diarrhoea, rash, thick vaginal discharge.

Abnormal bleeding

A normal period is 28-35 days / bleeding days 1-7(+), but there is huge variation from light to heavy. The definition of abnormal depends on woman's previous experience

Menorrhagia – heavy periods

Intermenstrural bleeding – bleeding between periods

Post-menopausal bleeding – bleeding after the menopause and usually means cancer

Chapter 29 Nuclear Biological & Nerve Agent Warfare

Biological Warfare

Aflatoxin (W)
Not contagious person to person but can cause poisoning if exposed to affected crops through Inhalation, eye, skin or ingestion this toxin is produced by fungus from the Aspergillus genus and can also be used in biological warfare. It causes cancer that particularly affects the liver. Symptoms are Pain, vomiting, fever, Jaundice which can be seen in the eyes or general complexion, swelling of limbs, an enlarged liver may also be felt during palpation of the abdomen.

Anthrax (W)
Anthrax is a bacterial infection, which is rare and mainly occurs in Africa, Asia, China and Eastern Europe. It has also been used as a bioterrorism weapon. Spread is by contact with the infected carcasses of hoofed animals such as goats and sheep. Three routes of infection;
- Through a cut or puncture in the skin.
- Inhaled spores through the Lungs.
- Through eating poorly cooked infected meat.

Black pustules form with swelling, fever, enlargement of liver and spleen, if inhaled can cause pneumonia and shortness' of breath, if swallowed can cause internal bleeding. Natural disease is relatively indolent and if recognised treatment is usually effective. Weaponised anthrax on the other hand is more virulent and harder to treat.

Brucellosis (W)
Brucellosis is an infectious disease passed from animals to humans usually through contaminated food. Common Symptoms include; Fever (sometimes re-occurring), headache and back pain, generalized weakness with joint and muscle pain. A general examination will show enlarged Lymph nodes and an abdominal assessment may also reveal enlargement of the liver and spleen. Can also cause localized infection in the testes, lungs and heart leading to endocarditis.

Cholera (W)
Cholera is caused by faecal-oral contamination and presents with copious watery stools, fever and vomiting, which leads to profound dehydration. The fluid loss can be 10-20 litres a day. Incubation ranges from a few hours to 5 days.

Clostridium botulinum – aka botulisim (W)
(See Infectious disease)

Diphtheria (W)
This is another disease caused by the toxin produced by the bacteria. It is best considered as a sore throat on steroids. The main problem is severe respiratory distress and asphyxia from a grey membrane of dead and dying cells from the throat.

Encephalomyelitis (W) (inflammation of the brain tissue)
Symptoms: Fever, headache, severe photophobia (aversion to light).

Primitive treatment: Supportive.

Alphavirus infection (Eastern, Western, or Venezuelan Equine Encephalomyelitis).

High mortality. If occurs outside endemic areas may indicate biological attack.

Meliodosis and Glanders (Burkholderia pseudomalleri)
This disease is endemic in northern Australia.

Symptoms: Pneumonia with associated septicaemia. Meliodosis may occur in the form of localised lesions.

Normal infection occurs via contaminated soil or water in endemic areas. Dispersal can be via aerosol in a biological attack.

This is a second line bio agent.

Plague (W)
Plague is caused by a bacteria that infects wild rats, it is rare but can be found throughout the world. Incubation period is 2 to 6 days. It comes in two forms, bubonic plague (spread by infected fleas) and pneumonic plague (spread by droplets from coughing).

Symptoms: Fatigue, fever, cough, shortness of breath, and malaise or fever with grossly swollen lymph nodes.

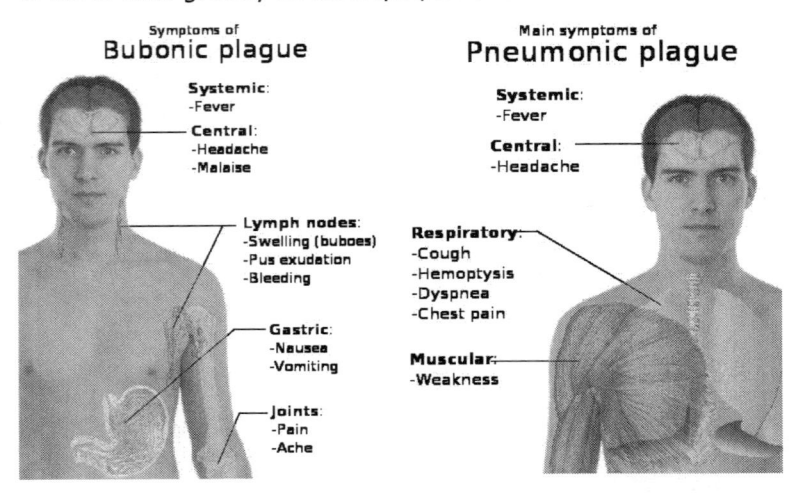

Symptoms of Bubonic plague

Systemic:
- Fever

Central:
- Headache
- Malaise

Lymph nodes:
- Swelling (buboes)
- Pus exudation
- Bleeding

Gastric:
- Nausea
- Vomiting

Joints:
- Pain
- Ache

Main symptoms of Pneumonic plague

Systemic:
- Fever

Central:
- Headache

Respiratory:
- Cough
- Hemoptysis
- Dyspnea
- Chest pain

Muscular:
- Weakness

© Mikael Häggström

Psittacosis (Chlamydia psittaci) (W)

Symptoms: Atypical pneumonia with fever and cough.

Rarely fatal. Transmitted naturally to humans after contact with infected bird droppings.

Q-Fever (Coxiella burnetti) (W)

Symptoms: High fevers, chills, sweats, headache.

Human transmission usually from inhaled dust infected with placental tissue or secretions from infected sheep, cows, or goats. Rarely fatal.

Rabies

Rabies is spread through the bite of an infected animal. Any bite in a high risk area from an unprovoked animal should be considered to be at the risk of being rabid.

Incubation is usually 1 to 2 months but can vary between months and years. Symptoms include headache, confusion, fever, hallucinations and hydrophobia (fear of water). Paralysis may also occur.

Salmonella (aka Typhoid) (W)
Transmitted through faecal-Oral contamination and presents as a gastroenteritis and occasionally septicaemia. The more severe cases present with headache, rigors, fever, decreased appetite, constipation or diarrhoea, backache, nosebleed and tender abdomen.

Typhoid is caused by a faeco-oral contamination usually through consumption of poorly cooked food or dairy products.

Incubation can be anything between 3 days and 3 weeks. Fever rises daily for 7-10 days, peaks for 7-20 days then drops over the next 7-10 days. In the first stage of the disease, rose-coloured marks appear on the patient.

Shigella sp (W)
Transmitted through Fecal-Oral contamination and presents as a gastroenteritis. It is highly Contagious

Smallpox (W)
Caused by the orthopox virus It is relatively easy to manufacture, infectious and can be administered by an aerosol effect making it attractive to terrorist as a weapon. In theory smallpox has been eradicated from the wild.

After an incubation period of 7-19 days, casualty become tired has a fever, rigors, vomiting, headache and backache. 2-3 days later, a rash appear on the face, hands and arms; these get bigger as disease progresses.

Initially it can be confused for chcken pox – however the lesions are bigger and tend to occur more on the face.

A vaccination is available, 30% of unvaccinated casualties will die. Diagnosis is clinical and treatment supportive. Smallpox can be prevented by vaccination. Death rate for unvaccinated casualties is 30%. Highly contagious both though contact and airborne.

Tularaemia (W)
Symptoms include Fever, shortness of breath, fatigue, malaise, cough, and abdominal pain.

Viral Hemorrhagic Fever
Symptoms: GI bleedings, petechia, bleeding from mucous membranes.

Other Diseases that can be weaponised are;
Jap B Encephalitis. Pneumoniae, Polio, Ricin, Rotavirus, Staphylococcal enterotoxin B (SEB), VEE, T2 Toxin, West Nile Fever

Chemical Warfare

Nerve Agents

Nerve agents work by interfering with the natural destruction of acetylcholine in our neural pathways this causes organ failure. They can enter the body through mouth, nose, eyes and skin. They are effect in very small doses and can kill in 30 seconds.

Effects of Nerve Agents

With all suspected nerve agents examine patient's pupils and note if normal, dilated or contracted (Pin Point), note colour of skin and if sweating, check mouth for (mucosal) secretions, record pulse and blood pressure.

Ricin

Symptoms: Block protein synthesis within the body. Abdominal pain, diarrhoea,

Nausea, vomiting and severe diarrhoea. Pneumonia if infection is by inhalation route, cause cardiovascular collapse. Derived from the castor bean, highly potent, inhalation following spraying is most likely route of spread.

BZ
Symptoms - Confusion, Hallucinations

Classic Nerve Agents

Nerve gas: GA(Tabun), GB(Sarin), GD(soman), GF(cyclohexyl Sarin) and VX

Nerve gas can cause sweating, excess saliva, excess respiratory secretions, tachycardia (fast heart rate) or bradycardia (slow heart rate), abdominal cramps, vomiting, muscle twitching, headache, seizures, confusion, and coma. They cause their effects by blocking the breakdown of acetylcholine – a communication chemical between nerves and muscles. When the enzyme, which breaks it down, is blocked, it accumulates, and causes the symptoms of nerve agent poisoning.

Blood agents

The most common of these agents is cyanide or its derivatives. They work by blocking cellular respiration. It is mainly spread by aerosol. If the patient survives the initial contact then it is likely that the patient will survive. The spectrum of symptoms runs from weakness, dizziness, and nausea through seizures and respiratory arrest.

Cyanide & Hydrogen Sulphide
Symptoms
Normal or Dilated Pupils, Pink or Cyanosed Skin, Normal Secretions, Decreased Respiration Rate, feels unwell

Blister agents

Blister agents include Lewisite and Mustard gas. These cause damage to the skin and when inhaled damage to the lungs. Mustard gas can also cause suppression of the bone marrow.

Lewisite
Symptoms
Stinging for 10-20 seconds, Deep Pain and Toxic Blisters

Vesicants (Mustard Gas)
Symptoms
Airway, Eye and Skin damage and systemic effects

Radiation Incidents

There have been around 100 civilian nuclear accidents in the last 15 years, fortunately only a few have resulted in a direct loss of life. Well known ones include the Chernobyl Disaster in 1986 where over 50 people died at the time off the disaster but several thousand are believed to have since died of cancer. This year (March 2011) in Japans Fukushima Daiichi nuclear disaster several explosions caused by an earthquake released radiation into the air creating a 20km exclusion zone around the nuclear plant. Two months later surveys recorded hazardous levels of radiation outside the exclusion zone.

The likelihood of being exposed to a nuclear explosion is extremely slim but I will detail the basic facts for completeness with more emphasis on the possibility of radioactive contamination from a civilian accident.

The effects and intensity of nuclear weapons vary considerably depending of the yield and the height at which it is detonated. This can be at ground level, in the air, underwater or in the up atmosphere. There is an optimum height at which a weapon is detonated for maximum blast damage. If the explosion occurs on or too near the ground, a large part of the force is reflects back up into the air, with less effects on ground targets.

The harmful effects of a nuclear explosion can be divided into the following categories;

Blast Wave

The blast wave will cause total destruction of people and property close to the explosion, with decreasing effect as it moves away from ground zero. As with a conventional blast serious injuries can occur at a distance away from ground zero.

Typical distances for blast waves are below;

- 0.7 km for 1 kiloton (kt)
- 3.2 km for 100 kt;
- 15.0 km for 10 megatons (Mt)

Primary injuries

Primary injuries are caused by shock waves, ear drums can burst, brain haemorrhages can occur, damage to lungs and other hollow organs such as the intestines, not all injuries may be immediately apparent. Injuries can result in shock and respiratory failure. Blast waves can exceed 1000 km/hr and can cause loss of memory, confusion, headache and disorientation.

As the blast wave will flatten and damage most building injuries and fatalities are commonly caused through structural collapse as much as primary blast damage.

Secondary injuries

Secondary injuries are caused by casualties being hit by debris, which is thrown by the explosion, some can cause blunt trauma whilst others will cause penetrating injuries.

Tertiary injuries

Tertiary injuries are caused by impact injuries from the casualty being thrown in the air and landing on or against a hard surface. Fractures and head injuries are common tertiary injuries

Quaternary injuries

Are other miscellaneous effects such as burns, contamination, retinal damage etc

Thermal Radiation (Heat)

At the centre of a nuclear explosion the temperature briefly reaches tens of millions of degrees. Close to the explosion the heat will vaporise everything, as it expands it causes fires, severe burns and eye injuries. If the blast is close to the ground it forms a fireball and a mushroom cloud.

As radiation covers the visible, infrared, and ultraviolet light burns can extend further than the blast radius. Two types of eye injuries occur the first is flash blindness this is usually temporary lasting 30-60 minutes.

Retinal burns can also occur and permanent damage can occur if the retina is scared and the casualty had looked directly at a fireball, else damage is likely to be minor at worst.

Ionizing Radiation

A relatively small amount of the blasts energy takes the form of ionizing radiation as neutrons, alpha particles, gamma rays and electrons, the greater the distance from the point of explosion the less the initial radiation effects. Dust and particles released during the initial blast are irradiated and become fallout, this can be distributed away from the original site of the explosion by weather patterns.

When an unstable nucleus decays, there are three ways that it can do so.
It may give out:-

- an alpha particle

- a beta particle

- a gamma ray

Many radioactive substances emit alpha particles and beta particles as well as gamma rays. In fact, you won't find a pure gamma source: anything that gives off gamma rays will also give off alpha and/or beta too. Alpha-decay occurs in very heavy elements, for example, Uranium and Radium. These heavy elements have too many protons to be stable. They can become more stable by emitting an alpha particle. Alpha particles have a large charge(+2), so they easily ionise other atoms that they pass. Ionising atoms requires energy, so alpha particles lose energy rapidly as they travel. Thus they have a range of only a few centimetres in air. The main danger from radioactivity is the damage it does to the cells in your body.

Most of this damage is due to ionisation when the radiation passes, although if levels of radiation are high there can be damage due to heating effects as your body absorbs the energy from the radiation, rather like heating food in a microwave oven. This is particularly true of gamma rays.

When Alpha or Beta particles pass another atom, they tend to pull electrons off it.

We then say that the atom is ionised.

If it has lost electrons, we call it a positive ion.
(Electrons have a negative charge, so losing electrons means the atom becomes positive).

When an alpha particle or beta particle ionises an atom, it slows the particle down. This is one reason that alpha particles have such a low penetrating power - they ionise other atoms strongly and thus get slowed down a great deal.

Alpha particles

Alpha particles are relatively slow and heavy. They have a low penetrating power - you can stop them with just a sheet of paper. Because they have a large charge, alpha particles ionise other atoms strongly.

Alpha particles are slow, have a short range in air, and can be stopped by a sheet of paper. You might therefore assume that alpha particles are the least dangerous of the three types of radiation. Whilst they cannot penetrate your skin, you could easily eat or drink something contaminated with an alpha source. This would put a source of alpha particles inside your body, wreaking havoc by ionising atoms in nearby cells.

If this happens to part of the DNA in one of your cells, then that cell's instructions about how to live and grow have been scrambled. The cell is then likely to do something very different to what it's supposed to do, for example, it may turn cancerous and start multiplying uncontrollably.

Thus alpha particles, whilst they have a low penetrating power, can be the most dangerous because they ionise so strongly.

Beta particles

Beta particles are fast, and light. They have a medium penetrating power and are stopped by a sheet of aluminium or plastics such as Perspex. Beta particles ionise atoms that they pass, but not as strongly as alpha particles do. The particles have a longer range than alphas, but ionise much less strongly, with the result that they do around 1/20th of the damage done by the same dose of alpha particles.

However, they do have more penetrating power, which means that they can get through your skin and affect cells inside you.

Gamma Waves

Gamma rays are waves, not particles. This means that they have no mass and no charge. Gamma rays have a high penetrating power - it takes a thick sheet of metal such as lead, or concrete to reduce them significantly. Gamma rays do not directly ionise other atoms, although they may cause atoms to emit other particles which will then cause ionisation. We don't find pure gamma sources - gamma rays are emitted alongside alpha or beta particles. Strictly speaking, gamma emission isn't 'radioactive decay' because it doesn't change the state of the nucleus; it just carries away some energy.

Gamma rays hardly ionise atoms at all, so they do not cause damage directly in this way. However, gamma rays are very difficult to stop, you require lead or concrete shielding to keep you safe from them. When they are absorbed by an atom, those atom gains quite a bit of energy, and may then emit other particles. If that atom is in one of your cells, this is not good!

Summary of the effects

The following table summarizes the most important effects of nuclear explosions under certain conditions.

	1 kT	20 kT	1 MT	20 MT
Complete Destruction	0.2	0.6	2.4	6.4
Destruction of most buildings	0.6	1.7	6.2	17
Buildings damaged	1.7	4.7	17	47
Fireball	0.5	2.0	10	30
Full Thickness Burns	0.6	2.5	12	38
Partial Thickness Burns	0.8	3.2	15	44
Superficial Burns	1.1	4.2	19	53

Fall-out

Fall-out is dust that is sucked up from the ground by the explosion. It rises high in the air and can be carried by the winds for hundreds of miles before falling to the ground.
The radiation from this dust is dangerous. It cannot be seen or felt. It can be detected only by Geiger counters. If the dust fell on or

around your home, the radiation from it would be a danger for many days after an explosion. Radiation can penetrate any material, but its intensity is reduced as it passes through - so the thicker and denser the material is, the better.

Radiation Poisoning

Rad = Radiation absorbed dose. Normal background radiation is 0.1 Rad / year. Maximum recommended dose for a nuclear worker is 5 Rads / year.

Radiation poisoning can be external through direct irradiation or internal through ingestion of contaminated foods or animal products. Symptoms vary in onset and intensity dependant on the total dose of radiation exposure the higher the dose the quicker and more intense the symptoms show. Relatively small doses induce loss of appetite, nausea, diarrhoea, abdominal pain, vomiting, headache, anaemia, infections and increased risk of haemorrhage where as larger doses see below are invariably fatal. Long term exposure at low doses can increase the risk of developing cataracts, cancers and birth defects in future generations.

When considering clinical radiation effects they are broken down into:

Immediate symptoms (0.5-6 hrs) – dose dependent

Nausea, vomiting, loss of appetite, and loss of energy

Symptom-free period (3 hrs – 3 weeks) – dose dependent

Second phase symptoms (1-2 days to 3 weeks) – dose dependent.

Recovery or death occurs in a further 3-4 weeks

GI symptoms – nausea, vomiting, diarrhoea

Bone marrow suppression – infection, bleeding

Cerebral and vascular – very high doses cause blood vessels to leak, and chemical mediators to activate causing oedema (fluid leaking from blood vessels) and shock. The brain is very sensitive to high doses and this leads to confusion, seizures, and coma. Patients presenting with cerebral and vascular signs and symptoms will die over a 1 to 2-week time frame.

Cumulative exposure will give the following timing of initial symptoms:

Rads		Death Rate
<150	Minimal initial symptoms only, increased long term cancer risks	OK
150		10% Mild Symptoms
250		50% Rad Poisoning
400	Median lethal dose with no medical treatment	25% Die
600	Initial symptoms can occur 1-4 hours post-exposure depending on dose, Symptom-free period of 10-20 days.	50% Die
800	Initial symptoms 30-60 minutes post exposure lasting 12-48 hours.	75% Die
1000	Incapacitation soon after exposure, and death within 1-2 days with no symptom-free period.	100% Die

Sterility

A dose of 100-200 rads in women will suppress menstruation for up to 3 years; only 10 rads will lower sperm counts in men and a dose of 400 rads will cause sterility in either gender.

Single Radiation Source

Initial radiation decrease in strength using the inverse square law, If it was 900 rads at 1km from blast, it would be 225 rads at 2km and 100 rads at 3km.

It also decreases in time by a using the seven, tenths rule. After 7 hours it will be at 10th of original strength, after 49 hours at 100th and after 343 hours at 1000th of original strength.

Multiple Sources

Although the same physical laws apply to multiple radioactive sources, changes in weather patterns and concentration of fallout make predication of radiation levels very difficult.

Radiation effects on skin

Following exposure to radiation itchy, reddened areas of skin occur within a few hours. This can last for several weeks during which time the skin will blister and become ulcerated. Healing occurs as with any burn although areas may remain damaged with loss of colour and hair growth

Chapter 30 Gunshot Wounds, Explosions & Tactical Considerations

Gunshot Wounds

Introduction

Gunshot wounds can be split into two groups depending on the muzzle velocity of the weapon. Generally handguns are considered as low velocity weapons with a muzzle velocity below 1000 ft/sec and can be fired with one hand, whereas a rifle is high velocity weapon with a velocity of greater than 1000 ft/sec.

Exceptions to this are high calibre handguns such as .357 and .44 Magnum, which are usually fired with two hands and are treated as high-velocity and .22 Rifles and Shotguns at long range that are considered low-velocity weapons.

The difference is mainly academic as the extent of wounds caused by firearms is determined by many factors including the deformation and fragmentation of the projectile, its entrance profile and the path travelled through the body.

Most handgun wounds can be treated without surgery and with careful wound care management; although fractures are likely if the projectile hits bone. Even if the wound appears clean contamination is common and prophylactic antibiotic therapy is recommended. If open fractures are present intravenous antibiotic therapy for 48 to 72 hours is preferred or a full course of oral antibiotics.

Rifles and shotguns at close range cause high velocity wounds. Due to the characteristics of high velocity rounds the chance of open fractures and wound contamination is much higher than with handguns. In high velocity injury tissues are pushed away around the projectile path this is known as temporary a cavity. The effect produces blunt trauma that extends beyond the tissue actually contacted by the projectile if the tissue retains its contractility this cavity will disappear when the tissue returns to its normal position. The pulsation of the cavity results in a strong negative pressure that draws contamination from both the entry and exit wounds along the entire wound tract.

However even with high velocity wounds if there is only a small amount of tissue damage, no fragmentation or fractures then simple wound care may be enough.

Ballistics

In addition to the range and calibre of the weapon we must also consider the type of ammunition that is used. A normal military bullet is coated with a solid metal jacket and is less likely to fragment when it passes through the body, additional fragments may occur when a jacketed bullet fragments when hitting bone or when a non-jacketed, soft-point, hollow-point, or composite bullet fragments when passing through soft tissue thus creating larger permanent cavities by mushrooming out. Fragmentation may significantly increase injury. Should the cavity at the point become plugged with clothing, wood or other debris it may fail to expand.

Some Military rounds are designed to tumble in flight and thus create a larger tract and more damage. Civilian rounds such as the Black Talon, Hydra-Shok, or Golden Saber are designed to ensure complete transference of the kinetic energy to the target. Whilst other rounds may achieve over penetration and pass through the body without fragmenting, thus not impart all of its energy.

A shotgun blast creates multiple projectiles creating numerous holes and significant tissue damage, especially at close range. A variant bullet is the composite round. These have a copper hollow point outer shell containing shot stabilised with epoxy resin which fragment upon hitting a surface, creating multiple projectiles once they enter the body. This dramatically increases the size of the permanent cavity.

Even blank ammunition containing powder but no bullet may cause injury or death at close range due to the gases, heat and packing released when fired.

Evaluating the Casualty

Both knowledge and practice is needed to properly assess a firearms injury, when evaluating a wound interview any witnesses to determine both the range and angle the bullet entered from and the type of weapon used. Ask how many shots were heard, as the bullets will need to be accounted for. Any bullets or fragments removed or found should be retained to try and ascertain if all parts of the round were recovered and nothing is left within the wound.

If there are any spent cartridges cases or shell casings around these can be examined to determine both the weapon used and its calibre

Carry out a full secondary survey and instigate any life saving measures as you progress. Whilst examining the body check for additional injuries as well as entry and exit wounds. Assume that there may be both fractures and neurological damage until proven otherwise.

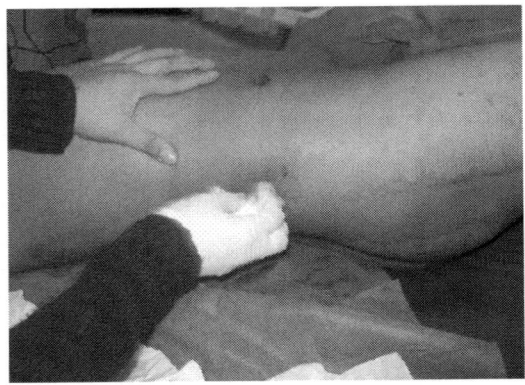

Bobjgaalindo

Types of Wounds from firearms.

The primarily mechanism of injury is the path the projectile takes when it passes through the body. A shotgun loaded with shot as opposed to a solid load fired at close will produce a large entrance wound, but will usually lack the energy to penetrate the body completely. The entry wound from a rifle or handgun may be more difficult to locate as the small diameter of a projectile and elastic property of the skin will close the wound once the bullet has passed through.

A shot fired at point blank range may exhibit charring to the clothing or skin from the muzzle flash and hot gasses escaping from the barrel when fired. A stellate, or star-shaped, wound is formed at the skin with a jagged appearance to the entrance wound and sometimes, an imprint of the barrel is left in the skin. Complications can occur from this as the gasses are transmitted into the wound making the temporary cavity larger and carrying soot and charred clothing into the cavity to further contaminate the wound.

Conversely exit wounds tend to be larger and will contain whatever debris the bullet has sucked through the body. Also even if only one shot is fired the bullet may have fragmented within the body and created more than one exit wound or propelled bony fragments through the skin.

The second injuring mechanism is the temporary cavity created by the kinetic energy of the projectile This can cause tissue to be forced from the projectiles path, causing stretching, tearing and concussive forces to the surrounding tissue. The cavity may measure 15 times the projectile diameter. During the first five minutes, the wall collapses and reforms (pulsates) several times. This additional sheering force can damage tissue some distance from the projectile tract itself.

Wounds to the chest or abdomen will frequently incur Organ damage, observe for signs of air *(pneumothorax)* or blood *(haemothorax)* in the space between the chest wall and the lungs, which may cause one lung to collapse or compression of the heart (Cardiac Tamponade) by the presence of blood or fluid in the sac surrounding the heart (*Pericardium*) or damage to the organs in the abdomen. Not forgetting to check under the armpit and in the space between the genitals and the anus (*perineum*) for entrance and exit wounds.

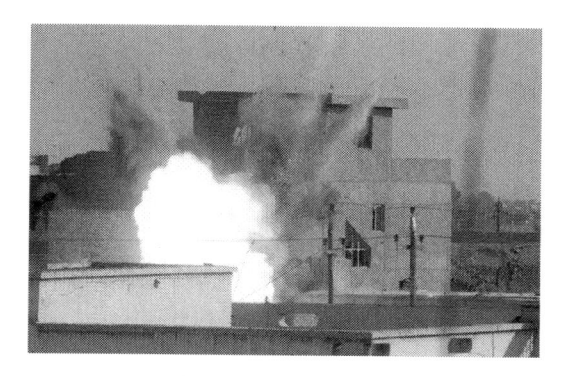

Explosions

Thomas D. Hudzinski

Primary injuries

Primary injuries are caused by initial explosion and shock waves, ear drums can burst, brain haemorrhages can occur, damage to lungs and other hollow organs such as the intestines, not all injuries may be immediately apparent. Injuries can result in shock and respiratory failure. Blast waves can cause loss of memory, confusion, headache and disorientation.

As the blast wave will damage structures injuries are commonly caused through structural collapse as much as primary blast damage.

Secondary injuries

Secondary injuries are caused by casualties being hit by debris, which is thrown by the explosion, some can cause blunt trauma whilst others will cause penetrating injuries.

Tertiary injuries

Tertiary injuries are caused by impact injuries from the casualty being thrown in the air and landing on or against a hard surface. Fractures and head injuries are common tertiary injuries.

Quaternary injuries

Are other miscellaneous effects such as burns, contamination and infection etc

Chapter 31 Triage

The word Triage is derived from the French 'to sort', it has been used in both military and disaster situations to prioritise the treatment of casualties. If the casualty is in cardiac arrest or severely injured and not expected to survive they may be left in favour of casualties that would benefit more from medical attention and evacuation.

In most triage systems casualties are sorted into categories based on an initial survey of their Airway, Breathing and Circulation. When dealing with a mass casualty incident the triage officer will give cards to each casualty showing their Triage Category, there level of consciousness, observations and treatment can be recorded on it. If there condition changes then their Triage Category may also change. The Cards can be folded in different ways to show the various categories.

The initial Sieve is designed to quickly establish priorities a more detailed sort can then take place when resources are available.

The adult Triage Sieve is one method of sorting casualties into one of four categories exist;

Category	Priority	Colour
Delayed	3	Green
Urgent	2	Yellow
Immediate	1	Red
Dead		

Dead : Casualty when checked is not breathing even after opening there airway.

Immediate: Unable to walk & (Respiratory Rate <10 or >29 and/or Central Capillary Refill > 2 seconds)

Urgent: Unable to walk & (Respiratory Rate >9 or <30 and Central Capillary Refill <=2 seconds)

Delayed: Walking Wounded

Triage Sort

The triage sort takes longer to complete as it requires further observations it can change a casualties priority so should be rechecked frequently as resources are available. Total points scored for Glasgow Coma Scale, Respiratory Rate and Systolic Blood Pressure as below.

Glasgow Coma Scale

13-15	4
9-12	3
6-8	2
4-5	1
3	0

Respiratory Rate

10-29	4
>29	3
6-9	2
1-5	1
0	0

Systolic Blood Pressure

90+	4
76-89	3
50-75	2
1-49	1
0	0

12 = Priority 3 — Delayed
11 = Priority 2 — Urgent
<11 = Priority 1 — Immediate
0 — Dead

Chapter 32 Nutrition

Food contains nutrients, some of which provide energy, while others are essential for growth and normal bodily function.

Food can be broken down into a number of building blocks Carbohydrate, protein and fat are need to be eaten in relatively large amounts whereas Vitamins and minerals are only needed in small amounts to keep the body healthy.

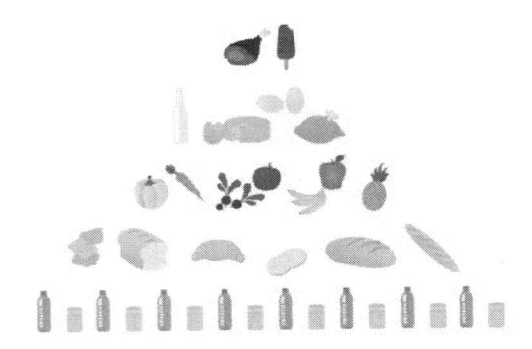

Food Pyramid by © Brailescu Cristian | Dreamstime.com

In order to provide a balanced diet the principal of the food pyramid is used.

At the top of the pyramid

(Group 1) fats, oils and sweets these should used sparingly.

(Group 2) dairy products, Milk, Yogurt and Cheese

(Group 3) meat, dry beans, eggs and nuts.

(Group 4) Vegetables

(Group 5) Fruit

(Group 6) Bread, Cereal, Rice & Pasta

(Group 7) Water (Drink at least 2 Litres a day)

Servings

1600 Calories for Women

2200 Calories for Children, Teenage Girls, Active Women and Men

2800 Calories for Teenage Boys and Active Men

Cal	Group 2	Group 3	Group 4	Group 5	Group 6
1600	2	2	3	2	6
2200	3	3	4	3	9
2800	3	3	5	4	11

One Serving Sizes

Group 2 dairy products, Milk, Yogurt and Cheese

1 Cup Milk or Yogurt, 2 oz Cheese

Group 3 meat, dry beans, eggs and nuts.

3oz Cooked Meat, ½ Cup Cooked Beans, 1 egg, 2 tbls peanut butter

Group 4 Vegetables

½ Cup raw or cooked Vegetables, 1 Cup leafy Veg, ¾ Cup Veg Juice;

Group 5 Fruit;

Fresh Fruit; ¾ Cup Fruit Juice; ½ Cup Chopped, Canned Fruit; ¼ Cup Dried Fruit.

Group 6 Carbohydrates;

One oz ready to eat cereal; Slice Bread; Half Cup of Rice, Pasta or Cereal; 4 Crackers.

Carbohydrate

Carbohydrates provide the body with fuel it needs for physical activity and for proper organ function.

Protein

Protein provides 10 to 15 per cent of its dietary energy, and is needed for growth and repair.

Fats

Fats allow the transport of fat soluble vitamins A, D, E and K around the body. Fat is easily stored in the body for later use as an energy store. Too much fat can contribute to unhealthy cholesterol levels.

Minerals

Calcium

Calcium helps build strong bones and teeth, regulating muscle contractions, including heartbeat and aiding blood clotting.

A lack of calcium could lead to a condition called rickets.

Food sources of calcium include: milk, cheese and other dairy foods, green leafy vegetables, such as broccoli, cabbage and okra, soya beans, tofu, nuts and fish where you eat the bones, such as sardines and pilchards.

Iodine

This helps make the thyroid hormones. These hormones help keep cells and the metabolic rate healthy.

Food sources include sea fish and shellfish, cow's milk and cereals and grains.

Iron

Iron is used in the manufacture of red blood cells, which transport oxygen around the body.

Iron Deficiency

A lack of iron can lead to iron deficiency anaemia.

Food sources include: liver, meat, beans, nuts, dried fruit, such as dried apricots, whole grain food, such as brown rice, watercress and curly kale

Spinach, tea and coffee contain a substance that limits the body's ability to absorb iron. Avoid Liver if you are pregnant.
Recommended daily amount of Iron are 8.7mg for men and 14.8mg a for women

Malnutrition

Malnutrition can be caused by a poor diet that is either inadequate or unbalanced. It can also have medical causes that affect digestion or absorption of food. Problems can occur even if you lack a single vitamin in your diet, it may be mild and have little short or long term effect or severe and leave permanent damage to your body after recovery

Symptoms vary but can include fatigue, dizziness, and weight loss.

Vitamin A

Vitamin A helps maintain healthy skin, teeth, skeletal and soft tissue, mucus membranes, and skin. It aids low light vision.

Vitamin A is found in eggs, meat, fortified milk, cheese, cream, liver, kidney, cod, and halibut fish oil, cantaloupe, pink grapefruit, apricots, carrots, pumpkin, sweet potatoes, winter squash, broccoli, spinach, and leafy vegetables.

Vitamin A Deficiency

Lack of vitamin A increases chances of acquiring infectious diseases and defective vision.

Folic Acid

Folic acid helps tissues grow and cells function. It helps the body break down, use and build proteins, form red blood cells and produce DNA.

Folic Acids are found in Dark green leafy vegetables, dried beans and peas (legumes) and Citrus fruits and juices

Folic Acid Deficiency

A lack of Folic Acid can cause spina bifida in new born babies is recommended that a supplemental dose of 400mcg is taken during pregnancy. It also may cause Diarrhoea, Gray hair, Mouth ulcers, Peptic ulcer, Poor growth, swollen tongue and anaemia.

Vitamin B1 (Thiamine)

Thiamine help convert Carbohydrates in the body into energy. It is important for healthy skin, eyes and hair.

Vitamin B1 is found in Asparagus, Avocado, Brown rice, rice bran, sprouts, egg yolks, fish, Leafy, green vegetables. Liver, mushrooms, peas, poultry, quern, spinach, wheat germ, bread, pasta and yeast.

Vitamin B1 (Thiamine) Deficiency

Lack of vitamin B1 can cause Cardiovascular and Neurological problems and Beriberi

Vitamin B2 (Riboflavin)

Riboflavin (vitamin B2) is used to help with growth and red blood cell production it also aids in converting carbohydrates into energy. B2 is water soluble so excess amounts are removed from the body each day in urine

Vitamin B1 is found in Dairy products, Eggs, Green leafy vegetables, Lean meats, Legumes, Milk and Nuts.

Vitamin B2 (Riboflavin) Deficiency

Lack of vitamin B1 can cause anaemia, mouth or lip sores, skin disorders, sore throats and swelling of mucus membranes.

Vitamin B6

Vitamin B6 is an important vitamin it helps the body produce antibodies to fight disease, is used in the production of haemoglobin, maintains nerve function, blood sugar levels and aids in the metabolism of protein. It's a water soluble so excess amounts are removed from the body each day in urine

Vitamin B6 is found in Avocado, Banana, Legumes, Meat, Nuts, Poultry and Whole grain Bread and Pasta.

Vitamin B6 Deficiency

Lack of vitamin B1 can cause anaemia, Confusion, Depression, Irritability, Mouth and tongue sores.

Vitamin B12 (cobalamine)

This helps in the formation of blood and in the maintenance of a healthy nervous system. Older people may require a supplemental dose as will those on a vegetarian diet and women who are pregnant.

Foods rich in Vitamin B12 are Liver, Sardines, Kidneys, Rabbit, Pate, Fatty Fish, Eggs, Muscles, Corned Beef, Lamb, Turkey and Hard Cheese.

B12 Deficiency

Prevent anaemia and problems with nervous system.

Vitamin C (ascorbic acid)

Vitamin C. Helps protect cells maintains connective tissue, which gives support and structure for tissues and organs.

Food Sources of vitamin C include; peppers, broccoli , sprouts, Citrus and kiwi fruits.

Vitamin C is water soluble, so you need40mg in your diet every day.

Vitamin D

Vitamin D helps regulate the amount of calcium and phosphate in the body to keep bones and teeth healthy.

Sources of vitamin D include the sun, oily fish, such as salmon, mackerel, sardines and eggs.

Vitamin D Deficiency

A lack of vitamin D can also lead to developing rickets (see) below

Vitamin E

Vitamin E aids the immune system and is an antioxidant that protects tissue from damage caused by free radical which damage cells, tissues, and organs. They are believed to play a role in certain conditions related to aging such as dementia. It is also important in the formation of red blood cells, dilates blood vessels and acts as an anti-coagulant.

It is found in vegetable oils, almonds, peanuts, hazelnuts, sunflower seeds, spinach and broccoli

Vitamin E Deficiency

Lack of vitamin E can cause problems with vision, muscle weakness and dementia.

Vitamin K

Vitamin K is vital in the blood clotting process it also helps maintain strong bones in the elderly.

Vitamin K is found in the following Green leafy vegetables, such as kale, spinach, turnip greens, collards, Swiss chard, mustard greens, parsley, romaine, and green leaf lettuce, Brussels sprouts, broccoli, cauliflower, cabbage, Fish, liver, meat, eggs, and cereals. Vitamin K is produced by bacteria in the gastrointestinal tract.

Vitamin K deficiency

Is very rare as it's naturally produced by the body. It occurs when it can't absorb the vitamin from the intestinal tract. Vitamin K deficiency can also occur after long-term treatment with antibiotics. Patients are usually more likely to have bruising and bleeding.

Recommended Daily Intakes for Individuals of Vitamins

	Vitamin A	Vitamin B1	Vitamin B2	Vitamin B6
0 - 6 months	400 mcg		0.3 mg/day	0.1 mg/day
7 - 12 months	500 mcg		0.4 mg/day	0.3 mg/day
1 - 3 years	300 mcg		0.5 mg/day	0.5 mg/day
4 - 8 years	400 mcg		0.6 mg/day	0.6 mg/day
9 - 13 years	600 mcg		0.9 mg/day	1.0 mg/day

Males 14 +	900 mcg	1.5mg	1.3 mg/day	1.3 mg/day
Females 14 +	700 mcg	1.5mg	1.0 mg/day	1.2 mg/day

	Folic Acid	Vitamin E	Vitamin K	
0 - 6 months	65 mcg/day	4 mg/day	2.0 mcg/day	
7 - 12 months	80 mcg/day	5 mg/day	2.5 mcg/day	
1 - 3 years	150 mcg/day	6 mg/day	30 mcg/day	
4 - 8 years	200 mcg/day	7 mg/day	55 mcg/day	
9 - 13 years	300 mcg/day	11 mg/day	60 mcg/day	
Males 14 +	400 mcg/day	15 mg/day	80 mcg/day	
Females14 +	400 mcg/day	15 mg/day	80 mcg/day	

Protein malnutrition

If treatment is not given or comes too late, this condition is life-threatening. Even with treatment it can cause permanent physical and mental problems, can also cause shock and coma.

Early Symptoms

- Changes in skin pigment
- Decreased muscle mass
- Diarrhoea
- Failure to gain weight and grow
- Fatigue
- Increased and more severe infections
- Irritability
- Large belly that sticks out (protrudes)
- Lethargy or apathy
- Loss of muscle mass
- Rash (dermatitis)
- Shock (late stage)

- Swelling (oedema)
- Enlarged Liver

Treatment

Increasing calorie intake will cure protein malnutrition if caught in early stages. However, children will never reach their full potential for height and growth and can be left with physical and mental problems.

Calories are given first in the form of carbohydrates, simple sugars, and fats. Proteins are started after other sources of calories have already provided energy. Vitamin and mineral supplements are essential. Since the person will have been without much food for a long period of time, eating can cause problems, especially if the calories are too high at first. Food must be reintroduced slowly. Carbohydrates are given first to supply energy, followed by protein foods.

Prevention

Ensure an adequate diet with enough carbohydrates, at least 10 percent fat and 12 percent protein.

Megaloblastic anaemia (Pernicious)

Megaloblastic anaemia is a blood disorder in which there is anaemia with larger-than-normal red blood cells which can be caused by a deficiency of folic acid or vitamin B12.

Symptoms include; tiredness, palpitations, shortness of breath, dizziness, red sore tongue and mouth, chest pain, weight loss, diarrhoea and in severe cases chest and leg pain and headache. It can also cause neurological symptoms.

Rickets

This is caused by a lack of vitamin D, calcium, or phosphate. It causes softening and weakening of the bones.

Vitamin D is absorbed from food or produced by the skin when exposed to sunlight.

You may not get enough vitamin D from your diet if you have trouble digesting milk products or have a vegetarian diet. Not getting enough calcium and phosphorous in your diet can also lead to rickets

Symptoms

Symptoms include Bone tenderness or pain, dental deformities, impaired growth, increased risk of fractures, muscle cramps and skeletal deformities.

Treatment

The goals of treatment are to relieve symptoms and correct the cause of the condition. The cause must be treated to prevent the disease from returning.

Replacing calcium, phosphorus, or vitamin D that is lacking will eliminate most symptoms of rickets. Dietary sources of vitamin D include fish, liver, and processed milk. Exposure to moderate amounts of sunlight is encouraged. If rickets is caused by a metabolic problem, a prescription for vitamin D supplements may be needed.

Scurvy (Vitamin C Deficiency)

Symptoms of Scurvy include general weakness, anaemia, gum disease, and skin haemorrhages.

Chapter 33 Mental Health

Psychological stress can be initiated by a number of stressors:
- Deaths or serious injuries of friends / family
- Fear at possible outcomes
- Grief at loss of "life-style" or changes to plans or expectations
- Constant high level stress

Situational crisis such as this can also bring any pre-existing psychological disorder on – depression, psychosis, anxiety, obsessive compulsive disorder.

Depression

This is big catch-all term with lots of subgroups within it – essentially it is low mood – but spectrum from feeling sad to being trapped in black hole with no hope and no pleasure from life.

The true clinical term applies to those at the more severe end of the spectrum and this is the end of the spectrum we are primarily talking about here.

Diagnosis requires a minimum of 2 weeks' duration of symptoms that includes depressed mood or loss of interest/pleasure and at least four other symptoms of depression. Individual symptoms should be assessed for severity and impact on Impairment of social, occupational or other areas of functioning, and be present for most of every day.

Major depression is characterised by feelings of hopelessness / low mood combined with a combination off:

Poor sleep

Poor appetite

Changes in Weight

Lack of enjoyment or pleasure in life / sadness

Moodiness

Fatigue

Feelings of worthlessness or guilt

Inability to concentrate

Thoughts of death or suicidal ideation, plans or actions.

Consider:

Onset, duration, fluctuations, past episodes, past treatment, medication, signs and symptoms, social support, cognitions, familial history, suicidal thoughts/actions (self-harm), social and occupational functioning, social situation, coping strategies, motivation

The less severe end of the spectrum is really not a lot different to an unhappiness with life – a significant number of people are unhappy with life, work, partners or friends and this will be exaggerated in a catastrophe. But this isn't true depression and it is important to make a distinction. Many people have found themselves on anti-depressants simply due to being unhappy with life and being unwilling or unable to make required changes to their lives. For these people generally support and a degree of understanding from their family group and friends will go a long way.

Suicide prevention

In situations of high stress it is important to have an increased awareness of the possibility of suicide. Early intervention with recognition and emotional support will frequently help.

The pneumonic SAD PERSONS provides a way to remember risk factors:

S – sex – male

A – age – older

D – depression – history of

P – previous attempts

E – ethanol abuse – heavy alcohol drinking

R – rational thinking loss – is unable to see things in a rational way

S – support – lack of

O – organised plan – of how they would do it

N – no spouse or partner

S – sickness – being chronically or disablingly unwell

To assess a patients risk of self harm or suicide a number of tools exist. Using the facts below add 1 pt for each fact present. Less than 3 indicates a low risk, 3-6 a medium risk, 7+ High Risk

Patient is Male

Age under 19

Aged over 45

History of Depression

Previous self Harm

High Alcohol / Drug Use

Loss of Rational thinking

Widowed, Divorced or Separated

Serious attempt at Suicide or Self Harm

No close family, friends or job

Determined to Repeat attempts

Ambivalent When questioned

Psychosis

Psychosis is an abnormal perception of stimulus / loss of contact with reality

A common feature are hallucinations – auditory and or visual.

It is a spectrum from a single episode (more common) to being a component of a broader illness such as schizophrenia, bipolar disorder or severe depression. Regardless of the under lying biochemical cause it can be precipitated by drug abuse, severe stress / exposure to psychological trauma, sleep depression

The diagnostic criteria are very variable and complex, but the basics of this diagnosis is the loss of touch with reality.

Dealing with someone who is psychotic can be very distressing to carers. It is also very disabling to the patient. The basic management of psychosis is aimed at calming the patients and frequent tethering to reality.

Most episodes self limiting and can be managed with support and minimising the stimulus which lead to the psychosis – drugs, alcohol, stress. Sedation may be useful in the short-term with benzodiazepine such as diazepam (valium).

Recurrent or persistent psychosis is much more of a problem. Historically "madness" or "insanity" wasn't uncommon and while this was a catch-all for a lot of illnesses a number would have been psychotic.

Reactions to loss and grief

Elizabeth Kubler-Ross in 1969 published a book on death and dying in it she discussed the stages people go through when coming to terms with an impending death usually from a terminal disease.

Although her work has been disputed since that time, the basic principals are widely accepted.

The same model of loss and grief can be applied to someone left behind after the death of a relative or close friend. The model consists of five stages there is no set sequence in which they may be experienced and a person may not experience all the stages or may move back and forth between stages as mood and experience change.

Denial

Where the person won't believe the situation applies to them.

Anger

The beginning of acceptance of the situation, the person becomes angry that the situation has happened to them. Feelings of anger and envy for those in a better position become evident.

Bargaining

In this stage the person try`s to negotiate to extend own or others life sometimes using religion as a support.

Depression

This is a feeling of hopelessness, it may bring on suicidal thoughts and the person detaches themselves from those around them.

Acceptance

The final stage when the person accepts the inevitable and both physically and mentally prepares for it.

Dementia

Dementia is an umbrella term used to describe a group of symptoms exhibited by patients with Alzheimer's, vascular dementia, picks disease, lewy bodies, Parkinson's and CJD. The symptoms of CJD don't occur for decades, so consequently the amount of cases that will arise from the BSE crisis of the 1990s is not yet known. dementia is a progressive degeneration of the brain which commonly affects the speech and language centres, thus patients often loose short and or long term memory, have difficulty understanding speech and communicating. They also can lose life skills such being able to care for themselves.

Statistically the likelihood of developing dementia doubles every 5 years after 65. By the age of 85, 20% of the population will have it.

There is no cure for dementia and it is a fatal disease usually within 10 years of first developing symptoms. However there are thought to be protective measures which will decrease the chance of developing it. As it is vascular in nature these measures are equally protective against heart attacks and strokes. They are in moderation drinking coffee and red wine. Low cholesterol, regular use of NSAIDs, eating oily fish and five to seven portions of fruit and vegetables a day especially those rich in vitamin E. Keeping your brain active by reading and doing puzzles is also helpful.

Chapter 34 ECG Interpretation

By Gareth J Mallon from "Let`s Make The ECG Easier to Understand"

You should be able to recognise the basic heart rhythm within 45 seconds, some can take just a bit longer others may take only a few seconds (we call these the Oh dear! rhythms, explained later).

The best way to start this is, to learn the basics about the activity of the heart, so please bear with me if we follow over old ground.

The heart as we know is the most effective mechanical pump known to us. It has never been synthetically replicated (copied to you and I!) to last as long or to work as effectively as nature's version since time began. True, surgeons have implanted many a mechanical heart, saving many lives, but they have yet to design something that is as effective in it's long term low maintenance, robust construction as the human heart. Something, which is capable of working 24 hours a day 365 days a year and if we are fortunate, quite efficiently for up to and over 100 years.

As for it's construction, it is a hollow muscular organ, about the size of the owner's fist in an adult and is located behind the sternum (or breast plate) and is actually upside down (the top, or apex is at the bottom and the base is at the top).I suppose it could be compared to, say a washing machine or car petrol pump. It works both mechanically and electrically and one can't work without the other, if there is a fault in either of them then the other becomes affected. The heart works on the same principle, if the wiring is faulty then this means the motor won't run smoothly, consequently if the motor is damaged (i.e. heart attack) then the wiring is put under a strain.

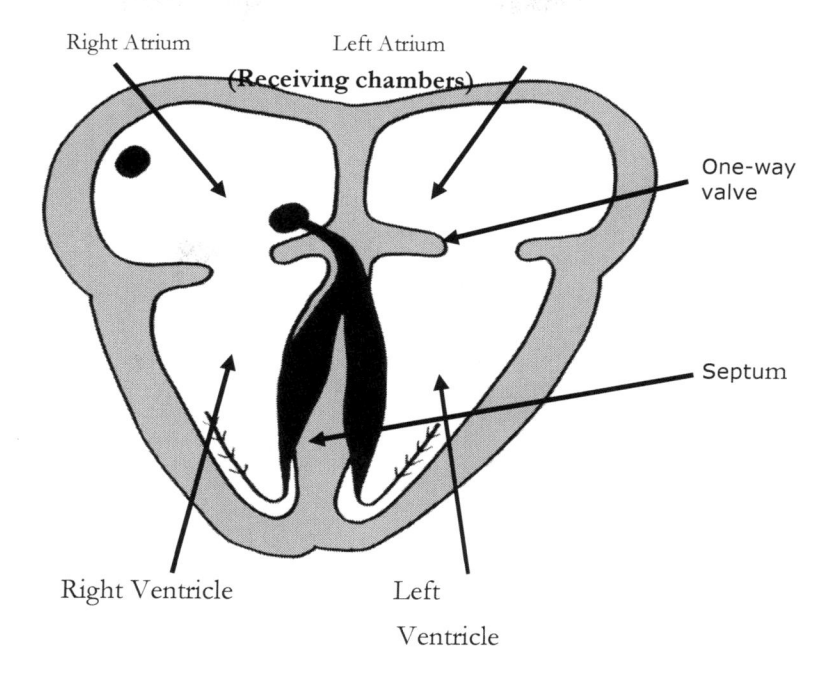

Diagram of heart showing: Right Atrium, Left Atrium (Receiving chambers), One-way valve, Septum, Right Ventricle, Left Ventricle

Lets Get Down To Basics

The basic heart construction consists of four chambers. The top two are the atrias (receiving chambers) and the lower two are called the ventricles (pumping chambers). The atrial chambers are separated and sealed from the ventricles by one-way valves to prevent any blood flowing back whilst lying down or doing handstands and things!

All four are divided down the middle by something called the septum, thus giving us four chambers. The right side of the heart deals with receiving deoxygenated blood from the body (**R**ight-**R**ubbish) in the right atria, and also for pumping blood to then to the lungs via the right ventricle. The left side deals with receiving oxygenated blood from the lungs to the left atria, and the left ventricle pumps blood to the bodies systems. Because the pressure needed to pump the blood throughout the whole body, the walls of the left ventricle are much thicker than the right.

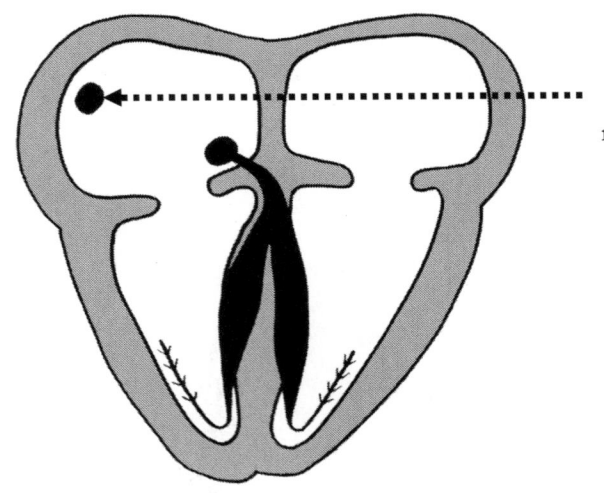

This is the Sino Atrial or "Start" node the heart's natural pacemaker.

Every muscle that contracts gives electrical changes. This is called "depolarisation" When they rest it is known as "repolarisation". These changes are detected and recorded on an ECG monitor.

The electrical impulses have a predetermined pathway to follow, which starts in the right atrium and is called the sinoatrial **(SA)** node (or the "S"t"A"rt node). This is the heart's natural pacemaker and like all nodes is made up of a mass of specialised cells embedded high up into the heart wall in the right Atria and under normal circumstances will fire at about 60 to 100 Beats Per Minute (BPM) controlled by nerves, but it can only handle a maximum speed of a about 140 BPM before it gives up and the cells in the Atria take over (see next).

Within the walls of the atria are millions of excitable cells each one capable of firing on its own accord or when linked together, spread to the next cell, then to the next and on down the line. When the impulse leaves the SA node it excites the nearest cell which in turn excites the next one to it and so on creating something very similar to a Mexican wave throughout the atrias. This in turn contracts the two atrias simultaneously, pumping blood through the one-way valves, down to the ventricles. Only 30% of the blood is pumped to the ventricles, the remaining 70% is passed down by gravity.

When the Atrial impulse reaches its end it is picked up by the AtriaVentricular (**AV**) node or the "A"rf "V"ay (Half Way node). This node is like a relay and holding station and holds on to this impulse for a brief moment before passing it down the **Bundle of HIS** and to the ventricles.

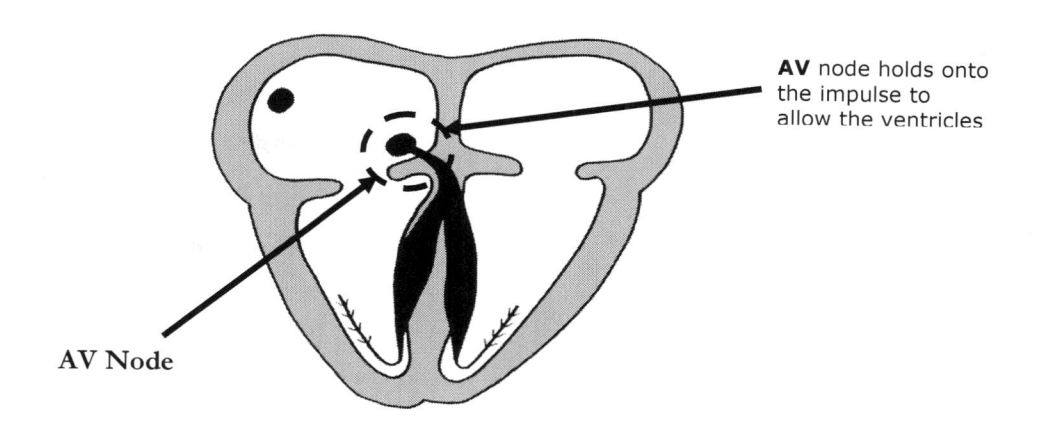

AV node holds onto the impulse to allow the ventricles

AV Node

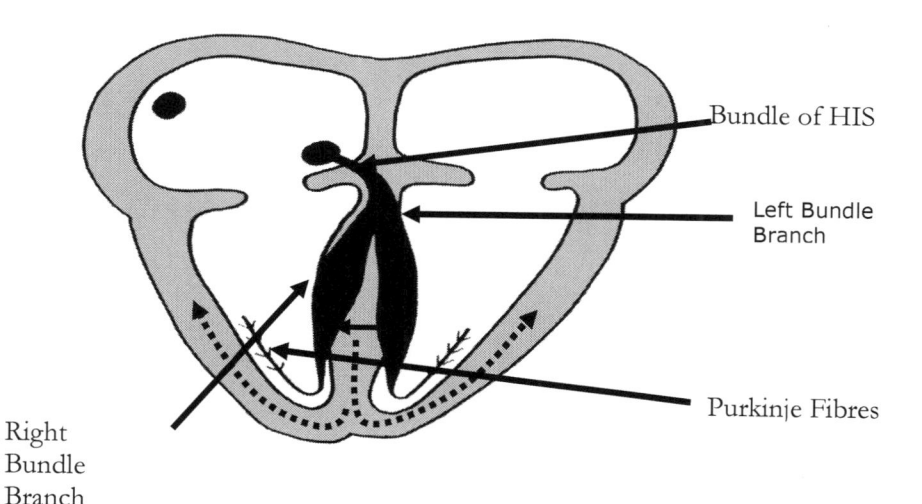

Bundle of HIS

Left Bundle Branch

Purkinje Fibres

Right Bundle Branch

It first passes it down the **Bundle of HIS** (named after a German gentleman call HIS) which looks like an upturned tuning fork called the **bundle branches**. The impulse starts in the left hand side, and then travels over to the right. The left bundle branch feeds the left side of the ventricles and the right branch feeds the right. They both travel down and around and down to the bottom of the heart (or the apex) to the spidery type nerves embedded in the ventricular walls known as **Purkinje fibres**. As with the atria these then excite the cells in the muscle and cause them to contract both ventricles simultaneously, pumping the blood again through one-way valves around the body through the arteries.

To Sum It All Up

So the electrical path followed from start to finish would be,

- **SA** node (the pacemaker).
- Mexican wave across the atrias (simultaneous contraction of both atrias).
- **AV** node
- Short delay (to allow the ventricles to fill).
- Down the **bundle of HIS**.
- Left and right **bundle branches** (Upside down tuning fork), first left side then right side.
- **Purkinje fibres.**
- Mexican wave across the ventricles (simultaneous contraction of both ventricles).

Let's Get Connected!

It's time to connect up our poor unsuspecting soul to the ECG monitor! Electrodes (or "dots" as they are often called) are used to transmit the electrical activity of the heart, from the skin's surface to an ECG monitor. But how do we do it and where do we connect the leads? Well fortunately a person who was mentioned earlier, a Mr Einthoven worked this one out for us and strangely enough he called it Einthoven's triangle. It goes as follows - You will usually find three leads coming from the machine, labelled RA (Right Arm), LA (Left Arm) and LL (Left Leg). These might also be colour coded as RA (red), LA (yellow) and LL (green or black). Some newer machines have **Four** leads just to confuse matters, if this is the case, connect up the three leads as shown (see diagram below), then place the fourth one on the spare part of the abdomen or leg. If you are still not sure, you may have to consult the machines manual for more details.

The leads are connected up using the electrodes to form a triangle on the body. The most common place is on the shoulders and the abdomen.

A NOTE TO REMEMBER - Before you start wiring up anyone to the monitor, please remember to tell them what you are doing at all times as not to alarm or upset them; the idea of being wired to a heart monitor can conjure up all sorts of fears about what could be wrong or what might be found. Also it will give you a better and more accurate reading, as hopefully they should be more relaxed.

Einthoven's Triangle

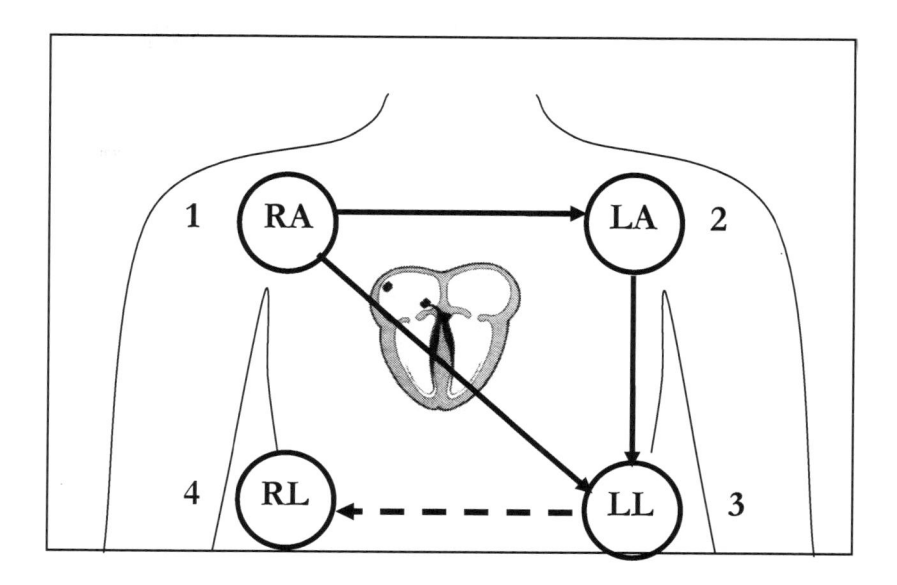

The **RA** lead (1) is placed on the **right shoulder** just below the collar bone.

The **LA** (2) on the **left shoulder** same position, and the **LL (3)** placed on the **left abdomen** or on the **left leg.** This should give us our Einthoven's triangle, now we can now look at the heart from three different directions.
Note: If you have four leads place the last one (4) on the **right abdomen.** You will find on your machine that there are three lead settings, **lead I, II and III** (these will view the heart from 3 different angles). We will concentrate on just these 3 lead settings from now on.

- **Lead I** will look at the heart from the **RA** to the **LA** lead (or R shoulder to the L shoulder).
- **Lead II** will look from the **RA** to the **LL** lead. As this direction follows the heart's natural electrical pathway then this is the most common one used for monitoring someone (R the L abdomen).
- **Lead III** is from the **LA** to the **LL** lead (the L shoulder to the L abdomen).

Don't Interfere Please

Quite often when monitoring someone, the quality of the ECG reading might not be very clear. The main reasons for this are usually poor or loose connections to the machine, the sticky electrodes have not stuck properly, or they may need moving to get a better reading. People with hairy chests may cause you a problem or two, as the sticky electrodes no matter how sticky, do not stick very well to hair, so the only way around this is to shave them and get down to skin, but having someone diving at your chest wielding a razor could be a bit alarming so please tell them what you are doing first. If all is well there, check the connections of your leads and stickiness of the electrodes, if they are ok then check your patient. See if they are moving around or shivering or they have difficulty breathing. Some people who are cold or agitated cannot control their shaking, all of these movements cause interference to your reading. If so, try to relax them as much as possible. If you can't then try moving the electrodes to places that don't move as much, try the RA and LA to the tops of the arms or to the wrists, and maybe moving the LL lead to the left thigh. This can sometimes solve your problem or may give you a clearer reading.

The rhythm below as an example is actually a normal rhythm but it has some muscle tremor on it, which could confuse you into thinking that it was a problem rhythm.

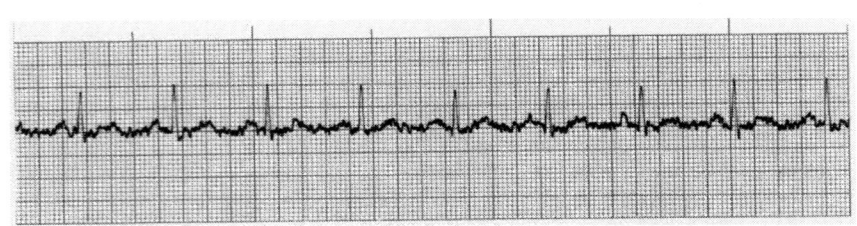

Another problem you may get is called the **"Wandering Baseline"**. When a patient has breathing difficulties then they tend to use their chest muscles a lot more, which can cause the reading to look rather wavy. You will see the rhythm rise up over the baseline on breathing in and down on breathing out.

Below is an example of "Wandering Baseline" rhythm (for baseline see page 19) rhythm, which can be caused by the chest, leads moving on a person with breathing problems. If you suspect that someone's breathing might cause a poor reading, try connecting the chest leads on the upper arms or the wrists and see if that helps.

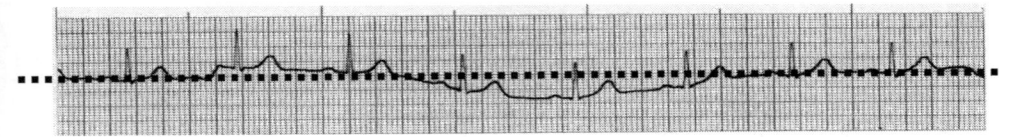

Sometimes overlooked is, the possible cause of interference by electrical appliances, like a syringe pump, mobile phone, fridge, television, or even table lamps. If you can keep the person you are monitoring away from electrical things (not easy sometimes!), or even try repositioning the electrodes or move the monitor further away from what you think is causing the interference. Also remember that the type of person that you are monitoring can influence the type of signal you may see. For instance when looking at an ECG from a large person you might see a small QRS complex due to the fact that the signal has to go through lots of fatty tissue before it is picked up on the body's surface. A person with emphysema will also give off a small QRS complex as the signal has to go through a lot of air pockets (due to the lung problem) before it reaches the surface.

The Paper Work

Seeing an ECG rhythm on a screen is ok if you are there to watch it all the time and have a photographic memory, but like the majority of us who can't, then the only answer is a hard copy for reference, analysis or for just putting into your pocket for a later date, then finding it after a 40 degree biological wash where everything, including the ECG strip is now whiter than white. What we can do is to link up this action to what comes up on the ECG screen. First lets run through a bit about the ECG machine itself. There are loads of different models on the market, so I won't be giving examples using on type of monitor or recorder but they all give roughly the same results anyway (see page 7).

To make life a bit easier all ECG machines use the same scale paper and all should kick this out at the same speed which is 25mm/sec, so no matter what machine you or anyone you know uses, you can be safe that there shouldn't be too many differences in the reading of the rhythm (but if in doubt then read the instruction manual that comes with your machine). Which means if you can get someone to get hold of as many different types of rhythms strips as you can and practice, practice, practice!!

The electrical side of the heart gives off an electrical signal picked up through the skin and is recorded on an ECG monitor either as a positive (+) or as a negative (-) signal, if it goes up it's positive if it goes down it's negative, simple really. The monitor is similar to the types used by electrical engineers to test printed circuits and components so we are not talking high voltages here.

As for the ECG paper, it is of a grid type construction and is split into two types of squares, either small or large.

The paper comes of the machine sideways, so along it's length is recorded the time. Then up and down the paper is recorded the voltage.

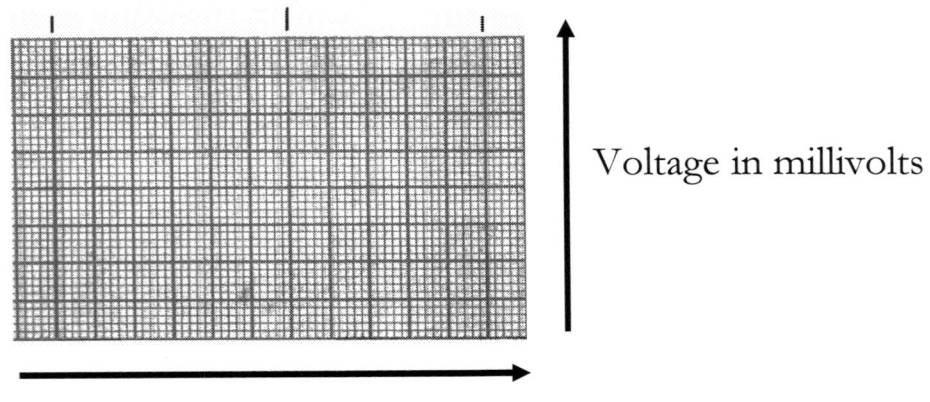

Time in milliseconds

Voltage in millivolts

Each small square on the paper is equivalent in time as 0.04 sec., and each large square (5 small squares) is equivalent to 0.2 sec. So 5 large squares would equal 1 second of time.

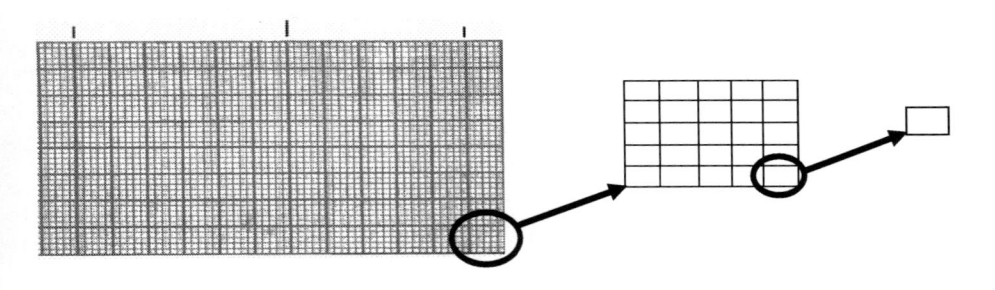

1 small square = 0.004 sec.

5 small squares = 1 **large** square = 0.2 secs.

It's As Simple As ABC

The letters used in describing each ECG heartbeat are **P, QRS** and **T** in that order, each one represents a different part of the complex.

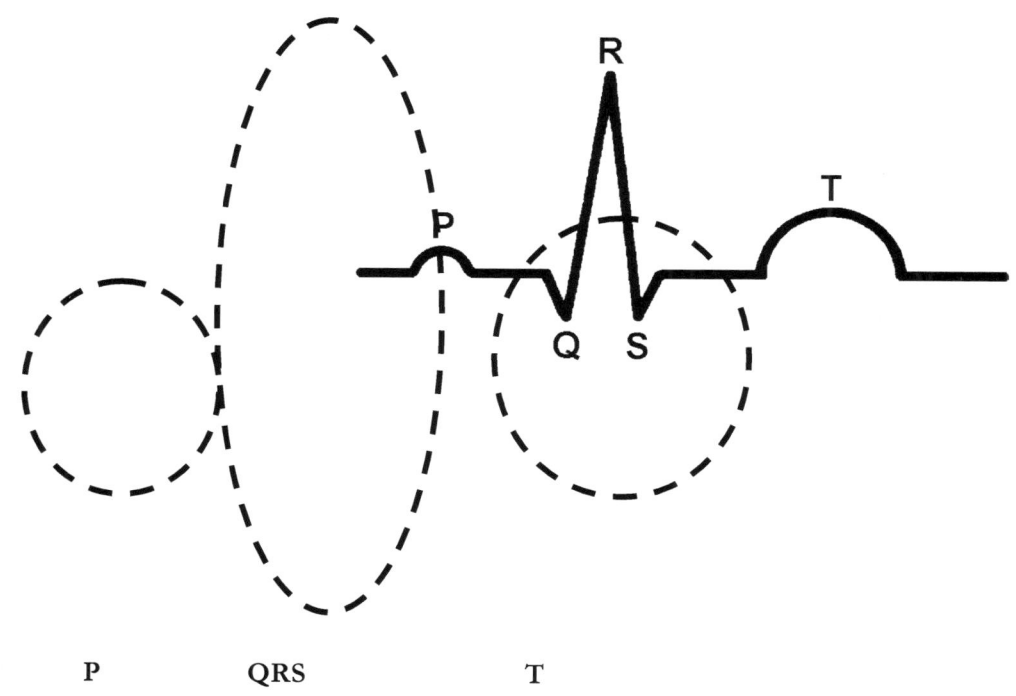

P   QRS   T

Before we begin, we should start with describing what's known as the "baseline" (or the iso-electric line as it is sometimes know as) of the ECG. This is an imaginary line drawn through the recorded ECG rhythm. All impulses should start and finish on this imaginary line. I.e. The normal P wave impulse should start on the baseline and also end on the baseline.

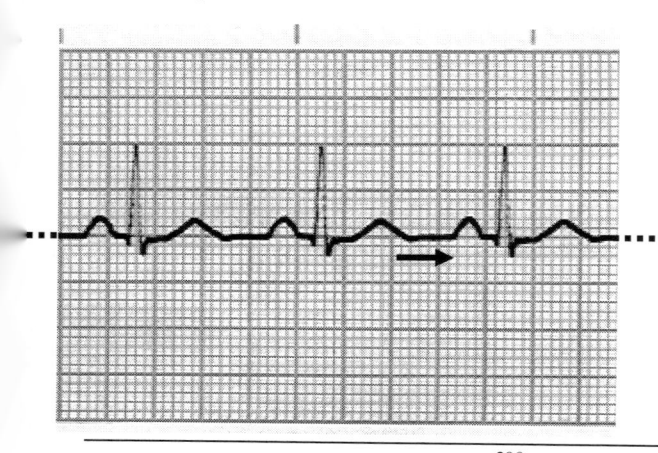

An imaginary line running straight through the rhythm.

The Normal P Wave

The first part of any complex should be the **normal P** wave. This shows up looking like a small hump and must be at the start of any complex, it should also be upright telling you that it is a positive signal. This is the Sino Atrial (or SA node) node and the atriums firing off and depolarising and contracting (the Mexican wave). All cells in the atria are capable of becoming the pacemaker, but the SA node has a higher frequency (or shouts the loudest!) so it overrides and controls all the others. As the P wave tails off, the impulse now reaches the AV node.

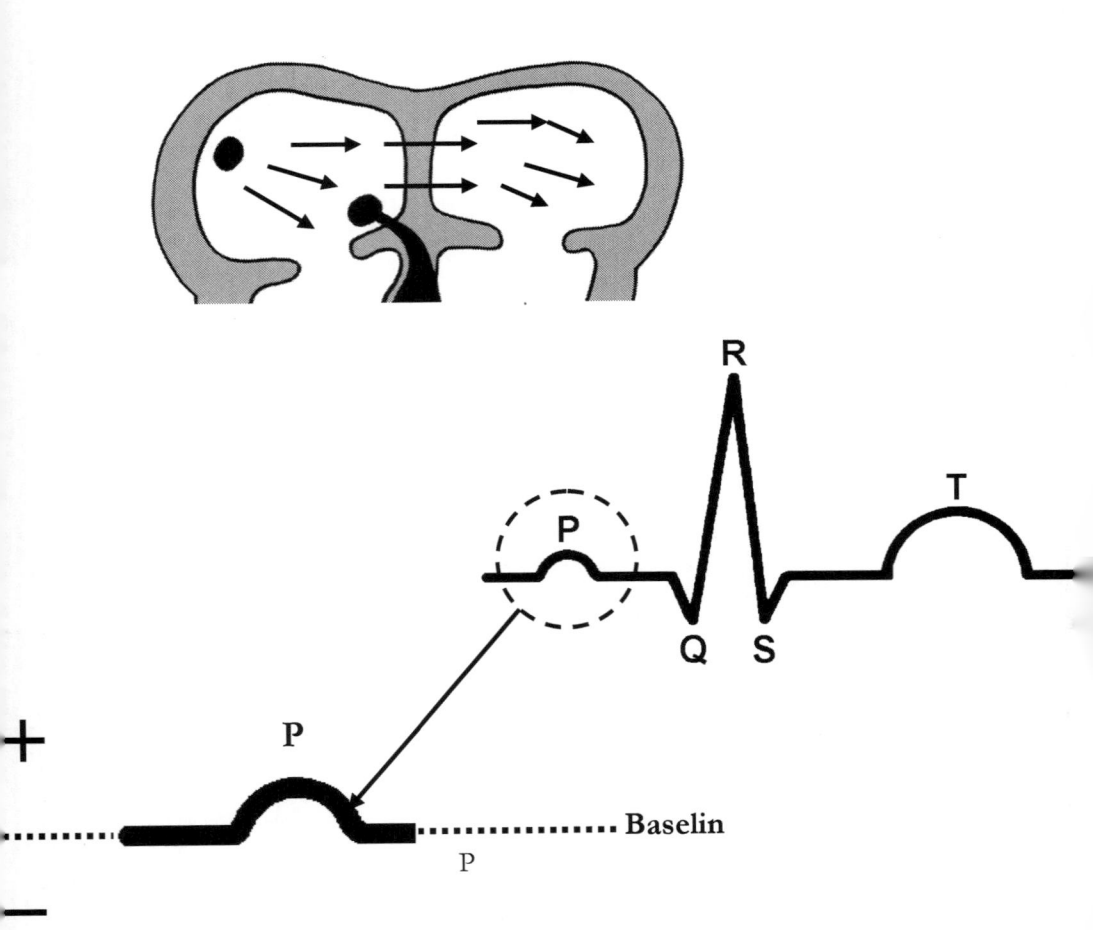

The PR interval

There is now a small delay in the conduction process in the AV node to allow the ventricles to relax and have time to fill with blood from the atrias. This shows up on the ECG as the **PR** interval. This should be **no longer** than 3 to 5 small squares from the **start** of the P wave to the start of the QRS complex, which is the QRS complex. If there is an excessive delay then there is a problem with the AV node, in which case the PR interval will be **longer** than 5 small square
or sometimes prescribed dr

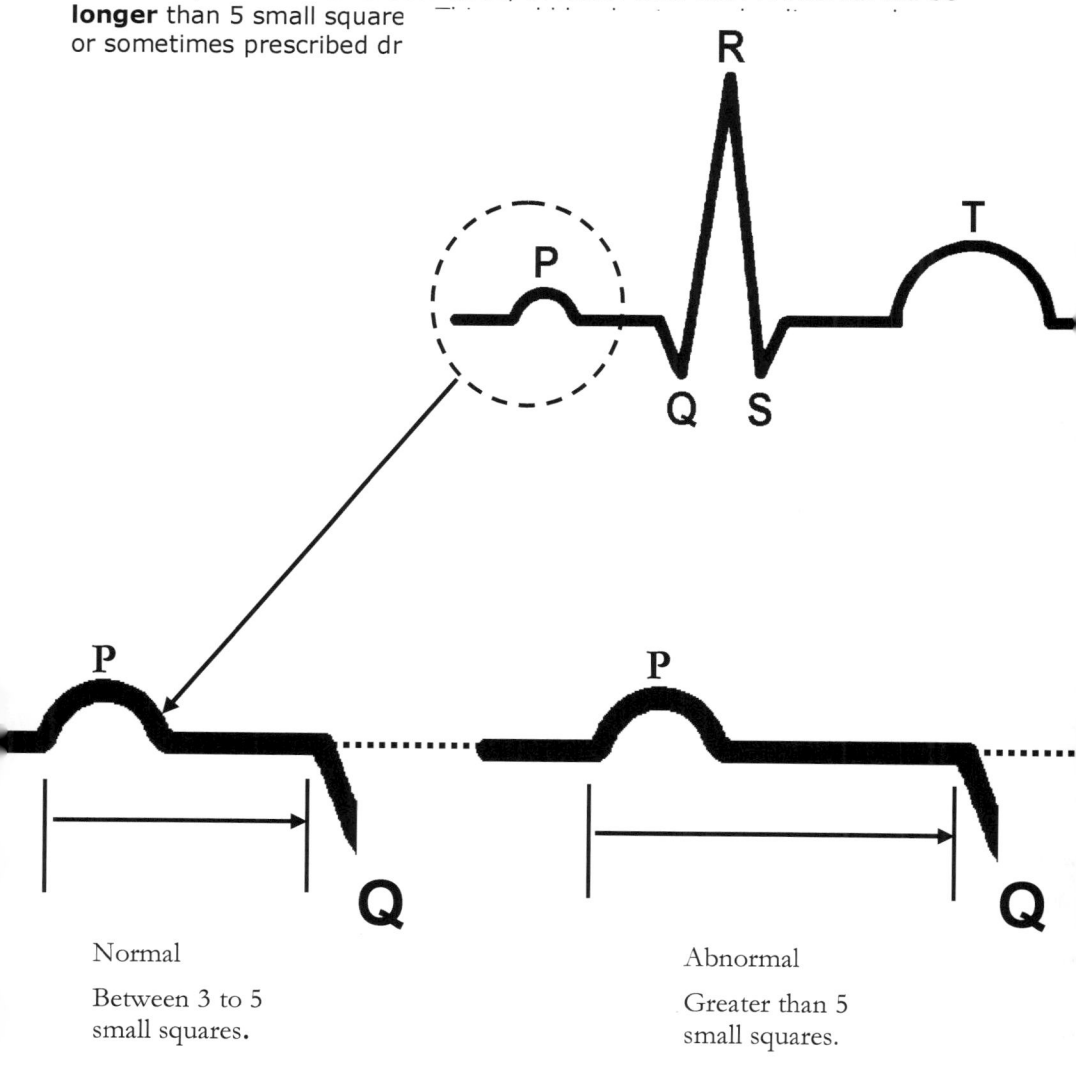

Normal

Between 3 to 5 small squares.

Abnormal

Greater than 5 small squares.

The QRS Complex

The next to come along is, the **QRS** complex. This is basically the straight up and down bit and is the impulse passing down through various parts of the ventricles. The first bit you might see is the **Q** wave, not always shown and if it is then it should be small and narrow (deep and wide Q waves usually indicate previous heart muscle death). This one is a downward, or negative deflection and is the impulse travelling from the left side bundle of HIS to the right side. Next we see a large deflection upward, or positive and this is known as the **R** wave. This one is the impulse reaching down into the heart muscle at the bottom and up into the purkinje fibres embedded in the heart muscle of the ventricles. The R wave then nosedives back to the baseline as the impulse reaches the purkinje fibres, it may dip slightly below or it may not. If there is one, then this is the **S** wave, which is a downward, or negative signal. After all this, the end of the QRS complex should return to the baseline again. All of the above should be **no wider** than 3 small squares if it is a normal complex. If it is wider than this then there is some sort of conduction problem in the ventricles.

As the ventricular problems are usually the most critical ones, the QRS complex can provide considerable clinical information about the condition of the heart and is therefore is one of the most important parts of the rhythm to be observed.

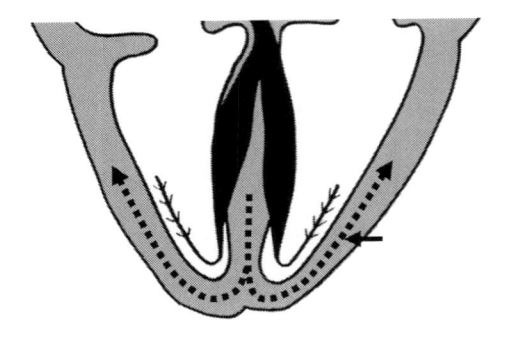

P

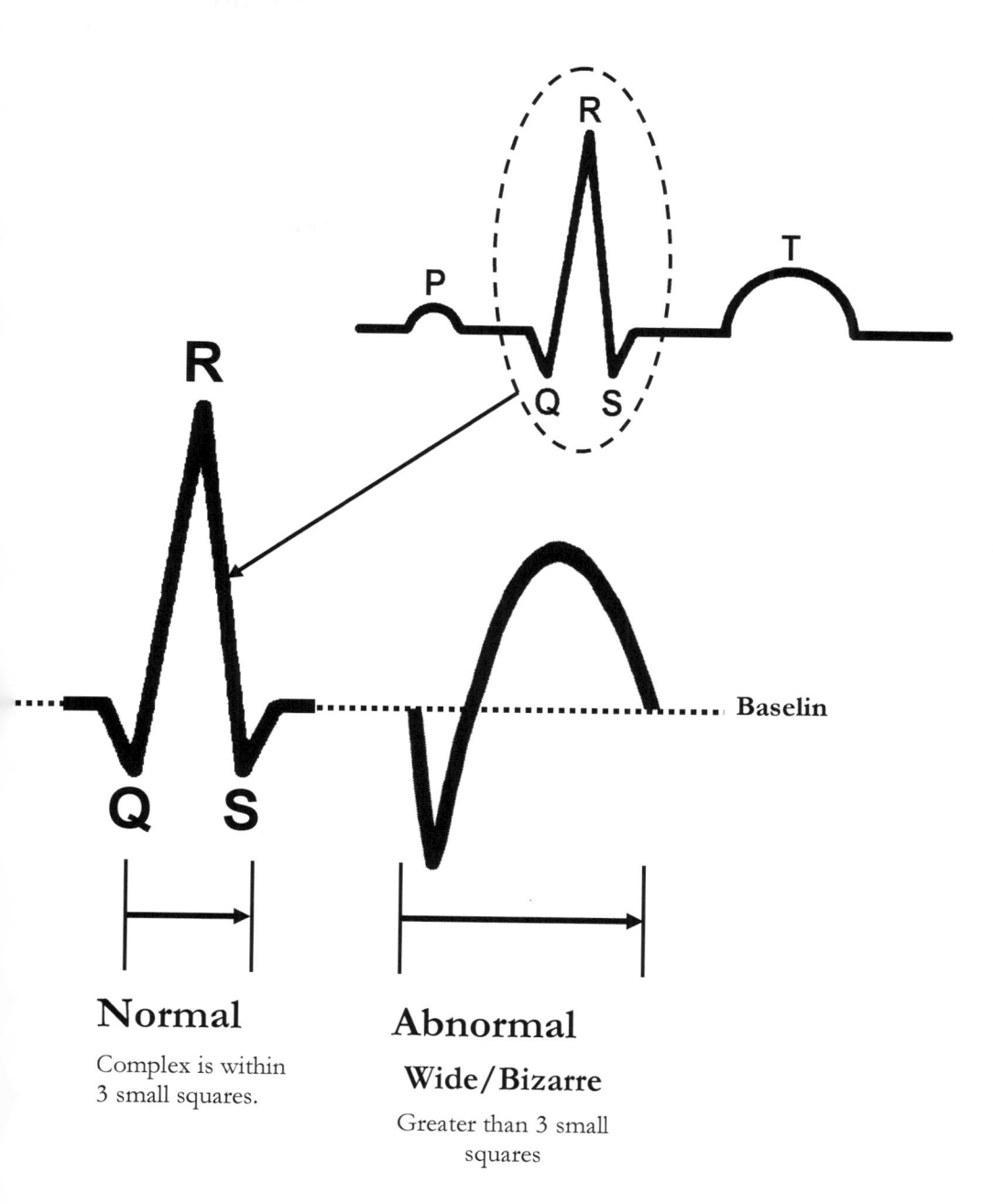

R

T

Q S

R

Q S

······· Baselin

Normal

Complex is within
3 small squares.

Abnormal

Wide/Bizarre

Greater than 3 small squares

The T Wave

Following the QRS complex should be the **T** wave, this again should be an upward, or positive signal. It is shaped like the P wave but only bigger. This is the heart repolarising, or recharging ready for the next impulse, I suppose like having a bit of a short breather before starting it all again. This is very sensitive and dangerous time in the ECG phase, as if you get any kind of impulse or stimulation then it could send the heart berserk and create all sorts of problems usually resulting in a cardiac arrest. The tail end of the T wave should finish on the baseline followed by a short pause until it all starts up again!

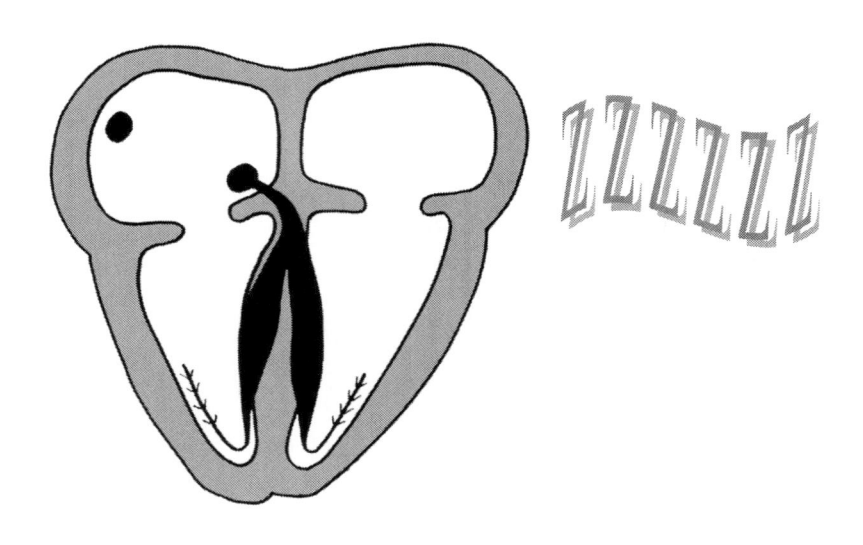

305

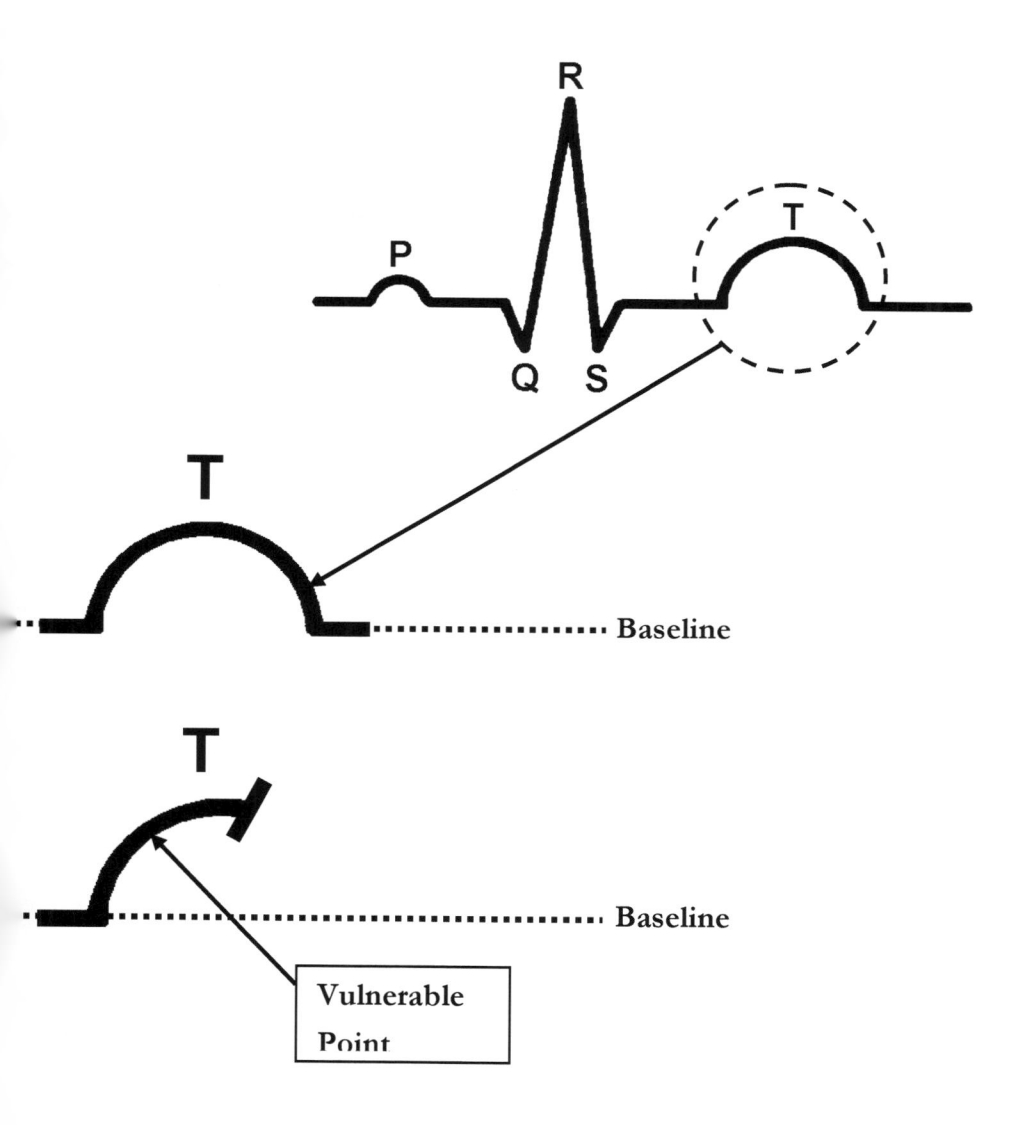

The things to look out for on an ECG are -

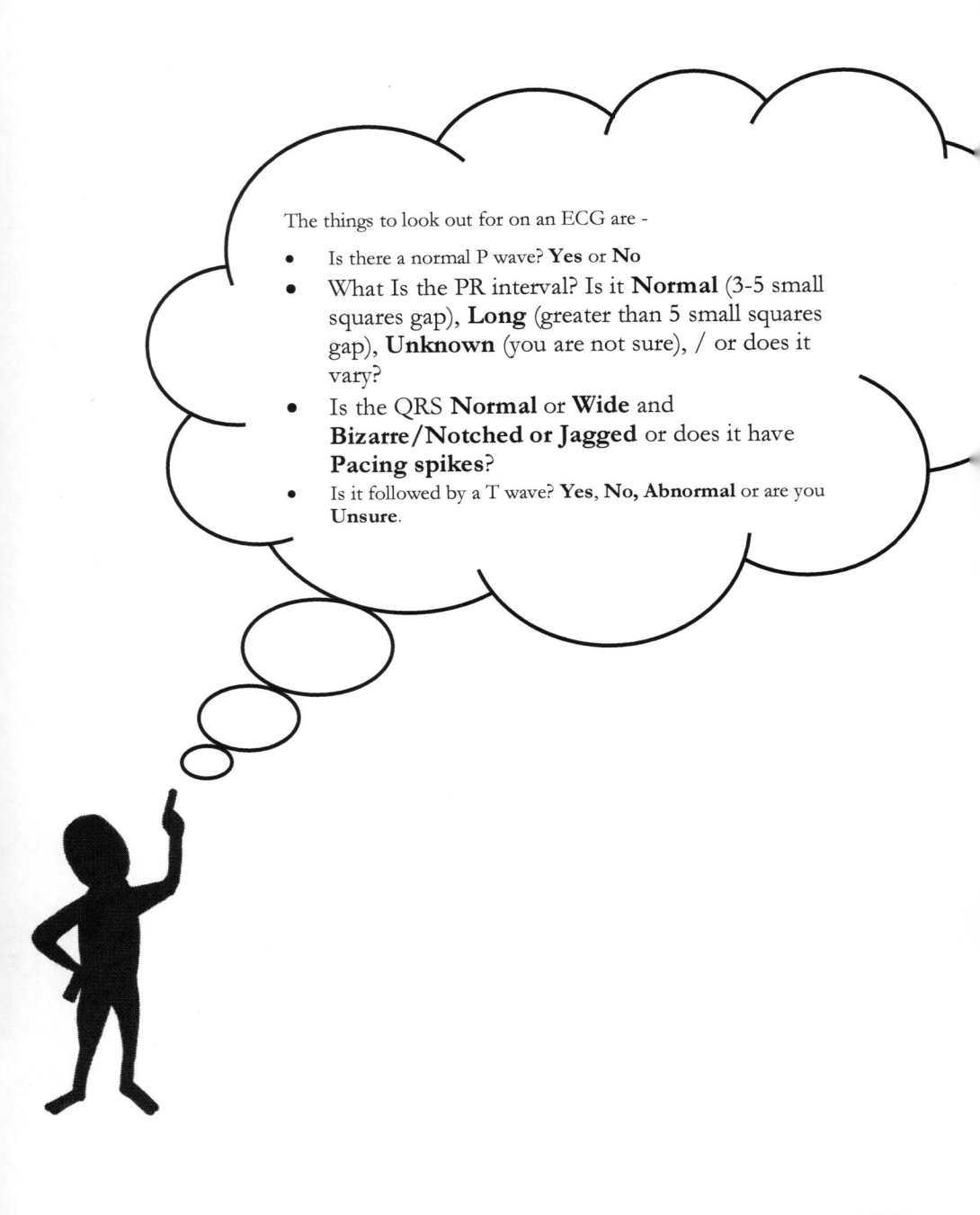

- Is there a normal P wave? **Yes** or **No**
- What Is the PR interval? Is it **Normal** (3-5 small squares gap), **Long** (greater than 5 small squares gap), **Unknown** (you are not sure), / or does it vary?
- Is the QRS **Normal** or **Wide** and **Bizarre/Notched or Jagged** or does it have **Pacing spikes**?
- Is it followed by a T wave? **Yes**, **No**, **Abnormal** or are you **Unsure**.

A Question of Speed

- **Question** - How on earth can you work out the rate of a rhythm?
- **Answer** - Cheat if you can and let the machine tell you, or if not then try this -

Remember-this only works out if the rhythm is regular but we can give a close guess if it is not.

The R waves are used for counting the rate, as they are the most prominent and easiest to follow.

1. Pick an R wave and count the number of **large** squares to the next one, and then divide that number by 300. For example: if there are 3 large squares between two R waves, then $^{300}/_3 = 100$ BPM.
2. Another way of doing it is slight less conventional and is only a rough guide. A quick glance will tell you if the rhythm is slow or fast. Look at how many **large** squares there are between two R waves.

- In a **normal** speed rhythm (60-100 BPM), there will be between **three** and **five** large squares between R waves.
- In a **slow** rhythm (30-60), there will be between **six** and **eight** squares.
- In a **fast** rhythm (100-150 BPM), there will be between **three** and **two** squares.
- In a **very** fast rhythm (150+ BPM), there will be **one** or less large squares.

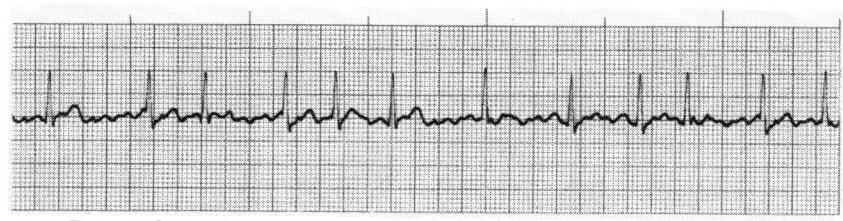

Irregular Rhythm (Above) Regular Rhythm (Below)

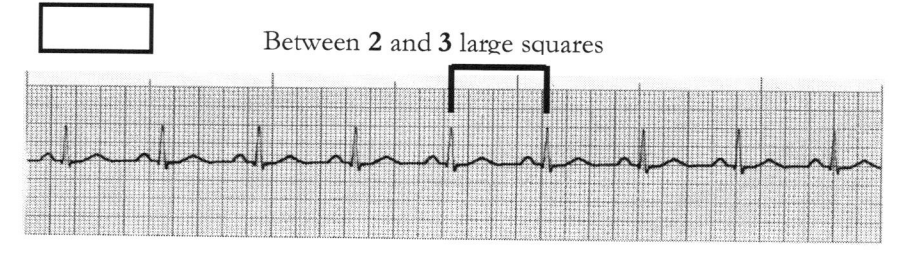

Between 2 and 3 large squares

Atrial Rhythms	P Waves	PR Interval	T Wave	Rate	Rhythm
Sinus Rhythm	Yes	Nml	Yes	Normal 60-100	Regular
Sinus Tachycardia	Yes	Nml	Yes	Fast 100-120	Regular
Sinus Bradycardia	Yes	Nml	Yes	Slow <60	Regular
Sinus Arrhythmia	Yes	Nml	Yes	Normal	Irregular
Atrial Tachycardia	Don't know	Don't know	Don't know	Fast 120-140	Regular
SVT	Don't know	Don't know	Don't know	Fast 140+	Regular
Atrial Fibrillation	F Waves	Don't know	Don't know	Fast 120+	Irregular
Atrial Flutter	Saw toothed	Don't know	Don't know	Normal or Fast	Regular
Atrial Ectopics (Sinus)	Yes	Yes	Yes	Any	Irregular
Junctional Ectopics	No	No	Yes	Any	Irregular
First Degree Heart Block	Yes	Long	Yes	Normal	Regular
Second Degree Type One	Yes	Lengthens	Not Always	Normal	Regularly Irregular
Second Degree Type Two	Yes	Sometimes	Not Always	Normal	Regular

Ventricular Rhythms	P Wave	PR Interval	T Wave	Rate	Rhythm
Ventricular Ectopics	No	None	Abnormal	Normal	Irregular
R on T Ectopics	No	None	Abnormal	Normal	Irregular
Bigeminal Ectopics	No	None	Abnormal	Slow	Regular
Third Degree Block	Yes	None	Abnormal	Slow QRS Normal P	Regular
Pacemaker	Maybe	Maybe	Abnormal	Normal	Regular
Ventricular Tachycardia	Maybe	None	No	Very Fast	Regular
Ventricular Fibrillation	Don't know	None	Don't know	Very Fast	Irregular
Asystole	No	None	No	None	None
Bundle Branch Block	Maybe	Maybe	Abnormal	Normal	Regular

And Now For Something A Bit Different

An interesting question that was mused over recently in the wee hours of a Sunday morning was, what if a person was buried up to their neck (feet first of course!) in something like a sand pit or tunnel cave-in or a similar accident, then where would you put the leads to monitor them? Well after many minutes of deep and meaningful discussions and many deep and strong cups of coffee it was thought the only way to find out is to have a go, so a cave in was simulated using two armchairs and a tea cosy (don't ask!) and it was found that in amongst the fits of laughter, spilt coffee and the occasional passing "what's the tea cosy for?" question, that it was actually possible to connect someone to an ECG monitor by wiring up their ears, nose or forehead to the machine as long as you get the LL lead (the green or black one) as far down the chest as you could reach. This created would you believe a perfectly normal looking ECG reading, but please kids don't try this at home!

A Little Bit Extra For The 12 Lead Addicts

As technology has now advanced considerably over the last few years, 12 lead diagnostic ECG machines have now become more common on the wards and departments and more common in A+E ambulances, so you are more likely to get the chance to use one of these.

The correct placements of these leads are far more important than the three or four lead ECG readings as the 12 lead reading takes an accurate reading of the heart, from all angles, left, right, up, down, top and bottom. With practice though you can put these on quite quickly and accurately. Before you dive into putting on these extra leads (they call it 12 leads but you only physically use 10 leads in total), connect up the normal chest and limb leads as described on page 16.

It is best to start with the V_1 lead. First, on the right hand side of the patient's chest find the Angle of Louis by sliding your fingers under both collar bones down to the notch just above the sternum (this is not easy to do, so you may have to practise to get the feel of this), then count another three rib spaces down then place the first electrode in this fourth intercostal space just to the right of the sternum. The V_2 lead then goes in the same intercostal space just to the left of the sternum. Place the V_4 lead next. Find the midway point between the clavicle that joins at the sternum and at the shoulder, draw an imaginary line straight down the chest to the fifth intercostal space (just count down one more space from lead V_2). Place the V_3 lead between V_2 and V_4 on the 5th rib. V_5 goes in a horizontal line from V_4 in line with the shoulder and finally V_6 is placed again level with V_4 in line with the crease of the armpit. So –

- V₁ – In the fourth intercostal space to the right of the sternum
- V₂ – In the fourth intercostal space to the left of the sternum
- V₃ – On the fifth rib in between V2 and V4
- V₄ – In the fifth intercostal space in the mid clavicle line
- V₅ – In line with V4 and in line down from the shoulder
- V₆ – Again in line with V4 and in a line down from the armpit crease

Dependant on where the changes occur on the ECG this indicates the area of the heart which is damaged. E.g. an inferior heart attack would show changes on leads II, III and aVF see table below.

I Lateral	aVR	V1 Septal	V4 Anterior
II Inferior	aVL Lateral	V2 Septal	V5 Lateral
III Inferior	aVF Inferior	V3 Anterior	V6 Lateral

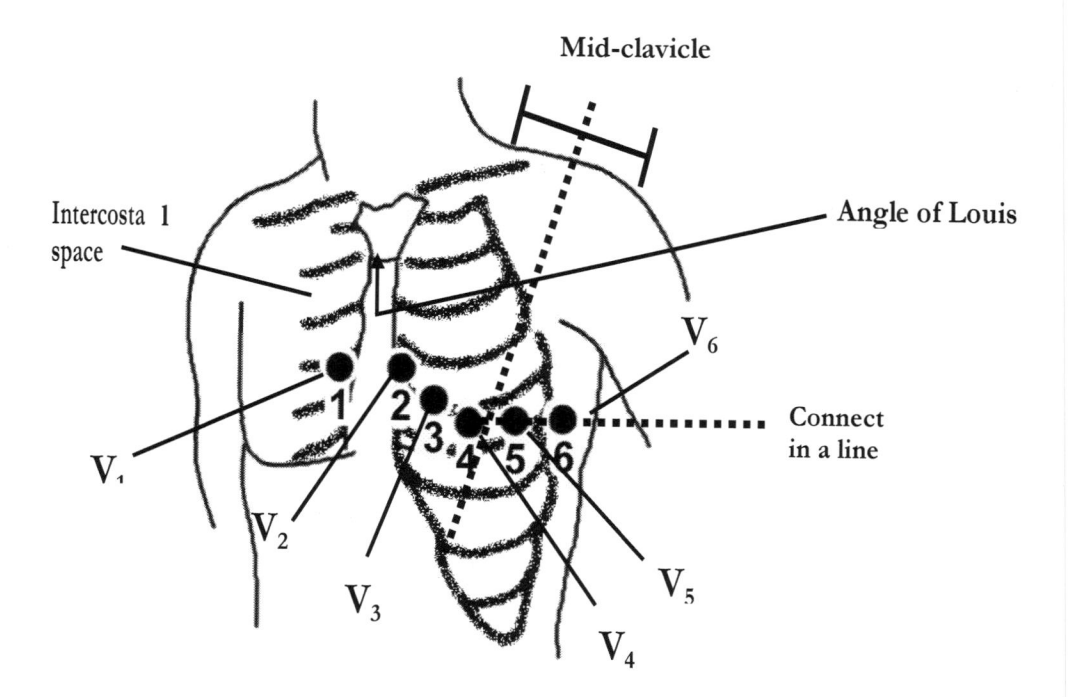

Below is a normal 12 Lead ECG.

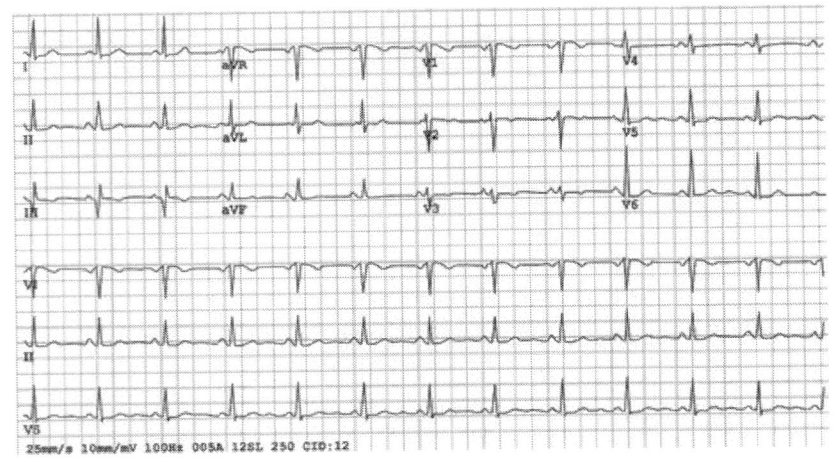

© Inna Ogando | Dreamstime.com

ECG images below reproduced with kind permission from ambulancetechnicianstudy.co.uk

Normal Sinus Rhythm

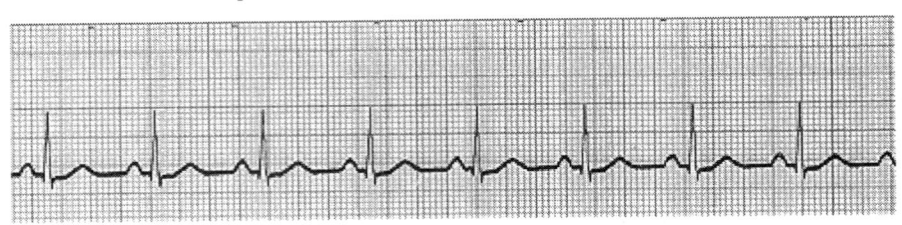

This is the Normal heart's rhythm, the heart can be seen to beat regularly with equal distance between each complex, and each complex is narrow with a rate of between 60-100 beats per minute.

Sinus Bradycardia

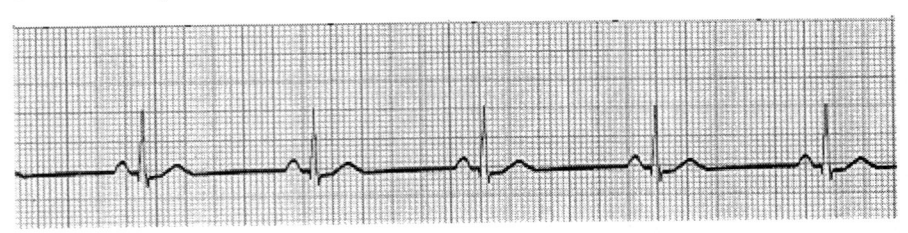

In Sinus Bradycardia, the heart can be seen to beat regularly with equal distance between each complex, and each complex is narrow with a rate of less than 60 beats per minute. Some fit people have a

natural heart rate of <60, there is a second level of <40 beats per minute, this is known as absolute Bradycardia. At this level the patient is usually in distress.

Sinus Tachycardia

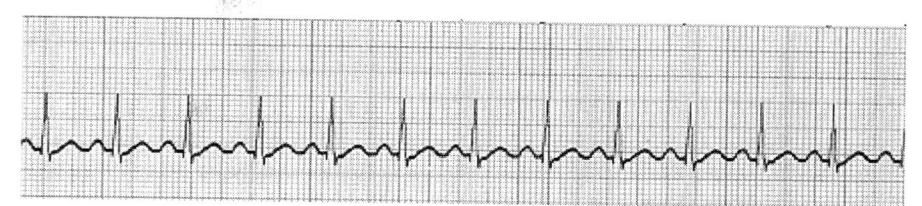

The heart can be seen to beat regularly, with equal distance between each complex, and each complex is narrow with a rate of >100 beats per minute.

Supraventricular Tachycardia (SVT)

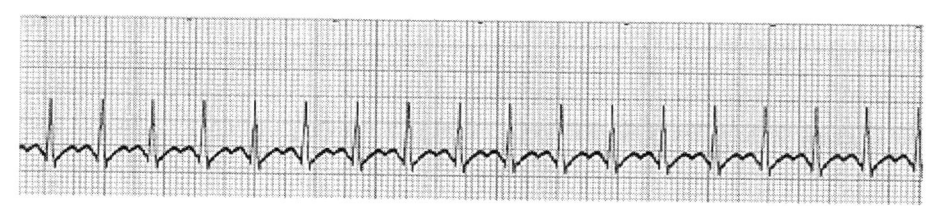

The heart can be seen to beat regularly, with equal distance between each complex, and each complex is narrow with a rate of >140 beats per minute.

Atrial Fibrillation

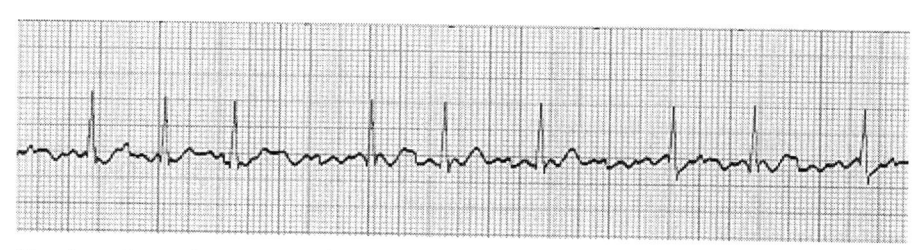

The heart can be seen to beat irregularly, with unequal distance between each complex. P Waves are not distinguishable as the base line is very uneven. Heart rate is usually between 100-140 beat per minute.

ST Elevation

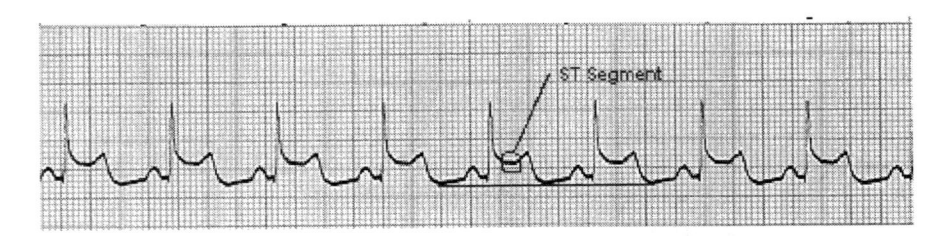

This is the rhythm most associated with a Heart attack, although is not diagnostic unless seen as part of a 12 lead ECG.

Bundle Branch Block

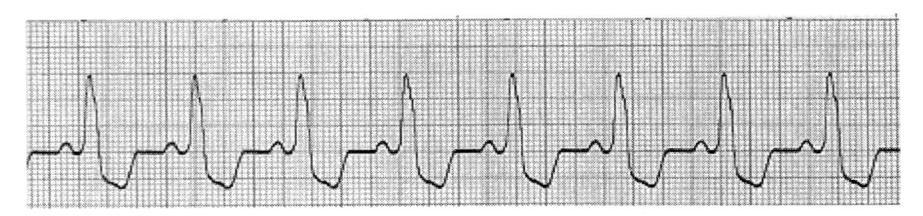

This indicates a problem with the bundles that carry electrical impulse through the heart. This is characterised by a 'rabbit ear' look to the peaks. Right Bundle Branch Block (RBBB) shows as positive changes whereas Left Bundle Branch Block (LBBB) shows as negative changes. A new LBBB may also indicate new damage to the heart.

Ventricular Fibrillation

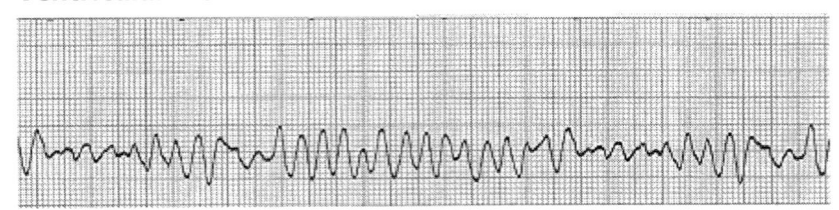

This rhythm is only found in patients in Cardiac Arrest, it shows uncoordinated electrical activity with the heart. These patients need to be immediately defibrillated.

Ventricular Tachycardia

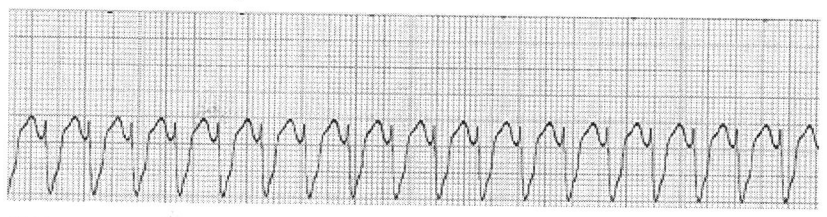

If the patient is in this rhythm and is in Cardiac Arrest. These patients need to be immediately defibrillated. Care must be taken as its possible to have this rhythm and be either conscious or unconscious but not in Cardiac Arrest. The defibrillator only measures electrical activity it doesn't know if the patient has a pulse or not. If it detects a Ventricular Tachycardia of over 180 beats per minute it will consider this as a shockable rhythm. A similar rhythm called Sinus Ventricular Tachycardia (SVT) is shockable if the rate is over 220 beats per minute. In this case the defibrillator may deliver a controlled shock on the R wave of the ECG to stabilise the heart rate.

Appendix 1 GCS

Glasgow Coma Scale for Adults

Glasgow coma scale 4+	
Response	Score
Eye Opening	
Spontaneously	4
To verbal stimuli	3
To pain	2
No response to pain	1
Best Motor Response	
Obeys verbal command	6
Localises to pain	5
Withdraws from pain	4
Abnormal flexion to pain	3
Abnormal extension to pain	2
No response to pain	1
Best Verbal Response	
Orientated and converses	5
Disorientated and converse	4
Inappropriate words	3
Incomprehensible sounds	2
No response to pain	1

Glasgow Coma Scale for Children <4 Years

Glasgow coma scale (<4 years)	
Response	Score
Eye Opening	
Spontaneously	4
To verbal stimuli	3
To pain	2
No response to pain	1
Best Motor Response	
Spontaneous or obeys verbal command	6
Localises to pain or withdraws to touch	5
Withdrawn from pain	4
Abnormal flexion to pain	3
Abnormal extension to pain	2
No response to pain	1
Best Verbal Response	
Alert, babbles, coos, words to usual ability	5
Less than usual words, spontaneous irritable cry	4
Less than usual words spontaneous cry	3
Moans to pain	2
No response to pain	1

Appendix 2 Medical Terminology

Although You may never hopefully need to know what all those long medical words mean. It is useful to have an understanding of the basics. It means you can converse with medics and if you intend to read more on medical subjects you will know some of the terminology already.

Like most words medical terminology are split into two or more parts, common suffix and prefix's are given below.

a-	Absence of	Oste(o)	Bone
-ab	Away From	Pneumo-	Lung
-ad	Towards	Thorac-	Rib Cage
Ante-	In Front off	-algia	Pain
Arthro-	Joint	-ectomy	Removed by surgery
Brady-	Slow		
Cardio-	Heart	-emia	to do with blood
Cholecyst	Gall Bladder	-itis	inflammation
Crani-	Skull	-oma	Tumour or swelling
Dys-	dysfunction, disorder, difficult or painful	-pathy	Disease
Gastr(o)	Stomach	-pepsia	Digestion
Glycol-	sugar	-plegia	paralysis
Heme-	Blood	-pnoea	breathing
Hemato-	Blood	-tension	Pressure
Hemi-	Half	-uria	Urine
Hepat-	Liver		
Hyper-	High, Above, Excess	i.e. A-pnoea breathing	is no
Hypo-	Low	Dys-pnoea) difficulty breathing	is
My(o)-	Muscle	Tachy- pnoea breathing	is fast
Nephr(o)	Kidney		
Neuro-	Nerve	Hypo-glyca-emia sugar in Blood	is Low
Onco-	Tumour		
Osseo	Bony		

Appendix 3 Further Reading

Medicine is a huge subject nobody knows everything which is why it is split into so many subjects.

Paramedic Texts
Admittedly I'm a little biased here but Paramedic text often contain a good variety of patient assessment, first aid, drug therapy, trauma and medicine, Paramedics being Jack of all trades in the medical world.

Oxford Handbooks
These are a comprehensive range of pocket books that cover a variety of medical subjects. Concise and very portable but presume some medical knowledge and few illustrations. The popular titles are also available in pdf and kindle versions.

Areas of Medicine
The following are areas of medicine where you may need some reference material to support treatment and care.

Recommended Books

Anatomy and Pathology
Ross and Wilson Anatomy and Physiology in Health and Illness
Principles of Anatomy and Physiology by Tortora

Dictionaries
Mosby's Medical Dictionary
Oxford Medical Dictionary

Dentistry
Where There Is No Dentist
Oxford Handbook of Clinical Dentistry
Pocketbook of Clinical Dentistry

Drugs
British National Formulary by Joint Formulary Committee
The Sanford Guide to Antimicrobial Therapy

Physicians' Desk Reference Publisher
MIMS
Rang & Dale's Pharmacology

ECGs
The ECG made Easy by Hampton

Emergency Care
Nancy Caroline's Emergency Care in the Streets
By British Paramedic Association. Published 2009, A heavy, large Format, Hardback book with nearly 1700 pages, contains a wealth of information on emergency care and is one of the core Texts for University Paramedic education in the UK.
Essentials of Paramedic Care by Bledsoe
Mosby's Paramedic Textbook by Sanders
Oxford Handbook of Emergency Medicine
Oxford Handbook of Pre-Hospital Care
Advanced Medical Life Support by Dalton
Includes assessment, diagnosis and treatment of adult medical emergencies

First Aid
First Aid Manual (St John Ambulance / British Red Cross)
The first book you should get gives good treatment advice and an introduction to how the body works.

Fractures
Pocketbook of Orthopedics and fractures by Ronald McRae

Medicine
Oxford Handbook of Clinical Medicine
Oxford Handbook of General Practice
A good book for anyone operating a clinic cover most non emergency problems
Kumar and Clark's Clinical Medicine
Merck Manual of Diagnosis and Therapy,

The Complete Idiot's Guide to Dangerous Diseases and Epidemics

Davidson's Principles and Practice of Medicine

Military Medicine
War Surgery, Field Manual by Hans Husum
Special Operations Forces Medical Handbook, by Steve Yevich
Emergency War Surgery by Thomas E. Bowen
US Army Special Forces Medical Handbook by Department of Army

NBC
The Survival Guide: What To Do in a Biological, Chemical or Nuclear Emergency by Angelo Acquista
The Nuclear Survival Handbook: Living Through and After a Nuclear Attack by Barry Popkess

Obstetrics and Gynaecology
Oxford Handbook of Obstetrics and Gynaecology
Oxford Handbook of Midwifery

Patient Assessment / Clinical Examination
There are some very good books on patient assessment, if you want a dedicated book on it try one from below.

Macleod's Clinical Examination by Graham Douglas
Medium Format, Paperback

Clinical Examination by Owen Epstein
Large Format, Paperback

Bate's Guide to Physical Examinations & History Taking
Large Format, Hardback

Oxford Handbook of Clinical Examination and Practical Skills
Small Format, Paperback, easy to transport but less pictures than other books

Special Groups
(PEPP) Pediatric Education for Prehospital Professionals by AAP
(GEMS) Geriatric Education for Emergency Medical Services

Trauma
68w Advanced Field Craft: Combat Medic Skills
by United States Army
A large Format, paperback book with 600 pages, mainly contains information on battlefield Trauma and covers some general health problems and CBRNE Incidents.
PHTLS Prehospital Trauma Life Support
by NAMET
International Trauma Life Support
by John R. Campbell
Oxford Handbook of Orthopaedics and Trauma

INDEX

12 Lead, 310, 311
abbreviated mental test score, 165
ABCDEFGHI, 8
abdomen, 82, 136, 137, 147, 229, 233
Abdominal Aneurysm, 151
Abdominal Assessment, 131
Abdominal pain, 132, 143, 146
Abdominal reflex, 157
Abducens, 161
Abnormal bleeding, 257
Abraisions, 71
Absences, 168
Absorption, 210
accessory muscles, 12
Acetylcholine, 213
Achilles reflex, 157
Achilles Tendon, 100
Acute Mountain Sickness, 230
Aflatoxin, 258
Aging patient, 45
Airway, 7, 10, 19, 103
Alcohol, 11
allergic reaction, 103, 236
allergies, 17, 24, 25
Allergies, 23
Alpha particles, 266
Alzheimer's, 288
amatoxin, 180
Amethocaine, 200
amnesia, 79
anaemia, 106, 283
Anaerobes, 218
Anal reflex, 157

Anaphylaxis, 103, 182, 232
aneurism, 50
Angina, 128
Ankle Assessment, 97
Anterior Cruciate Ligament, 96, 97
Anthrax, 258
antibiotics, 71, 72
Antibiotics, 73, 103, 216, 270
antihistamines, 103
anti-venom, 234, 235
Ants, 232
anxiety, 234, 235
Aorta, 82
Aortic Bruits, 136
Aortic dissection, 81
Aortic Pulsations, 135
APGAR, 256
Aphasia, 152
Aphthous Ulcers, 245
Apley's grind test, 97
Appendicitis, 140, 145, 237
appendix, 134, 144
ARDs, 122
Arteries, 64
arthritis, 88, 89, 90
Ascites, 139
Asthma, 114
Asystole, 309
Atrial Ectopics, 308
Atrial Fibrillation, 308, 313
Atrial Flutter, 308
Atrial Rhythms, 308
Atrial Tachycardia, 308
AtriaVentricular. *See* AV Node

Auditory Nerve, 163
Augmentin, 71
Aura, 168
Auscultation, 20, 111, 112, 136
AV node
    Atria Ventricular, 294, 300, 301
AVPU, 15, 36
Avulsion fractures, 52
Babinski, 157
Baby check, 43
Babycheck, 43
Back Pain, 91
Bacteria, 216
bag, valve, mask. See BVM
Ballistics, 271
baseline
    Wandering baseline, 299
Battle sign, 18
Bed bugs, 237
Bees, 232
Beta particles, 266
Biceps reflex, 156
Biliary colic, 144
Biliary Colic, 140
Biological Warfare, 258
Bird Flu, 120
Bites, 71, 232, 233
Black Widow, 233
Blast Wave, 264
Blister agents, 263
blisters, 205, 231, 235, 237
Blood agents, 263
blood glucose, 16, 38, 240
blood loss, 13
blood pressure, 13, 14, 16, 25, 80, 81, 178, 182, 234, 235
blood sugar, 178

Body Systems, 28
Bone Marrow, 53
Bone marrow suppression, 268
bowel obstruction, 148
bowel sounds, 136
box jellyfish, 235
brachial pulse, 13, 239
Brachioradialis, 156
Bradycardia, 14, 115, 308
Breathing, 7, 11, 59
Breech Presentations, 254
Bristol Stool Chart, 139
Brucellosis, 258
Bruits, 136
BSA, 77
bubonic plague, 259
bulbospongiosus Reflex, 157
Bulge test, 96
Bulla, 202
Bundle Branch Block, 309, 314
bundle branches, 294, See Bundle of HIS
Bundle of HIS, 293, See Bundle Branches
Burns, 75, 181
BZ, 262
Calf Muscle Rupture, 99
Campylobacter, 146
Cannabis, 11
Capillaries, 64
Capillary Refill Time, 13, 16, 106
Cardiac Tamponade, 19, 81, 273
Cardiogenic shock, 182
Cardiovascular and Respiratory Assessment, 104
Cardiovascular System, 28
Carotid pulse, 14

catfish, 234
cavity, 57, 74, 81, 270, 271, 272
Cellulitis, 203, 205
Cephradine, 71
cerebral spinal fluid. *See* CSF
cervical spine, 18
Chemical Warfare, 262
chest, 19
chest injuries, 57, 80
chest movement, 12
chest pain, 26, 28, 81, 231, 234
chest rise, 19
chest wall, 19
Child Birth, 252
Chlamydia, 248
Cholecystitis, 144, 147
Cholera, 146, 228, 258
circulation, 7, 8, 13, 21, 49, 56, 81, 149, 181, 231
citronella, 232
CJD, 288
Claudication, 129
clearing the C Spine, 58, 90
Closed fractures, 51
Closed Fractures, 51
Closed Pelvic Fracture, 53
Clostridium botulinum, 171, 259
Clubbing, 106
Comminuted Fractures, 52
common cold, 193
Compression, 78
Concussion, 78
Congestion, 193
Congestive Cardiac Failure, 118
Conjunctivitis, 199
constipation, 136, 143, 147
Constipation, 140

contraceptive, 211
COPD, 118
Corneal abrasion, 200
Coughs, 105
CPR, 13
cramping pain, 233
Cranial nerves, 159
Croup, 40
CRT, 13, 16
Crusting, 202
CSF, 18
CSM, 21, 49
Cullen's sign, 135
CUPS, 39
CVA. *See* Stroke, *See* Stroke
Cyanide, 263
Cyanosis, 21, 80, 122, 231
cystitis, 146
D&V. *See* diarrhoea and vomiting
Danger, 7, 8
DCAPBTLS, 17, 19, 20, 21
Death Cap, 180
Decerebrate, 37
decorticate, 37
Decreased urinary output, 150
Deep vein thrombosis, 125
DEET, 232
Defibrillation, 13
Deformity, 30, 51
De-gloving, 71
Dehydration, 25, 229
Dehydration, 17
Dehydration, 17
Dehydration, 150
Dehydration, 181
Dehydration, 229

delivery, 252, 253, 254, 255
Dementia, 288
Depression, 285
Dermatology, 201
destroying Angel, 180
diabetes, 177
diabetic, 25, 178, 179
Diaphragm, 59, 80, 81
diarrhoea, 17, 145, 149, 172, 180, 181, 207, 218, 234, 257, 261, 262, 268, 283
diarrhoea and vomiting, 180
Differential Diagnosis, 24
Digestive System, 28, 130
Diphtheria, 259
dislocation, 49, 50, 62, 63
displaced, 52
distended neck veins, 19, 80, 81
distension, 20, 136, 137, 138, 148
Distension, 136
Distributive shock, 182
diverticula, 147
Diverticulitis, 140, 147
DNA, 266, 279
dogfish, 234
Dorsalis Pedis. See Pulse
dressing, 64, 66, 67, 69, 70, 71, 74
DRS ABC, 7
Drug History, 23
Dupuytren's contracture, 107
DVT, 129, See Deep vein thrombosis
E coli, 171
Ear wax, 191
Ear, Nose and Throat, 187
ECG, 290

ElectroCardioGraph, 296
ECG Interpretation, 290
Eclampsia, 252
Ectopic Pregnancy, 50, 251
effusion, 96
ejected, 58, 84
elbow, 59, 63
Embedded Object, 68
emphysema, 118
encephalitis, 169
Encephalomyelitis, 259
end of bed', 6
Endocrine, Lymphatic and Skin, 28, 29
ENT. See Ear, Nose and Throat
entry wound, 272
Epidemic Parotis, 174
Epididymo-orchitis, 151
Epigastric, 134
Epithelial tissue, 74
Epithelialisation, 66
Erector spinae, 91
Erosion, 202
Erythema, 202
events, 9, 17, 24, 25
Examination of Injuries, 86
Excretion, 212
exit wound, 272
expeditions, 190
Expiration, 10
Exposure, 15
extremities, 21
Extrusion, 247
Eye Infections, 199
Facial Nerve, 162
Fahrenheit, 15
Fall-out, 267

Family History, 23
FAST, 152, 166, 167
Febrile Convulsions, 39
feet, 231
femoral. *See* Pulse
femoral artery, 55, 63, 82
Femoral Bruits, 136
Femoral pulse, 14
Femur, 53, 55, 56
fibula, 97
fingers, 10, 11, 13, 21, 49, 59, 63, 70, 89, 122, 235
first aid, 10, 25, 83
First Stage of labour, 253
FISHSHAPED, 9
fistula, 74
flail segment, 57
Flanks, 134
flapping, 107
Flapping Hands, 154
fleas, 236
Flucloxacillin, 71, 73
fluid requirement, 77
Fluorescein, 200
Focal, 168
fontanelle, 150
Food Pyramid, 276
foreign objects, 189
fractures, 18, 49, 50, 51, 53, 55, 56, 62, 63, 70, 78, 84, 270, 271
fragmentation, 270
Friction Rubs, 136
frostbite, 230, 231
Frostnip, 230
Full thickness, 75, 76
fungal, 203

Gait, 155
gallbladder, 147
gallstones, 144
Gallstones, 140
Gamma Waves, 267
Gastritis, 140, 147
Gastroenteritis, 140, 145
GCS, 15, 36
Generalised abdominal pain, 134
Genitourinary System, 28, 130
GERD, 148
German measles, 175
Glanders, 259
Glandular fever, 194
Glasgow Coma Scale, 9, 10, 275, 316
Glossopharyngeal, 163
Gonorrhoea, 248
GORD, 140, 148
Gout, 90
Granulation tissue, 67, 73
Greenstick Fractures, 51
Grey Turners sign, 135
Gunshot wounds, 270
Gynaecology, 256
Gynaecomastia, 135
H5N1, 120
haemoglobin, 240
haemorrhage, 19
Haemorrhagic, 181
haemorrhaging, 13
Haemorrhoids, 149
Hairline Fractures, 51
hand, 10, 63, 270
head injury, 58, 78, 79, 84
Headache's, 168, 207
Head-to-Toe, 17

heamothorax, 57, 81
Heart Rate, 14
Heat exhaustion, 229
Heatstroke, 229
heel to shin, 155
Heel to Shin, 153
Helmet Removal, 60
Hernias', 135
herniated, 78, 81, 82
Herpes Labialis, 245
Herpes simplex, 248
Herpes zoster, 176
high altitude, 230, 231
High altitude cachexia, 231
High Altitude Cerebral Oedema, 230, 231
High Altitude Pulmonary Oedema, 230, 231
high calibre, 270
high velocity, 56, 270
Hip, 56, 63
hip joint, 56
History, 17
History of Presenting Complaint, 23
homeostasis, 185
Humerus, 53
Hydrogen Sulphide, 263
hyperglycaemia, 178
hypertonic, 37, 185
Hypogastric, 134
Hypoglossal, 164
Hypoglycaemia, 179
Hypothermia, 77, 229
hypotonic, 37
Hypovolaemic, 36
Iliac Bruits, 136

immobilisation, 59
Impetigo, 205
incontinence, 20
Indigestion, 207
Induration, 202
Infected wounds, 73
Inferior vena cava obstruction, 135
Inflammatory Phase, 65
insects bite, 232
Inspection, 134
Inspiration, 10
Insulin, 178
internal injuries, 50
Intestinal obstruction, 181
intoxicated, 8, 26
Intra Veritable Disks, 92
Intrusion, 247
intubation, 19
Ionizing Radiation, 265
Iritis, 199
irregularities, 21
Irritable Bowel Syndrome, 140, 142
IV Fluids, 15
jaundiced, 18
jaw, 10, 62, 81
Jellyfish, 235
ketoacidosis, 178
ketones, 178
kidney stones, 144
Knee, 56, 63
Knee Assessment, 95
kneecap, 63, 97
labour, 252
laceration, 69, 78
Laryngitis, 105

Last Eaten, 24, 25
Lateral Collateral Ligament test, 96
Latissimus dorsi, 91
Left ventricular failure (LVF), 118
Level of Consciousness, 9, 15, 16
Lewisite. See Blister Agents
Lice, 235, 236
ligament Injuries, 87
lizards, 234
LLQ, 133
log roll, 10, 21
Lung Sounds, 111
LUQ, 133
Luxation, 247
Lymph nodes, 108
Macule, 202
Major nerves in the upper limbs and their functions, 158
Malaria, 172
malleolus, 53
malnourishment, 68
Malnutrition, 278
Malodorous wounds, 74
mantas, 234
Maturation Phase, 65
McBurney's, 137
Measles, 172
measure blood pressure, 239
medical, 8
Medical Assessments, 22
Medical Model, 22
medical terminology, 318
medication, 15, 17, 24, 25, 208
Melanoma, 204
Meliodosis, 259
Meningitis, 169, 174, 227, 228

Metronidazole, 72
Migraine, 169
Miscarriage, 251
mite, 235
movement, 10, 11, 21, 30, 49, 51, 59, 63, 80, 81, 145, 152, 181
Mucous in faeces, 143
Mumps, 174
Murphy's sign, 137
Muscle spasm, 233
Musculoskeletal Red Flags, 88
Musculoskeletal System, 28
mushrooms, 180
Mustard gas. See Blister Agents
muzzle velocity, 270
Myocardial Contusions, 81
nasal flaring, 12
nausea, 78, 145, 229, 230, 233
nausea and vomiting, 207
Neck, 19
Neck Pain, 90
necrotic, 72
NERVE AGENT TREATMENT, 262
Nerve Agents, 262
Nervous System, 28, 152
Nervous system assessment, 152
Nervous System Red flag, 165
neurogenic shock, 182
neutral position, 84
Nodule, 202
Normal Sinus Rhythm, 312
Normal Stages of Human Development, 40
Norovirus, 146
Nutrition, 276
Nymphs, 236

obstructed bowel, 136
Obturator sign, 138
Occulomotor, 161
Oedema, 186
Oesophagus, 80, 81
Olfactory Nerve, 159
On Arrival, 24
On Examination, 24
Open Book Pelvic Fracture, 53
Open Fractures, 51
open pneumothorax, 80
ophthalmoscope, 198
OPQRSTA, 26
Optic Nerve, 160
Oral Candidiasis, 245
orthopaedic, 30
Orthopaedic Assessment, 30
Osteoarthritis, 89
Osteoporosis, 50
otoscope, 188
Ottawa Ankle Rules, 99
Ottawa Rules, 53, 54, 55
Ottis Externa, 190
OTTOWA, 88
oxygen, 16, 64, 68, 80, 81, 122, 128, 230, 231
Oxygen saturations, 16
P wave, 299, 300, 301, 304
P Wave, 300
Paediatric Assessment Triangle, 32
Paediatric Trauma Score, 45
Pain, 9, 26, 28, 51, 58, 66, 81, 89, 90, 147, 318
palmar creases, 106
Palmar Erythema, 106
Palpation, 137

Pancreatitis, 148
pandemic, 121
Papule, 202
paralysis, 234, 318
Paraphimosis, 151
Parkinson's, 288
Partial thickness, 75
Past Medical History, 24, 25
Patellar, 156
pathogens, 234
patient examination, 6
Patient Position, 7
Peak flow, 115
Pear drops, 11
Pelvic pain, 256
pelvis, 20, 55, 56, 145
Penetrating wounds, 70
Peptic Ulcer, 140, 143
Percussion, 138
Peri-anal fissures, 149
Pericardium, 273
perineum, 273
Peripheral vascular disease, 129
Peristalsis, 135
Peritoneal pain, 132
Peritonitis, 136, 149
PERLA, 15, 152
Permethrin, 232
Petechiae, 202
Pharmaceutical science, 208
Pharmaceutics, 208, 209
Pharmacodynamics, 208, 212
Pharmacokinetics, 208, 210
Phrasing Questions, 22
pigeon chest, 110
pinworms, 236

Placenta Abruption, 252
Placenta Praevia, 251
Plague, 259
Plan, 24
Plantar reflex, 157
pleural cavity, 57
pleural space, 123
pleuritic, 231, 234
Pneumonia, 50, 81, 105, 111, 116, 120, 122, 132, 133, 259, 262
pneumonic plague, 259
pneumothorax, 19, 57, 80, 123, 272
Point-to-Point, 153
poisoning, 180
poisonous, 180, 233, 234
Portuguese man of war, 235
Post Ictal, 168
Posterior cruciate ligament test, 96
Post-Partum Haemorrhage, 255
Power, 153
PR interval, 301
Pre-Eclampsia, 252
pregnancy, 148
Pregnancy, 140
Pregnant Patient, 250
Presenting Complaint, 23
pressure, 13
Previous Medical History, 23
Primary Assessment, 10
Primary injuries, 273, See Blast Wave
primary intention, 66, 67
Primitive, 259
Prodrome, 169
Prolapsed cord, 254

Proliferative Phase, 65
prostate, 150
Protein malnutrition, 282
Providone iodine, 69
proximal interphalangeal, 63
Psittacosis, 260
Psoas sign, 138
Psychological Problems, 285
Psychosis, 287
Pulmonary contusion, 80
pulmonary embolism, 105, 125, 127
Pulmonary oedema, 235
Pulpitis, 245
Pulse, 13, 16
Pulse Oximetry, 240
pulse rate, 13
punctured lung, 50
pupil reactions, 18
Puritis, 149
Purkinje fibres, 293, 294
pus, 18, 73, 74
Pustule, 203
Q-Fever, 260
QRS complex, 296, 301, 302, 304
QRS Complex, 302
Quaternary injuries, 273, See Blast Wave
questioning, 22
Questioning, 131
Quinsy, 195
Rabies, 260
racoon eyes, 18
Radial pulse, 13, 14, 106
Radiation, 263
Radiation effects on skin, 269
Radiation Poisoning, 268

Rate, 308, 309
Reactions to loss and grief, 287
Red Flag indicators', 6
Referred Pain, 50
Reflexes, 155
rehydration, 211
Renal Bruits, 136
renal colic, 144
Renal Colic, 140
rescue hammer, 84
Respiration Rate, 12, 16
Respiratory System, 28, 104
Response, 7, 8
Retinal Haemorrhages, 231
Rhinitis, 196
Rhomboids, 91
Rhythm, 14, 308, 309
ribs, 26, 28, 57
Ricin, 262
Rickets, 283
RLQ, 133
road traffic collisions, 83
Romberg, 154
Root Fracture, 246
Rotaviru, 146
RTC, 58, 78, 83
Rubella, 175
Rule of 9s, 77
ruptured spleen, 50
RUQ, 132, 147
SA node, 292
   Sino Atrial node, 294, 300
   Sino Atrial Node. *See* sinoatrial
SAD PERSONS, 286
Salmonella, 146, 261
SAMPLE, 22, 24

Sarin. *See* Nerve Agent
SARS, 121
Scabies, 204, 235
Scaling, 203
Scarlatina, 195
Scarlet Fever, 195
Scars, 134
Sciatic Nerve stretch test, 93
Sciatica, 93, 170
scorpion fish, 234
Scorpions, 233
Scurvy, 284
sea anemones, 235
sea coral, 235
Second Stage of labour, 253
secondary assessment, 15
Secondary injuries, 273, *See Blast Wave*
secondary intention, 66, 67
seizures, 20, 167, 168, 234
sensation, 19, 21, 49, 50, 59, 79, 201, 230
Sensation, 157
sepsis, 9, 81, 122, 146, 147, 149
septic shock, 182
Septicaemia, 203, 230
Shigella, 261
Shingles, 176, 203
shock, 7, 13, 50, 81, 180, 181, 182, 183, 229, 238, 250
Shock, 36
Shortening of the limb, 55
shotgun, 271, 272
shoulder, 50, 62
Shoulder Dystocia, 255
Sick Child, 32
Signs, 8, 24, 25, 114, 230, 231

Simple Crown, 246
Simple Fractures, 51
simple pneumothorax, 80
sinoatrial. *See* SA Node
   SA Node. *See* SA Node
sinus, 74
Sinus Bradycardia, 312
Sinus Tachycardia, 313
Sinusitis, 196
skin colour, 16
skin grafting, 71
skull fracture, 18
Slough, 73
Smallpox, 261
smelly urine, 146
Smoke Inhalation, 76
Smoking, 68
Snow blindness, 200
Social History, 23
Solvents, 11
soman. *See* Nerve Agent
Sore throat, 193
sphygmomanometer, 239
spider, 233
Spider naevi, 135
Spinal Damage, 20, 57
Spinal Immobilisation, 10
spine, 10, 21, 57, 58, 84
Splenic Percussion, 139
sprain, 49, 87
Staphylococcus, 216
Sterility, 269
stethoscope, 20, 111, 136, 239
stingrays, 234
Stings, 232, 233, 234
strain, 49, 88

Streptococcus, 217
stroke, 166, 167
Subarachnoid haemorrhage, 170
subcutaneous emphysema, 19, 80
Subluxation, 247
Suicide prevention, 286
Sun damage, 204
sunburn, 229
Sunken fontanelle, 150
Superficial, 75
Supinator, 156
Suprapubic, 134
Supraventricular Tachycardia, 313
Surgery, 321
Surgical History, 23
Surgical Technique, 69
suture, 74
sweating, 229, 234, 235
Swelling, 19, 30, 51, 55, 231, 232
swelling of eyelids, 233
Swine Flu, 120, 121
Symptoms, 24, 25, 27, 29, 30, 58, 86, 89, 90, 104, 114, 121, 122, 126, 127, 130, 143, 146, 147, 151, 152, 182, 231, 234, 248, 249, 251, 252, 279, 282, 283, 284
Syphilis, 248
Systemic Inflammatory Response Syndrome (SIRS), 76
T wave, 304
T Wave, 304
Tabun. *See* Nerve Agent
Tachycardia, 14
TB. *Tuberculosis*
Temperature, 16
temporal. *See* Pulse
temporomandibular joint, 62

tenderness, 21, 51, 58, 75, 88, 90, 145
Tension Pneumothorax, 19, 80, 109
Terminology, 318
Tertiary injuries, 273, See Blast Wave
Testicular torsion, 151
Tetanus, 176
Thermal Radiation, 265
Third Stage of Labour, 255
Thirst, 150
thoracic cavity, 82
Threadworms, 236
three P's, 8
Throat, 193
thrombophlebitis, 128
Thrombophlebitis, 129
TIA. See Stroke, See Stroke
Ticks, 232
Tone, 153
Tonic Clonic, 168
Tonsillitis, 194
Torticollis, 91
Tourniquet, 13
Toxic Shock Syndrome, 257
trachea, 81
Tracheal deviation, 19
traction, 55
Trapezius, 91
Trauma, 5, 7, 48, 78, 86, 123, 246
traumatic injury, 7, 49
Triage, 274
Triage Sieve, 274
triage sort, 275
Triceps reflex, 156
Trigeminal, 161

tripod Position, 12
Trochlear, 161
Tuberculosis, 105, 176, 228
Tularaemia, 261
Tumour, 203
turgo, 150
Turgor, 16, 17
Typhoid, 228, 261
Typhus, 236
Ulcer, 143, 203
Umbilical, 134
Umbilicus, 134
unconsciousness, 9
unstable fracture, 51
Urethritis, 146
Urinary retention, 150
Urinary tract infection, 146
Urinary Tract Infection, 140
Urine Dip Sticks, 242
Urine pregnancy test, 250
Urology, 150
Urticaria, 203
UTI, 146, 151, 217
vaccine, 121, 122, 227, 228
Vaginal Discharge, 248
Vagus Nerve, 163
Varicose Veins, 128
Veins, 64
Vena Cava, 82
Venous Skin Ulcers, 128
Ventricular Ectopics, 309
Ventricular Fibrillation, 309, 314
Ventricular Rhythms, 309
Ventricular Tachycardia, 309, 315
Vesicle, 203
Viral Hemorrhagic Fever, 261

Visceral pain, 132
vital signs, 16
vomiting, 17, 145, 181, 230, 233, 234
Wandering Baseline
    Baseline, 296
Wasps, 232

Water on the knee, 96
weakness, 103, 233
whiplash, 91
Whooping Cough, 122
wound closure, 67
Wound healing, 65
Wryneck, 91

Printed in Great Britain
by Amazon